THE INNER POWER OF STILLNESS

A practical guide for therapists and practitioners

THE INNER POWER OF STILLNESS

ALEXANDER FILMER-LORCH
State Approved Graduate Diploma in Dance CertEd
Movement Senior Yoga Teacher SYT
Founder/Director Inside Meditation, CranioSacral
Practitioner, Teacher, Author and Artist
London, United Kingdom

CAROLINE BARROW
BSc CST MCSS
Managing Director Upledger Institute UK & College of Body
Science, Upledger trained CranioSacral Therapist and Teacher,
Wrington, United Kingdom

MAGGIE GILL
MBA, Cert Ed, CST-D, MCSS
CranioSacral Therapist and International
Teacher for the Upledger Institute
Brighton, United Kingdom

Forewords by
John Matthew Upledger, Lauren Walker and Charles Ridley

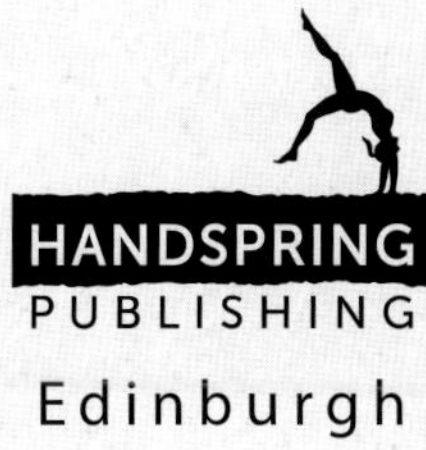

Edinburgh

HANDSPRING PUBLISHING LIMITED
The Old Manse, Fountainhall,
Pencaitland, East Lothian
EH34 5EY, United Kingdom
Tel: +44 1875 341 859
Website: www.handspringpublishing.com

First published 2016 in the United Kingdom by Handspring Publishing

ISBN 978-1-909141-33-9

British Library Cataloguing in Publication Data
A catalogue record for this book is available from the British Library

Library of Congress Cataloguing in Publication Data

A catalog record for this book is available from the Library of Congress

Notice
Neither the Publisher nor the Authors assume any responsibility for any loss or injury and/or damage to persons or property arising out of or relating to any use of the material contained in this book. It is the responsibility of the treating practitioner, relying on independent expertise and knowledge of the patient, to determine the best treatment and method of application for the patient.

Commissioning Editor Sarena Wolfaard
Copy-editor Margaret Hunter
Design and illustration Bruce Hogarth
Cover design Victoria Dokas
Index Aptara
Typeset DSM Soft
Printed Pulsio, Bulgaria

The Publisher's policy is to use paper manufactured from sustainable forests

CONTENTS

There is a channel between voice and presence

A way where information flows

In disciplined silence the channel opens

With wandering talk it closes

Rumi

(translation© Coleman Barks)

FOREWORDS

It is amazing how life happens. As I was reading this book, I realised that I have been an unwitting advocate for better understanding and acceptance of Alternative and Complementary Medicine my whole life.

In one of my earliest childhood memories, I remember running home to take a vitamin. I wanted to take the vitamin because I was about to get into a fight with a neighbourhood kid (Winchester) and I felt I needed some type of an edge. I was about 5-years-old and he was 2 years older and much bigger. I'm not sure if I really believed that the vitamin would help me win, or if it was more of an attempt to stall the inevitable beating I was about to face. Either way, I knew I needed to get home and take it.

Truth be told, I really did not want to fight Winchester. He was one of my best neighbourhood friends … but I was being egged on to fight in order to defend my family's honour. You see, Winchester was telling everyone that my Dad was not a real doctor. This was the mid 1960s and my father, Dr. John E. Upledger, was a fully licensed Osteopathic Physician and Surgeon who had a private practice in Clearwater Beach, Florida.

I now know that in different parts of the world, an 'Osteopath' can have various levels of training and licensure … but in the United States, an Osteopathic Physician attends a fully accredited medical school and receives the same training as a traditional Medical Doctor. The difference is that in addition to the full medical school curriculum, the Osteopathic Physician also receives the Osteopathic Philosophy and Manual Therapy training. And the Osteopathic Physician has a D.O. (Doctor of Osteopathy) after his name instead of the traditional M.D. (Medical Doctor). So I did not understand why a D.O., having had more training than an M.D., would be considered inferior. This did not make any sense to my 5-year-old brain and thus began my unwitting lifelong quest to educate people and professions about the validity of various alternative and complementary therapies, philosophies and ideas.

I suppose the quest was further fuelled by my father's unique, open and inquisitive approach to health and healing. Although he was internationally revered by many and was eventually named an Innovator to watch in the new millennium by TIME Magazine for his development of CranioSacral Therapy. And although he spent several years researching and developing his therapies at Michigan State University Department of Biomechanics and teaching his work at their Allopathic and Osteopathic Medical Schools, served on the National Institutes of Health Committee for Alternative Medicine, testified before the United States Congress as an expert witness and received numerous other awards and accolades … there have always been people who were not open to his beliefs and practices.

Luckily for me I am now able to use words, research, patient experiences, science and common sense to educate people rather than my 5-year-old vitamin infused fists. And I am also extremely fortunate that I have not been alone in this mission to broaden the understanding of health and healing. Over the past 50 years, more and more people have contributed greatly to support this quest. So while at times it has seemed frustratingly slow and like reaching for the unreachable star, I do believe we are part of an overall shift in views and understanding about health and wellness which seems to be gaining momentum. It is books like *The Inner Power of Stillness* that continue to help forge this path.

It was through a hugely challenging personal health experience that Alexander discovered another facet of his own potential hidden within his years of experience of meditation and study of the ancient knowledge. After going into anaphylactic shock during a routine angiogram and nearly dying, he found a place within that he described as 'stillness'. Holding on to this place kept him alive. Reflecting on this experience he found that not only did the place of stillness hold much power but it also seemed, somehow, to be familiar. He began exploring the idea of 'stillness-memory' being inherent within us all. What he found of course is that the idea of stillness is not at all new, but that there are many ways we can cultivate our connection to it. Doing so is not only beneficial for our own personal journeys but also for our growth as practitioners of any kind – this book is therefore for anyone who works with others.

What you will find in its pages is an exploration of stillness over the centuries and many ideas and 'experiments' to help you find and deepen your own connection to your stillness-memory. Extraordinarily, I found the depth of Alexander's understanding of this can be perceived both from the words and from the space behind and between the words – watch (or feel) for what happens as you read and hear his voice.

For those who also like exploring the scientific research that might add to our understanding of what is happening as we develop these parts of our practice there is an intriguing section written by Caroline Barrow. The importance of this section for the book as a whole is both as a bridge between the ancient knowledge and where we are in today's world, and as a place from which we can hold the space for the huge potential of future understanding if we can be open minded enough to expand our scientific horizons.

Those who want to deepen the ways they prepare and hold awareness as a practitioner will find the section written by Maggie Gill invaluable, contributed from her own experience, much of which, I am proud to say, has been with CranioSacral Therapy. There is much here that I believe my father would have been honoured to see that his work has contributed to.

There are many of us now walking the path towards a greater understanding of ourselves and we are often also drawn to help others in our own preferred and ultimately unique ways. This book will help us personally, will support an important plane of our development as practitioners and ultimately enable us to better hold a deeply healing space to serve our clients.

John Matthew Upledger, CEO of Upledger Institute International

Savasana, corpse pose, lying down at the end of yoga class, is considered the most difficult pose. This is because so many people struggle with being still. It is sleep with a trace of awareness. So while most of the body is still, the mind is conscious of this stillness.

In Energy Medicine Yoga, we do many poses in long, deep holds, where we hold specific points on the body. This is also a time of deep stillness, when we tune in to the energy pulses of the body and entrain with them. It is one of the most exciting parts of the class for many students who have never listened to the language of the body before. This deep listening and then learning to communicate with the body is a two-way street that leads us deeper into oneness with ourselves.

It is in these moments of stillness, of repose, of caesura – a complete pause in the motion, movement and action of the body – that true healing occurs. It is in these still moments that repair, growth, transformation and cleansing occur. We do not build muscle while lifting weights, we build muscle during the nighttime sleep after we lift weights.

It is this magical, quiet and potent time that *The Inner Power of Stillness* illuminates for us.

This book is a wonderful companion for the seasoned practitioner or teacher who wants to understand the often overlooked science behind the practices of meditation, stillness and repose. Bringing us fascinating insights into biophotons, water and light, it helps us understand what is happening beneath the surface that allows healing, and sometimes miraculous healing, to occur.

There are so many links between the physical body and the mind and the ability to become 'still', and *The Inner Power of Stillness* incorporates physiological science and simple exercises to connect us to the body in ways that are easy to practise but perhaps not so obvious. There is surely something for everyone seeking this place of peace and healing within, no matter where you are on the spectrum of client to advanced practitioner.

Something that really caught my attention, and is typical of how this book makes you look at your accepted ideas in a new light, is this sentence: 'If we work through intention, we are "in tension" stemming from our will.' So many of us in the somatic healing world use that word, intention, hoping that corralling our will can bring us into the highest place from which to work and change. And yes, intention is powerful and necessary in many situations. But if we are working solely from our 'will' and not allowing a spaciousness to enter our work and our bodies, we are overlooking a powerful flow of energy that is waiting just below the surface. This idea continues: '… the very first objective of our work is to gradually undo the default mechanism of doing and knowing, which takes us into allowing and being'. It is this state of allowing and being that leads us directly into healing, and peace.

Beginning with his own incredible healing journey, Alexander and his co-writers illuminate a path through our busy and frantic world, to help you, the reader, find ways to bring ease, calm and yes, stillness into the midst of your life. From that place of stillness, your deepest and best self, replete in peace and joy, can easefully manifest.

Lauren Walker
Creator of Energy Medicine Yoga
Author of the best selling *Energy Medicine Yoga* and *The Energy Medicine Yoga Prescription (Sounds True)*
Whitefish, Montana

The Inner Power of Stillness has arrived and now we can enjoy a book dedicated to Stillness. This book is chock-full of Stillness practices that you can seamlessly integrate into your daily life and work. All three authors share their extensive insights into Stillness from their personal experiences, professional practices, and research.

Quotes that illuminate the spectral nature of Stillness are from the likes of Pantanjali, Meister Eckhart, Ramana Maharshi, Krishnamurti, Sri Aurobindo, Zhou Xuanjing, T.S. Elliot, Shakespeare, Herman Hesse, and Wilhelm Reich. There are supportive articles gleaned from disciplines that range from the scientific, therapeutic, to the mystical; and if you want to dig more deeply you can use the provided links in the chapter references.

A few of my favorite topics in *The Inner Power of Stillness* are Trimetric Awareness, Stillness Memory, and Solace Stillness; you get to discover the sections that touch and inspire you. Stillness is characterized so clearly by the three authors that it is easy to segue from the personal to the universal. For example, ceasing objectification during a session frees a practitioner's awareness to expand from sensing a client's local stillpoint to the realization of Stillness as portal to infinite non-separate consciousness.

When teaching biodynamic cranial work, classrooms come alive with consciousness that evolves the teaching content. Such a class ignites when teaching is based on Stillness, without position, and is offered from 'don't know.' The living content will then inherently meet the receptive students and evolve them. The transmission of consciousness, from teacher to student and back to teacher, is by entrainment.

The living transmission in a classroom also applies to sessions: by applying those same principles, a practitioner avoids falling unconscious in a technique routine. The lead author summarizes this principle in his dedication: "to inspire you to treat or teach from a place of 'no position,' a point of convergence where conscious actions arise."

I savored the sections where Stillness is at the center of the therapeutic process and the fulcrum for the evolution of consciousness. The chapter on the heart is special because practitioners in my biodynamic cranial school are taught to access their heart field as an organ of perception, which evolves the consciousness of the client and practitioner alike.

The final touch is in the last chapter where the lead author presents Stillness in an enlightening way by summarizing the entire book from a single line of Rumi's poetry!

Let me not keep you from this exciting journey into *The Inner Power of Stillness*.

Charles Ridley
Author of *Stillness: Biodynamic Cranial Practice and the Evolution of Consciousness*
Founder of DynamicStillness.com
San Francisco, Nayarit, Mexico

ACKNOWLEDGEMENTS

The ancient teachings state that the work can't be done alone. Whatever knowledge, skill or expertise might be lacking in ourselves can be easily compensated by someone else or a group of people, provided everyone is truly working towards the same objective, with the same intentions and each individual's full potential, capacity and being. This book is the result of a real group effort, and if only one of the many genuinely dedicated contributors were missing, *The Inner Power of Stillness* would not have come into manifestation.

Our thanks and gratitude go to the following **contributors:**

John Matthew Upledger, Charles Ridley and Lauren Walker, for believing in the potential value of this book for practitioners, therapists and teachers, as well as taking the time to write and contribute their thoughts and precious insights through their forewords to this book.

Ann-Margaret Whittle, who contributed the beautiful and thought-provoking Chapter 29: Solace stillness – at the end of life and the final transition.

Dave Mason, who contributed the literally mind-blowing subchapter 'Quantum physics on consciousness – the brain in quantum space' in Chapter 12.

Sarena Wolfaard, our publisher, who, first of all, offered us a publishing contract and made us a part of the Handspring Publishing author team, who responded to all our creative ideas with such an open mind, who gave us the space to get on with our writing, yet was there the moment her valuable input was needed. Sarena truly is a joy to work with.

Hillary Brown (Handspring marketing consultant), for marketing the book and working with us on getting the name out in our respective fields of work.

Morven Dean, for seamlessly project managing the process from manuscript to the final book.

Michael Hill, for promoting the book in North America.

Robert Filmer, whose incredible support throughout the whole writing process cannot be put into words. It was Rob who brought everything together in the final stage, and kept us all on track with his infinite patience, eye for detail and gentle humour. He ensured everything was presented, filed and delivered on time and, most importantly, within the publisher's specifications.

Margaret Hunter (Daisy Editorial), our truly gifted book editor, who copy-edited and did the final mark-up on the book. She is a master in dealing with massively complex sentences, as well as sustaining the voice of the individual author.

Bruce Hogarth, our illustrator, for his fabulous illustrations and line drawings.

Victoria Dokas (ariadne-creative.com), who designed our stunning book cover, and created the stillness-inducing artwork for all the text bites that enhance the meaning of the respective text in different chapters.

Cristiana Canzanese, who gave permission to use her beautifully abstract paintings displayed at the beginning of each of the seven sections of the book.

Dr Natasha Curran, for taking her precious time to review specific chapters and for providing invaluable advice and expert knowledge.

Valerie James, for her amazing support, for patiently working with Alexander on the refinement of the introduction, as well as reviewing specific chapters and offering her wealth of experience on so many levels.

I personally want to thank my co-authors, Caroline and Maggie, for their truly inspiring and insightful contributions, without which this book would not have formed a coherent whole.

My gratitude goes to all of my former and current students, clients and colleagues who have been and always will be my special gateway to the force of meaning. They truly hold the most powerful source of wisdom, and are my real teachers of the work.

Maggie wishes to join with Alexander in acknowledging all of the above. Additionally, to honour Dr John Upledger for his legacy of a global community who practise his CranioSacral Therapy, changing so many lives every day. John Page, her first Upledger teacher, for bringing Dr John's work to the UK. Suzy Steiner, Sanno Visser, Tim Hutton, Avadhan Larson and Chas Perry – all of whom are truly remarkable and inspiring teachers of CranioSacral Therapy worldwide. John Stirk, whose extraordinary movement classes are about so much more than yoga, and who helped her regain not simply mobility but grace, poise and strength.

Caroline would also like to add thanks and appreciation to all mentioned above and all the other teachers who have shared their wisdom. Additionally to Alexander for inviting her contribution here. It would be unthinkable not to also offer deep thanks to Alasdair Morrison, for his ongoing love and support, and to her children Max and Theo for ensuring she stays grounded and connected to the world – if not the stillness! Gratitude also to Carolyn O'Neill, Jo Harris and Susie Watkins for their resolute belief and Christopher Potts for his time and helpful comments. Finally, to Sally Allnutt, who kept the office running whilst she all but vanished for the months it took to write.

Finally, thanks to each and every reader for their time spent within these pages and for taking into their practices and the world whichever ideas they most resonate with.

Alexander, Caroline and Maggie

DEDICATION

This book is dedicated to inspire you to treat, facilitate or teach from a place of 'no position', a point of convergence where conscious actions arise.

This inspired book invites us in to the enduring and transformational power of stillness. The authors combine experiential, esoteric and scientific resources in order to share their understanding of this most fundamental element in healing, personal growth and life itself.

Our attention is drawn to the dynamic, fluidic and spatial qualities of stillness as we re-discover that stillness lies beneath, and can dissolve from within, the acquired tension, stress, confusion and the other impediments that inhibit us from remembering our truer nature.

***The Inner Power of Stillness** reminds us of a potency found at the core of our physiology and our being that waits in the wings. This book, while acknowledging that stillness cannot be practised or methodised, introduces simple and effective 'ways in' that awaken this inherent entity to awareness.*

A refreshing and well-researched presentation on an ancient realisation, this book has more relevance than ever in our modern world. **The Inner Power of Stillness** *is an essential read for all those involved in the body–mind arena. Stillness speaks and beckons from our fundamental depths underpinning the invisible yet powerfully potent core of being on all levels.*

John Stirk, author of *The Original Body*

A gentle revolution is unfolding in the world of bodywork, yoga and movement therapies as more and more practitioners hear of the transformative power of stillness. Alexander Filmer-Lorch is one of the few people with a mind disciplined enough to understand the teachings behind this idea, a body awake enough to integrate them and an inner self stilled enough to transmit them. Read and learn.

Howard Evans, author of *A Myofascial Approach to Thai Massage*

Alexander Filmer-Lorch is carrying a lantern for the holistic healing world, his creative lightness guides the mind to settle, like a great bird finding her nest. There is astonishing wakefulness and refreshing insight in his and his co-authors' work.

Liz Lark, author of eight books on yoga, www.lizlark.com

This powerful book is a much-needed gift of insight and transformational tool for our inner body–mind that is yearning for stillness in this day and age.

Katy Appleton, author of *Yoga in Practice* and director of appleyoga

A beautifully researched and written tour de force of stillness. An in-depth empirical, scientific and philosophical study with the firm foundation in the practical. An unmissable opportunity to find out how and why we should be moving through our life, to stillness.

Kat Farrants, founder and CEO of Movement for Modern Life

Slip into this beautiful tapestry woven with strands of ancient wisdom, cutting-edge science and the authors' profoundly practical and original approach to life, rooted in their deep knowledge of the human being; allow yourself to ponder, wonder, be surprised and let stillness be your ultimate guide.

Veronique Ryan, MD and founder of Mindful Family

If you are holding this book in your hand you have found a precious and illuminating piece of work. The combined experience and wisdom of the authors in their respective fields shines through and will become an invaluable toolbox and guide for a wide spectrum of therapists, teachers and bodyworkers.

Linda d'Antal, founder of Treehouse Yoga, senior yoga teacher–trainer

The simplicity of the original concept of ***The Inner Power of Stillness*** *is carefully explained by a clever weaving of fascinating science, ancient philosophy and practical suggestions. It encourages you to cross the line from mechanical protocol to a place of quiet coherence.*

Tracey Mellor, editor of *Pilates for Children and Adolescents*

REVIEWS

The passion and dedication with which this book is written shines through, being one of the loveliest impressions to emerge from its many facets, investigating the next evolutionary step with huge potential, holding many possibilities for personal transformation through a commitment to stillness within.

Gillian Gill, author of *Take Control and Live*

The Inner Power of Stillness *is the work of much gravitas and insight, illuminating beautifully that which is deeply embedded within all of us – an inner stillness serving as a healing dimension. It is essential reading for therapists and practitioners alike who wish to draw from a higher wisdom in order to move into the deeper realms of healing.*

Jennifer Ellis, director of Yoga Wellness

Alexander is like a pocket poet, weaving the most magical of ideas and concepts into the most accessible language and movement. Every Stillness Workshop with Alexander has been a real joy and I am thrilled that the powerful teachings of this book will extend beyond the limitations of the Yoga Studio and into people's otherwise fraught everyday lives.

Lucy McNeill, co-founder of Flow Tunbridge Wells

We all need to find stillness in our lives these days. Let the authors guide you there in this book.

Martin D. Clark, editor of *Om Yoga and Lifestyle* Magazine

'Stillness is where I come from, and where I go to, and what I try to come in touch with in the time in between.' Alexander Filmer-Lorch experienced the importance of it during the time his health was attacked by a medical intervention. In this book the authors show us that in letting go of the convictions we have and allowing ourselves to come in contact with our inner truth, life-changing things can happen. Worth reading for everybody, but an essential read for people working in the healthcare and therapy sector. Impressive by the pureness.

Sanno Visser, DO CST-D

Alexander Filmer-Lorch, Maggie Gill and Caroline Barrow have produced an insightful and inspiring workbook which will resonate with therapists and practitioners from all disciplines. Shedding light on that which is within us all and yet at times seems so out of reach in today's world. By bringing together ancient teachings and melding them with today's science they have given us a book to treasure and come back to again and again.

Caro O'Neill, CST-D MCSS

In this book, Alexander Filmer-Lorch brings together the latest scientific research and the wisdom of ancient teachings that he himself has lived and breathed for many years. He and his co-authors Caroline Barrow and Maggie Gill offer us an understanding and very practical tools to develop our 'inner self', and to grow as a person, as well as a therapist or teacher.

Franziska Rosenzweig, cognitive hypnotherapist, founder of Holistic Ballet

Thought-provoking, inspiring and always practical. The authors have the gift of being able to give verbal shape to the most elusive of ideas to allow their simplicity to shine through and their truth to be learnt. A must-read.

Claire Carrie, actress, mindfulness and meditation teacher

STILLNESS CAN INCREASE AND MULTIPLY ITSELF INDEFINITELY,
PROVIDED OUR MIND BECOMES GENUINELY ATTENTIVE
TO THAT STILLNESS FOR LONG ENOUGH, AND TO SUCH AN
EXTENT THAT IT BECOMES AS STILL AS
STILLNESS ITSELF

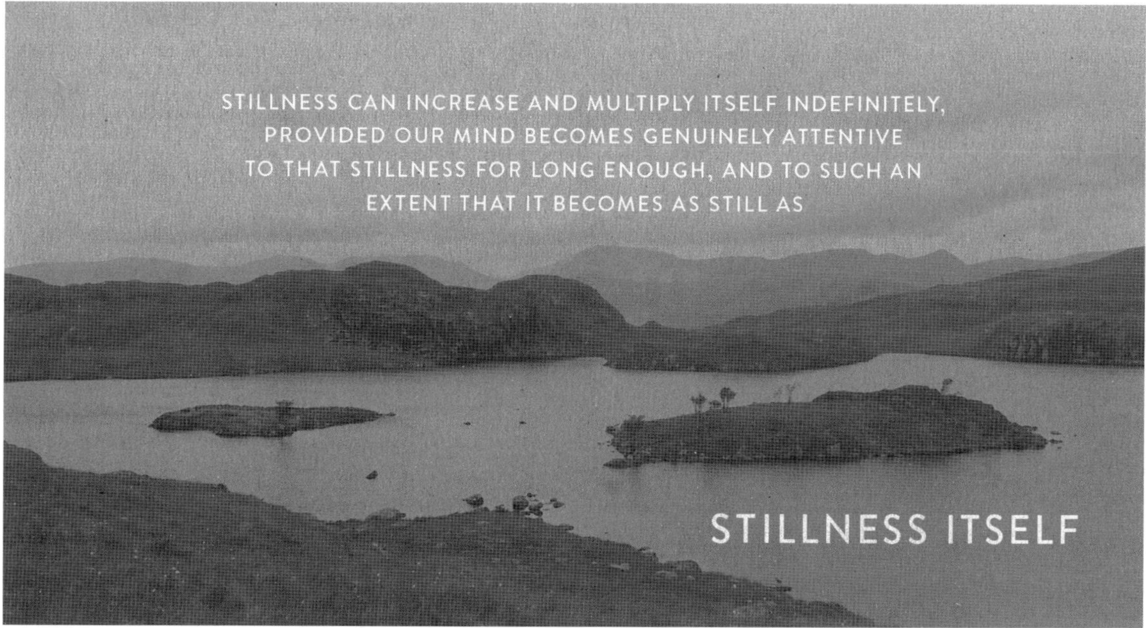

Artwork Victoria Dokas; photography Alexander Filmer-Lorch

Thursday 13th February 2014

The surgeon decided to put the catheter through the radial artery, using an entry point at the inside of my right wrist. I was undergoing an angiogram, throughout which things went terribly wrong. Little did I know at this point that this life-threatening situation would turn out to be an entry point to the actual experience and true understanding of 'the inner power of stillness' in action.

The cardiac registrar was far too busy to look into my medical file. If she had done so, she would have discovered my hypersensitivity and strong allergic reactions to drugs. Her lack of time led to my having an anaphylactic reaction caused by the iodine-based dye used in the process. The moment the dye was released into my bloodstream, it felt like it shot straight up into my brainstem and all the way down into my groin. Initially it caused temporary blindness, but the full consequences of what took place in hospital only became clear when I was considered stable enough to be discharged. Back in the safety of our own home, the inexorable battle between my immune system and the allergen started to unfold. Totally unprepared, I suddenly felt the poison attacking every cell of my body, with its epicentre located deep within my brainstem. Whilst trying to get safely back into bed, I lost my vision again. This time, however, it occurred alongside a whole range of other effects. First, the right side of my body went numb, then without any warning I lost all sensation in my left hand and arm, making both feel like heavy lumps that could not be used and no longer belonged to my body. My tongue, face and ability to speak followed, which made me feel so desperately sick, causing me to vomit compulsively. Whilst my physiology went into survival mode and tried to fight these powerful invaders, the dreaded pain arrived. It is a kind of pain that goes far beyond any kind of description. It attacked my brain with razor-sharp knives, leading to more and more vomiting and further loss of sensation until all connections to the external world ceased to exist, turning me into a prisoner in a body that had lost its sensory functions.

This went on for hours, with a few intervals in which things calmed down between these terrible episodes.

I was taken to A&E. The registrar simply prescribed a saline infusion to flush out more of the residue of the dye before sending me back home again. I was told that there was nothing else they could do. The episodes continued, triggered by any kind of sensory impression or stimulus, and usually lasting for many hours. I clearly recall the circumstances of two near-death experiences in the first two weeks. I sensed my closeness to the beginning of what is seen as our final departure, which was gradually pulling me further and further in. The merciless pain and violent sickness in every part of my body had finally become too much, so I was actually relieved, because dying seemed a far better solution than living with this, day in and day out. There was no space for fear or sadness, only a deep sense of relief that this torture would end.

Yet, a different destiny was waiting, and whatever I felt was about to happen was prevented by my body suddenly cramping and contracting to rid itself of more of the poison by violently vomiting again. After three weeks of consultations with NHS doctors, we decided to go private and consult a highly recommended neurologist. Two MRI scans and a whole range of blood tests later, the neurologist presented us with the results, stating that I had had a lucky escape this time. However, any further contact with iodine dye in the future would likely be fatal. 'Unfortunately,' he said, 'the allergic reaction, and some residues of the dye in your brain, affected your reticular alarm system badly, throwing it completely out of sync.' He explained more: 'We don't know how and when it will go back to its normal function', pointing out that this might take many months or even years, if at all. 'What we know is that something needs to happen to break this cycle, yet we don't know what that something could be.' During this meeting I saw my whole life falling apart, seeing myself during the past three weeks wobbling through the house depending on sunglasses and painkillers, all curtains closed, and as little noise and disturbance as possible around me.

The dreadful episodes continued and could last for hours, draining my body of the last of its reserves. However, I soon came to realise that the more I resisted and fought against them the worse they got. I clearly remember one particularly bad episode in which the penny suddenly dropped. Many times before I had found myself completely locked into a non-functioning body within which I was experiencing myself being fully conscious, yet feeling helpless and fearful of the next wave of excruciating pain. I knew that meditation practice was of no use in this situation because I had unsuccessfully tried it several times before.

This time round, however, I felt so extremely and unbelievably tired that I stopped resisting and simply surrendered into the pain. Following my *gut* feeling, I instinctively knew that I simply had to allow myself to become utterly still and motionless until only inner stillness remained. I could feel the poison and residue of the dye in my cells and tissue, yet I could sense living imprints of stillness that have been accumulating for over thirty years of stilling practice in there as well. That I could truly feel and experience this deeply engrained, inconspicuous, yet so active memory of stillness in my brain, cells and connective tissue caught me by surprise. Yet it was exactly this stillness-memory in the tissue, which felt like a

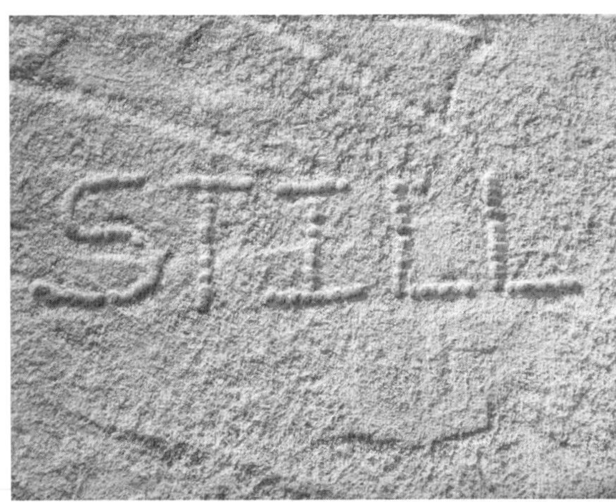

Photography Alexander Filmer-Lorch

soothing vibration or a kind of a subtle frequency, that turned out to be an incredibly powerful and life-saving remedy.

From that day onwards, the episodes became shorter, less frequent and less painful. One month later, during my last visit to my neurologist, he was not surprised at all about the changes. He backed up my experience by outlining how the autonomic nervous system and central nervous system respond to stillness, and that, considering how stillness leads to profound changes in brainwave patterns, he had no doubt that this deep inner memory of stillness played a major part in getting my reticular alarm system back into sync. After almost four challenging months, which turned out to be one of the most insightful and reaffirming times of my life, consolidating and completely transforming my view of a lifelong passion for stilling and meditation practice, the cycle was broken, and the fundamental idea of a possible new modality called stillness-memory – the basis of this book – was born.

I asked two friends and colleagues to write this book with me. They are my great friend and colleague Maggie Gill, a teacher of the Upledger training modules, who played a major part in the above healing process, and my lovely friend and colleague Caroline Barrow, the director of the Upledger Institute UK, without whom the courses that complemented the cranial work would not have been so much fun or filled with so much value. They both agreed to add their wealth of experience to this book, and I am delighted to have them as co-authors.

I trust you will find reading this book as inspiring as we found the whole process that led up to its writing.

With gratitude

Alexander Filmer-Lorch

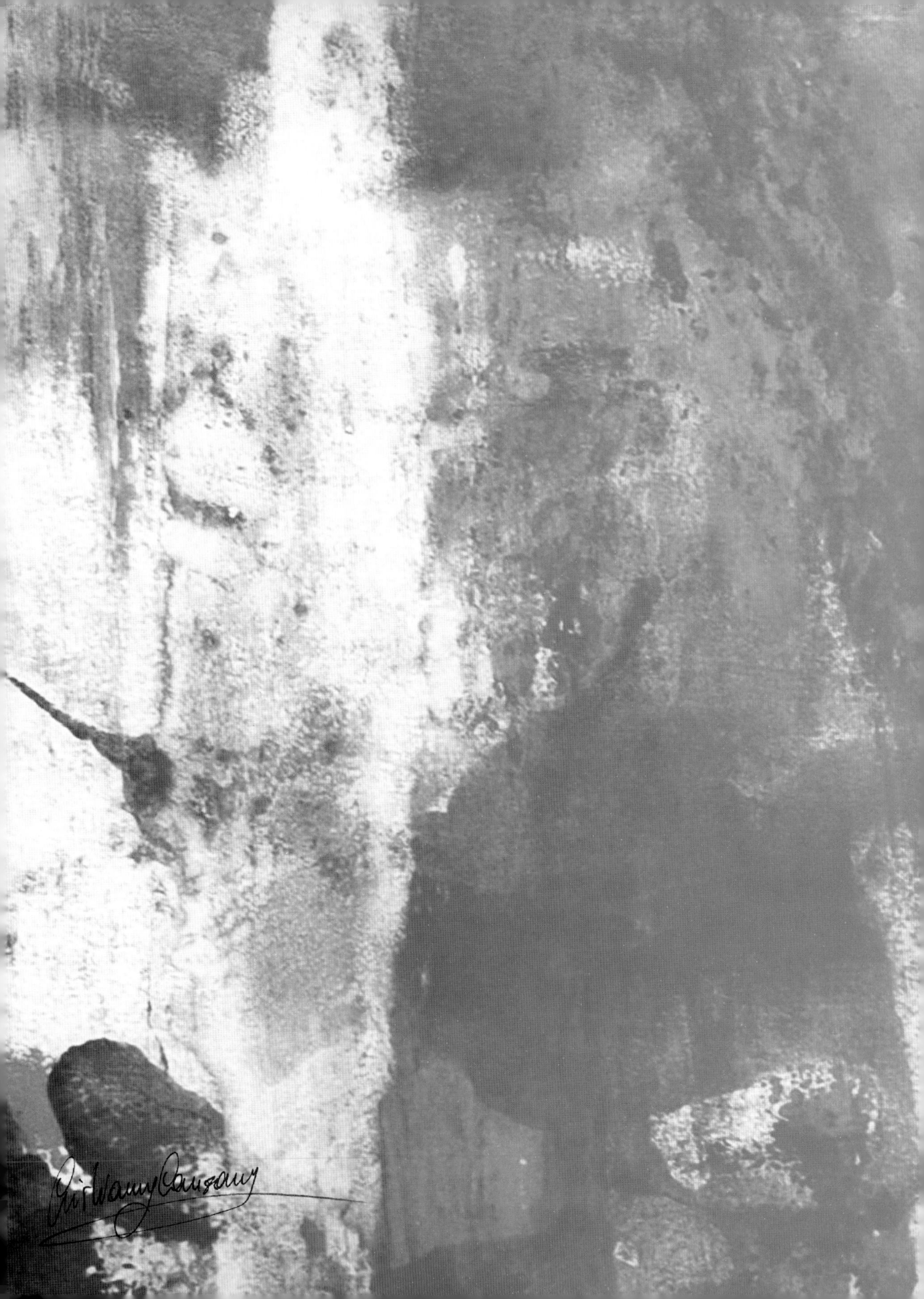

1

The lost value of stillness

Stillness 1

To best serve our clients is to best serve the moment. However:

> *In order to best serve the moment, you have to be still long enough to hear what it is saying.*
>
> Michael Jeffreys*

Jeffreys' quote offers a seemingly simple solution to a whole series of questions and situations that we, as therapists, teachers and practitioners, meet in our daily practice. For the majority of us, the most logical solution to this frequently recurring question of how to best serve our clients is by becoming more specialised and acquiring new knowledge, skills and qualifications. It makes sense that the more knowledgeable we become, the more we will know how to best serve, help and even heal our clients.

However, it is also important to remember that 'the moment' is not *only* about our clients. Each moment includes us too – our being, everything we are composed of physically, emotionally and intellectually, as well as the world and space that is surrounding us.

Our desire to best serve our clients often means that we are focusing and working mainly on one aspect of our practice, namely working with others, and this is perfectly illustrated by the levels of expertise that professionals and practitioners are trained for on a global scale today. The ethos of our practice and the approach to how we treat, teach and facilitate our clients or students are predominantly informed by formative ways of thinking, intellectual discourse and academic knowledge, including technical and practical skills, techniques and codes of conduct. This gives rise to the conclusion that the importance of knowledge has superseded the development of 'being' to a great extent.

In other words, we have acquired a great amount of expert knowledge, intending to best serve our clients, but at the expense of knowing how to simply 'be' in the moment with both ourselves and the people we are working with. Knowing how to simply be with clients is vital, especially at the crucial points just before the possibility of change occurs.

Yet, *in order to best serve the moment,* we first need to know and learn how to truly *be* in the moment. Additionally, we need to fully understand what pure 'being' really is in relation to every other facet of our makeup. Knowing how to be in the moment means, therefore, that *we have to be still long enough*, and only then will we be able *to hear what it is saying*.

The main objective of this book is to provide practitioners with a straightforward and easy-to-use toolkit for helping and facilitating others, and evolving our own being, as well as offering a variety of pointers towards possibilities that will gradually enable us to clearly hear what the present moment in our work with others is actually saying.

Overview

> *Only in quiet waters do things mirror themselves undistorted. Only in a quiet mind is adequate perception of the world.*
>
> Hans Margolius*

There is no real accepted place for philosophy and universal teachings in the field of science. At least that is what many scientists, medics and academics still think. From many a scientist's point of view, very little importance is given to the purpose and value of 'know thyself', the scale of meditation practice, contemplation, ancient psychology and the extensive work on 'being'. This standpoint undervalues the place and role of the philosopher in our modern world. However, since 2002, when the Dalai Lama and

* All quotations marked with an asterisk* are taken from the website effortlesspeace.com/stillness-quotes.

neuroscientist Richard Davidson brought the nature of stillness and the power of meditation into the limelight amongst the neuroscience community, scientists have started acknowledging the work of mystics and philosophers, and the inestimable impact that stillness and meditative practices can have on people and their wellbeing (provided that they are thoroughly researched and tested in the health and therapy sector). Unsurprisingly, a massive amount of serious research into the scope and benefits of stilling, meditation and mindfulness on our body, mind and emotions has been done since then, which has given us a strong foundation to build on.

But this book is not just another book about therapeutic presence, mindfulness and meditation. It explores and highlights the next evolutionary step, leading us beyond the already well-researched teachings of therapeutic presence, mindfulness and meditation, by looking at the multidimensional scale of stillness from an entirely different point of view. The focal point is the inner development by therapists and practitioners of the mainly dormant potential of stillness and the storage capacity of stillness-stimulus and imprints in our tissue, neurons and body fluid, as well as their benefits, use and application in a treatment or teaching environment.

The Inner Power of Stillness endeavours to illuminate the lost value of stillness for the therapist and practitioner, both as a person and as a professional.

We are anchoring the possibility of this inner evolution of the power of stillness on the latest research into water, tissue and cell memory. We also introduce the concept of a potential new modality called 'stillness-memory', and build upon this new understanding a logical and practical framework in which science and philosophy truly inform each other. This opens up access to a much larger scale of new ideas and possibilities that (providing the transformative teachings they embody are put into practice) carry the potential for us as practitioners to be the best person *and* the best professional we can be, without compromising our own overall health and wellbeing.

In-depth knowledge of how to arrive at this promising new modality, as well as how to apply it in our everyday work and life, is at the heart of the book, including topics such as working from our inner power of stillness, the insightful self and, most importantly, the practitioner's toolkit. Some thought-provoking themes that might be of great value to therapists and practitioners who are intending to dedicate some of their time to working for the greater good can be found at the end of the book. There we look at a universal view on compassion and the solace that stillness can bring to people who are nearing the end of their life and final departure.

The book concludes with a philosophical note acknowledging the timeless nature of ancient wisdom, and the ever more important relevance and role of the philosopher in our modern world today.

Before you start diving into this book, please keep in mind this one simple request on behalf of the authors: don't try to explain, analyse or replace new knowledge, insights and ideas you come across with what you already know.

Stillness-memory

When mind is still, then truth gets her chance to be heard in the purity of the silence.

Sri Aurobindo*

Experiment

Be fully present to your very existence for 2½ minutes. During that time, stay put and do not allow your mind to wander or respond to any distractions.

The stillness experiment gives us an idea of our actual ability to be genuinely present, and the amount of energy and willpower it would require to stay in that state for a more prolonged time. The experiment becomes even more challenging if we repeat it a second time, or whilst we are going about everyday things.

According to the National Centre for Biotechnology Information (Statisticbrain.com, 2015), the average attention span of a human being has dropped from

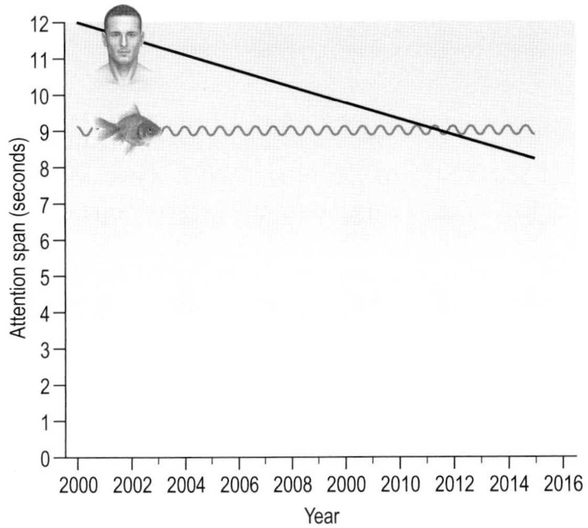

Figure 1.1

Decline of human attention span

12 seconds in the year 2000 to 8.25 seconds in 2015. This is almost one second less than the attention span of a goldfish.

This significant decrease in our attention span is due to the ever-increasing external stimuli we are exposed to in our daily lives, as well as the imbalance and disproportion between our knowledge and our being.

Unfortunately, unlike in some other cultural backgrounds, the great value of inner stillness, and learning how to be comfortable in stillness and silence, do not usually form part of our upbringing. *The ancient teachings point to the fact that dwelling in inner stillness is always accompanied by a deeper sense of being, and a stronger sense of self, from which we gradually disconnect the more we mature and start deriving our sense of 'I' (identity) through what we do and what we know.* Sadly, for most of us, we experience very few conscious moments of inner stillness and silence in our daily routine or at work. Modern life does not provide enough opportunities to enable us to create a reference point of inner stillness that we can instantly access, and that would hold enough gravitas to withstand the continuous stimuli we are exposed to every millisecond of the day.

However, it is interesting to note that these various stimuli can also create our knowledge. The sheer multitude of knowledge we have acquired on all levels is in actual fact composed of memory. That is, each piece of our knowledge is stored and held as memory that has been formed by repeated external stimulus (consisting of the same or a related impression), which was then processed through memory encoding and memory consolidation until it became indelibly imprinted in our brain as groups of neurons (nuclei), waiting to be activated and remembered.

So how can we reduce and neutralise the impacts of these ever-increasing stimuli of external impressions?

Our contention in this book is that we can do this by acquiring and developing memory of a completely different kind and quality – which we (the authors) call stillness-memory – and this provides us with a new modality that we can choose to work from. Using this new modality, stimuli that enter via our five senses are met by inner stillness, and they will not have the same effect as they normally do on other kinds of memory.

As long as external stimuli do not threaten our survival, genuine inner stillness renders them, and consequently the respective memory, knowledge or default response they would trigger, more or less passive, without diminishing them. That is, impressions and events are recognised for what they are, whilst our attention remains undistracted and devoid of the need to instantly spring into action.

An increasing depth of stillness within us will give rise to different brainwave patterns, and recent research has shown that we respond differently to external circumstances when we are regularly exposed to brainwave patterns that are normally not active in our everyday life (see Part 1: Chapter 4). Therefore, a repeated change in our response to stimuli and consequent behaviour (stillness as opposed to intent/action) will gradually lead to neurogenesis (the growth of new brain cells) and neuroplasticity (changes in neural pathways and synapses), as well as stillness-memory imprints in our cells and body matrix. Ultimately this will give rise to the subtlest and most refined levels of perception and an exchange of

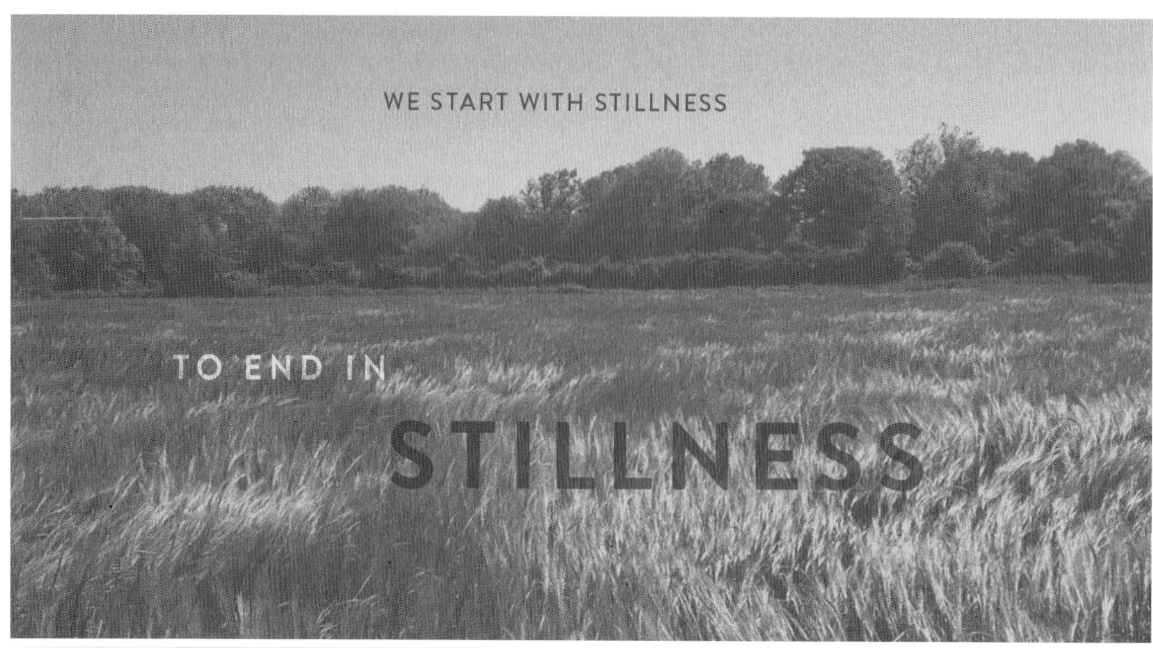

Figure 1.2

Artwork Victoria Dokas; photography Alexander Filmer-Lorch

information beyond our normal ways of communicating and how we perceive things. Such is the inner power of stillness.

The reflective practitioner

> *Within you there is a stillness and a sanctuary to which you can retreat at any time and be yourself.*
>
> Herman Hesse*

Working from our inner power of stillness means that our work has to come directly from the 'self'. Like the unknown and the beyond, the self can't be objectified, yet the great teachers and philosophers of this world say that the formless self resembles silence and stillness. In actual fact, it comprises a depth of silence and stillness that is transcendental:

> *Your innermost sense of self, of who you are, is inseparable from stillness.*
>
> Eckhart Tolle*

Hence, the gateway to self is first and foremost through inner stillness, which is the primary source and resource for the experienced reflective practitioner. That means working in three directions simultaneously (trimetric), the first two being horizontal and the third being vertical (see Part 3: Chapter 11). This will allow us to work from a multidimensional perspective that sheds light on the whole as well as the parts, and to respond to the cause and not only to the effect. We are usually taught to work with our clients from a place of *knowing* and *doing*, as well as *focusing* our attention on our clients and their pathology, which means we are only working from one end of the scale of possibilities. Reflective practitioners, however, aim to work with the whole scale of possibilities by profoundly increasing their field of awareness, implementing and utilising ideas such as *allowing* and *listening*, as well as working from and through the unknown.

> *The self must know stillness before it can discover its true song.*
>
> Ralph Blum*

Learning to work using the trinity of directions simultaneously gives rise to a truly self-reflective practice that no longer takes place at the expense of the self but instead is informed by the inner power of stillness that continuously radiates from the innermost depths of our self.

> Stillness and silence require a certain level of inner acknowledgement to be recognised for what they are. That is, we need to be connected to a far deeper sense of self to be naturally present to stillness and silence than we are in our ordinary or relative state of consciousness.

The scope of stillness

> *Nothing in all creation is so like God as stillness.*
>
> Meister Eckhart*

Stillness can increase and multiply itself indefinitely, provided our mind becomes genuinely attentive to that stillness for long enough, and to such an extent that it becomes as still as stillness itself. This is the beginning of our connection with the infinite, just like the reach and scope of stillness is infinite. In this dynamic stillness we can experience that all higher forms or manifestations of states of consciousness are merely different facets or expressions of different depths of inner stillness. The ancient teachings describe this spontaneous deepening as a process called the *expansion of consciousness*. That is, the subtle power of stillness induces consciousness to expand, which opens the doors to a much larger scale of possibilities, as well as different ways of perception.

However, for us practitioners, it is far more important to look at ways in which stillness can be utilised to benefit the physical, mental and emotional health of ourselves and our clients, which leads us to the scope of stillness in our work. As mentioned above, we are more conscious of and receptive to impressions and information when we are still. Our actions and responses are less driven by default and our palpation and listening abilities become significantly refined, leading to a much more objective and direct way of perception, which in turn gives rise to actions that are not created by any internal intent, impulse or active thought. This different kind of action rises from the depth of inner stillness and silence and meets us in the form of intuition and inspiration derived from and informed by the actual requirements and needs of our clients, within the dynamic of a much more undiluted exchange of information. Hence, it is our clients' inherent wisdom of what is asking for change within their own body/mind unit that is in charge and directs the process, supported by the background current of stillness continuously radiating from the depth of the practitioner's inner self, and through which whatever needs to happen is allowed to happen.

> *The secret of the receptive must be sought in stillness. Within stillness there remains the potential for action.*
>
> Zhou Xuanjing*

However, the true magic within this process is that as practitioners we are as much contained and safeguarded through the influence of stillness as our clients. Through stillness we are not losing our connection with a deeper sense of centredness, thus our physical and mental equilibrium and wellbeing are sustained.

Krishnamurti on 'Silence in the brain'

'The complete stillness of the brain is an extraordinary thing; it is highly sensitive, vigorous, fully alive, aware of every outward movement but utterly still.' Krishnamurti describes this state as an openness without any boundaries, intentions and frictions. 'It is utterly still in emptiness; this emptiness is not a state of vacuum, a blankness; it is energy without a centre, without a border.' He tells how he experienced how his brain had a much more refined and increased awareness of all the different sensations caused by the walking motion of his body down the street, the traffic around him, including smells, sounds and taste, without (in his own words) a 'centre from which watching, directing, censoring took place'. Furthermore, he describes that, throughout the whole duration of this rare experience, there was no movement in his brain, and although this has happened to him several times before, it was still a strange phenomenon, which kept surprising him once it was over.

(quotations from Jkrishnamurti.org, 2015)

Pure stillness:

- is ever present around all things observed and unobserved (sounds, objects and space)
- encompasses both the parts and the whole ('global and local') (Maggie Gill, SER workshop UIUK, June 2014)
- spans the macrocosm and the microcosm
- when the mind meets it leads us to perceive death / God / the presence / the unknown / the beyond as infinite, empty stillness
- resides between the gaps of our thoughts
- lives within the natural pause after the inhalation and the exhalation
- plays a major part in the healing process of the body
- can multiply indefinitely
- enhances and refines our palpation and listening skills
- is the most non-invasive and all-encompassing place to work from
- takes us out of our mainly linear ways of perception
- transforms each and everyone that meets it, including our non-conscious states
- is the remedy for stress
- activates different brainwave patterns
- gives rise to a natural state of effortless presence
- neutralises incoming stimuli and impressions
- leads to self-consciousness
- allows us to act and respond more consciously
- gives rise to insight, inspiration and creativity
- resembles pure self
- is the gateway to neutral
- neutralises opposites
- acts as a conscious shock
- is the key to our inner work
- creates stillness-memory
- is the common denominator in all world religions, schools of thought and philosophical teachings
- is free of charge, limitless and available to everyone.

References

Jkrishnamurti.org (2015). Krishnamurti's Notebook. J. Krishnamurti Online, www.jkrishnamurti.org/krishnamurti-teachings/view-text.php?tid=2372&chid=70770&w=Bombay+and+Rishi+Valley&s=Text [accessed 16 Jun. 2015].

Statisticbrain.com (2015). Attention span statistics. Statistic Brain, www.statisticbrain.com/attention-span-statistics/ [accessed 17 Jun. 2015].

Origins 2

What today's scientific research is discovering and proving about the impact of the stilling process has been known to the rishis, munies and yogis since long before the development of writing (around 3000 BCE).

Cristian Violatti, a scholar of archaeology at the University of Leicester, states that ancient teachings have come down to us from prehistoric times. He explains that,

> *The foundations of Hinduism can be found in the teachings of anonymous ancient sages or rishis, which were originally transmitted orally. We know very little about Hinduism beyond what can be learned from the Vedas, a collection of hymns and other ritual texts composed in different periods. These texts contain a lot of material including the teachings of the early sages. The oldest evidence of religious practices in India date back approximately to 5500 bce. It is a mistake to reduce all early Hinduism to Vedic religion: there were many other non-Vedic religious traditions in early Hinduism which have left no early texts and that can be known to some extent by archaeological evidence.*
>
> Violatti, 2013

It is great news that today's scientists have acknowledged the great potential in ancient teachings and that new discoveries and ancient teachings are starting to inform each other. In turn, these will gradually inform us, and ultimately the whole environment we live in. The almost forgotten wisdom of the past is now transforming into active knowledge for our times, and will perhaps be the beginning of a new cycle, leading to a new proposition from which we can work with or treat our clients.

The Yoga Sutras of Patanjali

The Yoga Sutras of Patanjali is an ancient scripture consisting of possibly the most comprehensive collection of knowledge texts ever written. This historical wisdom is transmitted through 196 sutras, which, based on research by Philipp A. Maas (2006), were written around 400 CE by Patanjali. However, it is supposed that the practices and techniques described in the sutras date back as early as 3000 to 4000 BCE. Most of the sutras in the first chapter of the Samadhi Pada focus on the process of stilling, which means that everything else, such as the different states of consciousness, presence and mindfulness, as well as meditation explained in subsequent chapters, naturally arise out of this initial process of stilling.

Patanjali's genius lies in not wasting any precious time, miraculously revealing only the relevant truth. The essence of the knowledge contained in all subsequent sutras is expressed right at the beginning of the text in his second sutra (1.2), which states: 'Yoga (yoking) is to still the pattern of consciousness' (the mind or citta) (Hartranft, 2003 p. 2). That is, the majority of patterns held in our mind are created by the active nature of our attention, which continuously responds to external stimuli and the constant flow of incoming impressions. However, the moment our attention is increasingly exposed to the influence of stilling, the energy of the pattern currently active in our mind dissipates, just like the energy that dissipates during a tissue release, or the energy of stress releases the moment we are back in the tranquillity of our home after a stressful day at work.

Sutra 1.12 informs us that: 'Both practice and nonreaction are required to still the patterning of consciousness [mind]' (Hartranft, 2003 p. 5), which does not mean to completely refrain from responding, but to first pause and listen, out of which a less mechanical and much more conscious and appropriate response can arise that does not originate from a pattern generated by the mind. We can find another pointer towards the objective of non-reaction in sutra 1.13, which says: 'Practice is the sustained effort to rest in that stillness' (Hartranft, 2003 p. 5). At first, this seems to be a paradox, taking into consideration that *sustained effort* is an activity that is based on doing, as opposed to *resting in that stillness*. Yet, the hint that leads to resting in stillness lies in the word 'practice', which stands for a series of practical exercises and techniques that give rise to inner stillness once put into action. The knowledge and instructions for these particular stilling techniques can be found in other parts of the Yoga Sutras, but some of them are not suitable for our modern times, especially if the reader takes them too literally.

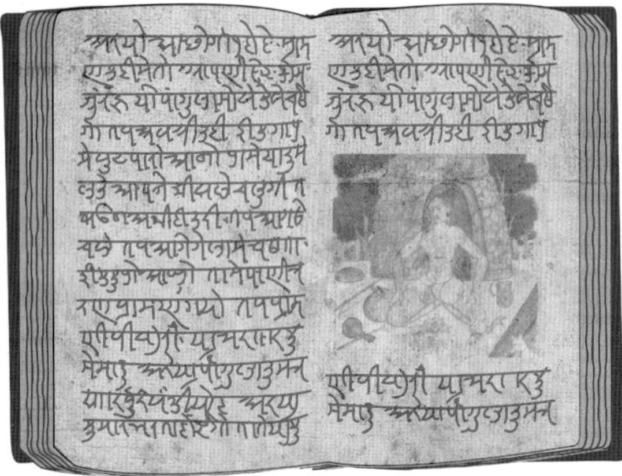

Figure 2.1

Stillness at the heart of all ancient teachings

Patanjali describes the process of reaching inner stillness in more detail in sutra 1.17, pointing out that, 'At first the stilling process is accompanied by four kinds of cognition: *analytical thinking*, insight, bliss and feeling like a self' (Hartranft, 2003 p. 8). This means that the first cognition of analytical thinking will gradually satisfy the mind, because regardless of what we want to achieve in life, we need our mind to be on board, otherwise it will interfere with our efforts and intentions. The initial friction created by critical thinking and continued questioning, as well as regular attempts to apply the practice, take us towards a deeper exploration of what we are enquiring into. That is, we are gaining a greater understanding by illuminating all aspects of the subject, which will lead to the second kind of cognition, that of *insight*.

A real insight gives rise to a true 'Aha' moment that effortlessly dissolves all friction, induces our consciousness to expand and leads to the third kind of cognition, that of *bliss*. This third insight is the actual experience of the initial idea, which in this case is the complete experience of stillness. This might instantly be followed by the fourth kind of cognition, the *feeling like a self*, which according to the universal teachings is the gradual realisation of our true self (purusha), possibly by self-remembering, and ultimately leading to full realisation. The self needs to be remembered because most of us have forgotten this essential part of us that we were born with.

However, sutra 1.18 reveals that, 'Later, after one practices steadily, these four kinds of cognition fall away, leaving only a store of latent impressions in the depth of memory' (Hartranft, 2003 p. 8). This means that the four kinds of cognition have served their purpose, becoming more or less passive because the initial theoretical knowledge of stilling has turned into actual experience.

Many recent research programmes on tissue memory, neuroplasticity and neurogenesis, as well as the inspiration to write this book, are based on the knowledge in the next sutra. According to sutra 3.9, at this point, 'The transformation toward total stillness occurs as new latent impressions fostering cessation arise to prevent the activation of distractive stored ones, and moments of stillness begin to permeate consciousness [mind]' (Hartranft, 2003 p. 48). These latent impressions are created by inner stillness continuously creating new impressions of stillness-memory, generated by the practice of stillness, which ultimately render all other forms of active memory passive, so that 'These latent impressions help consciousness [mind] flow from one tranquil moment to the next' (Hartranft, 2003 p. 48). By naturally flowing from one moment of tranquillity to the other, more prolonged stillness imprints are created, forming a permanent centre of gravity within our mind/body unit (fascia, cells and new neurons) (sutra 3.10). 'In other words, the mind is transformed toward focus as continuity develops between arising and subsiding perceptions' (sutra 3.12, Hartranft, 2003 p. 48).

At this stage in our practice, the mind greatly values the influence and benefits of stillness and stops opposing the true self, which draws its focus through attention even further into stillness. Then (sutra 1.41), 'As the patterning of consciousness [mind] subsides, a transparent way of seeing, called coalescence, saturates consciousness [the mind]; like a jewel, it reflects equally whatever lies before it – whether subject, object, or act of perceiving' (Hartranft, 2003 p. 15). This means all facets of the mind (including memories, 'I-believes', subpersonalities and personal philosophies) become utterly still and coalesce, giving rise to a new kind of perception in which subject, object and act of perceiving are simultaneously recognised for what they are with no filter. The common act of cognition, of thinking through from one thing to the other and having to recognise each of them separately by adding a name and meaning to them, is being omitted. That is, we purely perceive.

From a universal teaching point of view, this is called 'direct perception' or 'lucid cognition', in which things are not seen as separate from each other but rather experienced as being a part of one frictionless whole. Here (sutra 1.47), 'In the lucidity of coalesced, reflection-free contemplation, the nature of the self becomes clear' and (sutra 1.48) 'The wisdom that arises in that lucidity is unerring' (Hartranft, 2003 p. 18).

The best example that describes the beginning stages of direct perception (lucid cognition) we practitioners can relate to is the exchange of information that occurs whilst we are palpating and melding. Through the process of melding, the palpating hand becomes one with the body of the person we are treating and opens up a channel in which information can flow and be perceived in a way that would not be possible without having gone through the process of melding. Simply palpating would not do the job because of the subject–object dynamic, and the fact that as practitioners we experience ourselves as distinct from the palpating hand. Hence, the idea of 'me' distinct from the 'other' still exists. However, complete and direct perception (lucid cognition) occurs the moment the melding is informed by a lucid and coalesced, reflection-free contemplation that arises from the innermost nature of the self, through which the idea of 'me' distinct from the 'other' in the context of melding ceases to exist. That is, the practitioner perceives each element of this interchanging dynamic as one whole truth or reality through the true self (purusha), as opposed to separate truths or realities commonly perceived through the mind (citta), such as the reality of the palpated body, the reality of the client, the reality of the practitioner palpating the client, to the reality of the environment they work in.

Sutra 1.49 goes on: '... this wisdom has as its object the actual distinction between pure awareness [purusha] and consciousness [citta/mind]' (Hartranft, 2003 p. 19), which means that in time the work of the practitioner is not only informed by knowledge (mind), but comes directly from the true self (being) by means of the inner power of stillness.

Sutra 4.26 states: 'Consciousness [mind], now orientated to this distinction, can gravitate toward freedom ...' (Hartranft, 2003 p. 68), which, Patanjali concludes in sutra 4.34, is at hand when 'pure awareness [true self] ... stands alone, grounded in its very nature, the power of pure seeing [lucid cognition]. That is all' (Hartranft, 2003 p. 70).

World religions and different schools of thought on stilling

The knowledge in the most ancient teachings that were orally transmitted by the rishis 9,000 years ago, and which formed the basis of Hinduism, undoubtedly informed and influenced all our existing world religions, their founders and the many different schools of thought that have gradually evolved ever since. What all of them have in common are their in-depth teachings on stilling and the importance placed on reconnecting to the self.

Stilling forms the basis of the second direction of work in Buddha's threefold teachings, expressed in Kornfield's (2012) words as follows: 'The essential path taught by the Buddha has three parts to it. The first is kindness of heart, a ground of fundamental compassion expressed through virtue and generosity. The second is inner stillness or concentration. The third aspect of all Buddhist practice is the awakening of liberating wisdom.'

The Christian Bible refers to the importance of stilling in Psalms 46:10, 'Be still, and know that I am God', whilst Exodus 14:14 leaves no room for misunderstanding by saying, 'The Lord will fight for you; you need only to be still', which is a pointer towards the practice of non-reaction we previously looked at in sutra 1.12. Jesus's command to '… go into your room, and when you have shut the door, pray to your Father who is in the secret place' was directed at his disciples to encourage them to pray by connecting with the stillness within (Matthew 6:6).

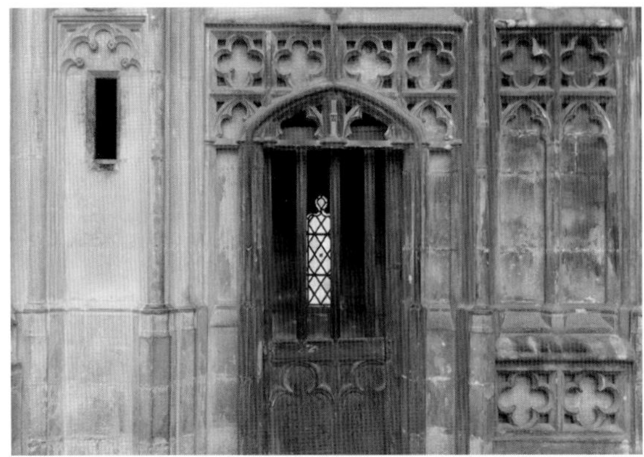

Figure 2.2

Photography Alexander Filmer-Lorch

The great teacher Sri Ramana Maharshi summarises the practical aspects of his teachings in just four lines. Godman (1991) says: 'The method is summed up in the words "Be still". What does stillness mean? It means destroy yourself.' He further explains what we need to do: 'Give up the notion that "I am so and so".' This leads to the conclusion that 'All that is required to realize the Self is to be still. What can be easier than that?' (Godman, 1991). How we can neutralise all ideas of 'I am so and so' is expressed by the simple words of Sri Nisargadatta: 'No particular thought can be mind's natural state, only silence.' (Dikshit, 2012).

The initial means towards this objective can be found in the Tao Te Ching, which states: 'Attain the ultimate emptiness. Hold on to the truest tranquility. The myriad things are all active. I therefore watch their return' (Lin, 2006 chapter 16). The Tao then explains: 'The Tao is constant in non-action. Yet, there is nothing it does not do' (chapter 37), which describes the process of yoking or coalescence of the opposites forming one whole truth. The very same truth is expressed by this final thought:

> *Where past and future are gathered. Neither movement from nor towards,*
>
> *Neither ascent nor decline. Except for the point, the still point,*
>
> *There would be no dance, and there is only the dance.*
>
> T.S. Eliot, from *Burnt Norton, Four Quartets*

To conclude we can say that stillness seems to be the pivot point around which all manifested and unmanifested things and ideas evolve, and the inner power of stillness seems to be the key that gives us access to a far greater insight into the truth of things, as well as into ways that information flows, whether that is within and through us or through others, and possibly even through the whole world around us.

References

Dikshit, S. (2012). *I Am That: talks with Sri Nisargadatta Maharaj.* 2nd ed. Durham, NC: Acorn Press.

Godman, D. (1991). *Be As You Are: the teachings of Sri Ramana Maharshi.* New Delhi: Penguin Books.

Hartranft, C. (2003). *The Yoga-Sūtra of Patañjali.* Boston, MA: Shambhala Publications.

Kornfield, J. (2012). *Bringing Home the Dharma: awakening right where you are.* Boston and London: Shambhala.

Lin, D. (2006). *Tao Te Ching: annotated & explained.* Woodstock, VT: SkyLight Paths Publications, www.taoism.net/ [accessed 18 Jun. 2015].

Maas, P. (2006). *Samādhipāda: the first chapter of the Pātañjalayogśāstra for the first time critically edited.* Aachen: Shaker.

ReligionFacts.com (2015). *History of Hinduism.* ReligionFacts.com, www.religionfacts.com/hinduism/history [accessed 17 Jun. 2015].

Violatti, C. (2013). Hinduism. *Ancient history encyclopedia,* www.ancient.eu/hinduism/ [accessed 17 Jun. 2015].

Stillness is universal 3

Transmission of universal knowledge in today's world

Finland has branded itself as the country of silence. In its Country Brand Report it says that 'Silence is a resource' and 'In the future, people will be prepared to pay for the experience of silence'. Gross (2014) comments that 'It could be marketed just like clean water or wild mushrooms'.

However, if the whole world starts holidaying in Finland, that would destroy the wonderful silence in this beautiful country, so we need to explore possibilities nearer to home.

We are usually exposed to two streams of influences in life. The first is directed at the mind and our personality, and the second is directed at the 'self'. That is, the former keeps us randomly engaged with all sorts of things in life, which we respond to mainly by default, whilst the latter touches us on a deeper level and makes us pause and listen to a greater truth that lies beneath. Why? Because this second influence transmits universal knowledge or truth that deeply resonates with the truth that makes up the nature of our self. This higher knowledge exists beyond us, and can be an incredibly potent resource, without which change and our realisation of truth and an objective outlook on life would be impossible. We are in fact surrounded by this knowledge in the form of specific impressions all the time, but are usually not receptive to them because of the 'noise' created by the overpowering stream of other influences.

Alongside the knowledge derived from religious scriptures, philosophy and psychology, most of the transformative impressions reaching us today are generated by the creative potential of artists, scientists, architects, photographers, writers and poets, etc. who are attuned with influences of higher knowledge themselves. Universal knowledge transmitted through the arts and sciences aims to fully awaken us to the omnipresent stillness at the core of all things visible and invisible. When our latent inner truth in our true self and the truth revealed in external impressions align, this triggers a reciprocal recognition in which opposites coalesce, leading to a brief but profound experience of eternal stillness. That is, the inner stillness of the self is reflected back to itself for a short time the moment it comes into contact with these other influences.

Examples of how these impressions can act on us in real life, and how profoundly they can change us internally, can be found in the works of minimalist artist Lee Ufan. He says his sculptures and paintings 'lead people's eyes to emptiness and turn their eyes to silence' (Compton, 2015), and provide 'an open site of power in which things and space do vividly interact' (Gary Tatintsian Gallery, 2015). In a similar vein, James Turrell's 'works radiate silence – but that of a particularly welcoming and appealing type – the one you desire the most while caught in the midst of a swarming megalopolis' (Urazmetova, 2014).

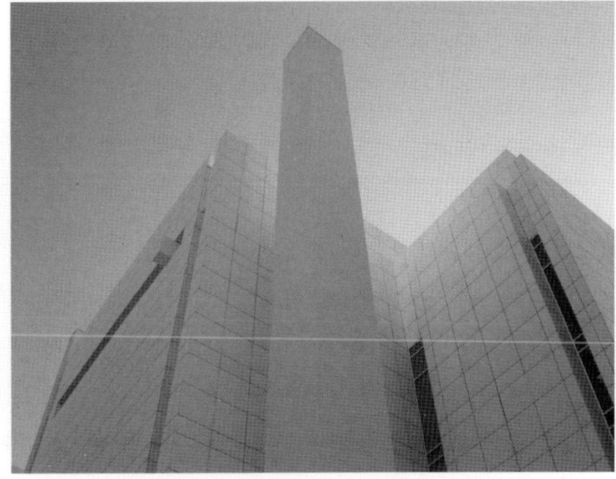

Figure 3.1

Grand architecture as an example of a second influence. Photography Alexander Filmer-Lorch

The works of philosophical artists – such as Anish Kapoor illuminating the dynamics of opposing forces and their neutralising element, and Richard Long's silent walks, where magnificent landscape sculptures rise out of his footprints left on the ground, as well as Mark Rothko's paintings, which are spaces within which we can contemplate the stillness at the core of who we are in essence – have induced a state of awe in millions of people, connecting them with a deeper sense of self. And, without a doubt, the same is true for countless other artists of all different genres.

However, any such impressions can connect us with our insightful self, including awe-inspiring architecture like the 'skyspaces' of Turrell, the Lilja Chapel of Silence, the Sacred Museum of Adeje and many other great public spaces that we can visit and experience, films such as *Waking Life* by R. Linklater and *The Fountain* by Darren Aronofsky, or the works of choreographers Wayne McGregor, Russell Maliphant and William Forsythe. The possibilities are many and have even caught the interest of the world of science. Recent studies in the field by Royal College in London have uncovered hidden dimensions that show a far-reaching connection between architecture and the nature of our existence (AIDEC World, 2012).

Entirely new influences generated by science, cosmology, quantum physics and psychology are transforming what has been taken as the truth in the past (ancient and contemporary alike), and are illuminating new possibilities, suggesting that there is an existing interconnecting and silent power behind all things. Take, for example, the proof of the existence of the Higgs Boson particle (dubbed the 'God particle') in 2012, or Das and Bhaduri's paper (2015) on quantum fluid, which proposes that the Big Bang never happened, based on a new model in which the universe has no beginning and no end.

But far more important is how these influences make us aware of our own insignificance in this incomprehensible cosmological play, and the feeling of astonishment and awe it gives rise to by simply contemplating it.

People spend decades trying to live their lives according to ancient belief systems, but there is no need to replicate or imitate these, nor try to fit or impose something on our life today that was designed for people who lived at a particular time in the past. Why not? Because the power within the timeless nature of the universal teachings forever transcends our self. The inherent wisdom of a mandala, a specific ritual or a scripture created 4,000 years ago, transmitting knowledge in a way that could be grasped by the people of those ancient times, evolves and transforms through millennia and presents as many different expressions of the same truth. Ultimately it may manifest as an earth circle created by an artist of our modern times; it is transmitting the very same knowledge but in a way that can be grasped by the people of today's world. This is how the eternal truth that existed before the existence of time morphs to meet the requirements of all times, ensuring that the essence of the teachings is being kept alive for eternity, which lies beyond time.

So, as our mind and body are increasingly fed and nourished by the second stream of influences, the latent impressions of universal truth they leave in our psychology and physiology will naturally transform us into a different kind of influence. This silent transmission that discreetly radiates through our being can be accessed and utilised by the people we work with, if they wish to do so. That is, through our own effort, and by applying and utilising the second stream of influences, we naturally evolve into a third stream that differs from the other two, since it emanates from a silent place somewhere deeply internal that is independent of anything external.

Utilising stillness in sports, dance, martial arts and yoga

Most athletes and sports enthusiasts are very familiar with an extraordinary occurrence called 'the second wind', which clicks in once we have reached the end of our physical and mental capacities and suddenly gives us the strength to continue with a top level of performance. It is described as a place of utter stillness and balance in which everything works together in perfect harmony, accompanied by the feeling that we can keep going forever. A similar level of performance can be achieved by implementing stilling techniques into our daily training programme. Today, most professional athletes are utilising scientific research on stilling to enhance their performance, and to maintain their equilibrium during stressful competitions.

Dancers and gymnasts have mastered their craft once they have established a still-point or centre of gravity deep within themselves. This inner still-point, out of which all movement arises, enables them to almost defy gravity. At this stage, they have established a level of concentration and stillness that transcends all technique, so that body, space, ground and gravity support each other, and work together in perfect balance. Throughout their performance, the dancer or gymnast experiences a great sense of inner stillness and tranquillity, as if the movements are coming from somewhere beyond, and not from a place of personal effort or intent. The Tao, martial arts, chi gong and tai chi have developed a whole science that focuses on the hara (Sea of Qi), a point along the *linea alba* on the lower abdomen below the navel. Settling into this still-point will ultimately enable practitioners to move from the centre of our very being. Most of us are familiar with yoga, which comprises a collection of teachings and practices (the eight limbs of yoga) that enable practitioners to gradually channel the energies of body and mind towards inner stillness, by means of a stilling process that acts on our physiology and our psychology, as well as on our everyday life.

These different examples demonstrate that, in all these different disciplines, inner stillness is the basis for and the means to ultimately attain mastery, enabling a congruency between the actual action, the person in action and the interaction between the two, which would not be possible otherwise. No knowledge, technique, aim, intent or the greatest will in the world would be able to achieve this with the same effect.

The relevance of stillness in medicine

A significant number of healthcare organisations and hospitals have started to implement mindfulness practice and a compassion-centred approach to working with patients. According to DasGupta (2007), the experiences of severely ill patients and their families 'hold unique insights for physicians in how to engage in an ethical, empathetic, and self-reflective practice'. He further highlights that not only story but other narratives like stillness or silence are of great importance to the practice of medicine. 'The voices of patients and their families hold both literal and allegorical lessons for physicians in how to move toward a medical practice' (DasGupta, 2007). According to his research this does not only involve different forms of diagnosis and treatments, but also includes and recognises the power of healing.

EVERY DAY I RENEW MY EFFORTS TO WORK FROM
BEING AND ALLOWING
OPPOSED TO KNOWING AND DOING

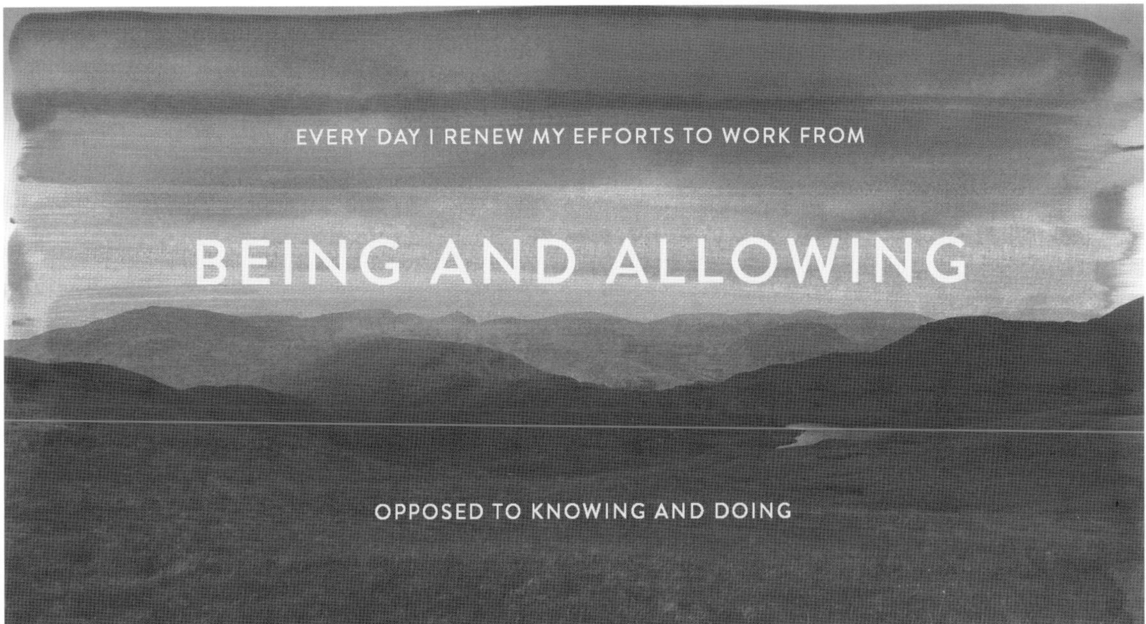

Figure 3.2
Artwork Victoria Dokas; photography Alexander Filmer-Lorch

It has become very clear that 'there is a strong need for more comprehensive training during medical school and residency for the application of mind–body methods such as meditation [stilling]' (Fortney and Taylor, 2010). However, to prevent interns and trainees from developing immunity to suffering and distress, these methods have to be taught at the early stages in each training programme. We now know that 'meditation can help foster present-moment awareness that may reduce medical error and improve patient care' (Fortney and Taylor, 2010). This is backed up by additional research that shows that 'patients of interns who received mindfulness training did significantly better than those patients treated by interns who did not receive mindfulness training' (Fortney and Taylor, 2010). Dobkin (2009) points out that Michael Kearney, the author of *A Place of Healing*, suggests that providing a safe place in which patients can regain a sense of integrity and wholeness is part of the healthcare mandate. In other words, reflective practice can be characterised by 'attentive observation of self, patient, and context; critical curiosity; beginner's mind (that is, viewing the situation free of preconceptions); and presence'. Kearney then defines presence as 'connection between the knower and the known, undistracted attention on the task and the person, and compassion based on insight rather than sympathy' (Dobkin, 2009).

> *Quiet is a part of care, as essential for patients as medication or sanitation. It's a strange notion, but one that researchers have begun to bear out as true.*
>
> Daniel A. Gross (2014)

Practising medicine accordingly – that is, to cure when possible and to promote healing even if there is no cure – the practitioner needs to add reflective practice, with emphasis on compassion, to the traditional ways. It can be studied and acquired by every dedicated practitioner, through regular practice and conscious effort. Many medical training centres throughout the world are acknowledging the importance and requirement to broaden training 'such that curing and caring are equally valued and simultaneously provided in the best interest of the patient. Outcomes may depend upon it' (Dobkin, 2009).

We trust that this book is encouraging practitioners, teachers and therapists to do just that.

References

AIDEC World (2012). *Sacred Architecture: designing for cosmic energy*. AIDEC World, www.aidecworld.com/cosmology/sacred-architecture-designing-for-cosmic-energy/#sthash.iEVsFbQF.dpuf [accessed 19 Jun. 2015].

Compton, N. (2015). Trauma and tranquility: Anish Kapoor and minimalist Lee Ufan take over London's Lisson Gallery. *Wallpaper Magazine*, www.wallpaper.com/art/trauma-and-tranquility-anish-kapoor-and-minimalist-lee-ufan-take-over-londons-lisson-gallery/8644#Sy11ZymOYS4SG1xF.99 [accessed 19 Jun. 2015].

Das, S. and Bhaduri, R. (2015). Dark matter and dark energy from a Bose-Einstein condensate. *Classical and Quantum Gravity*, 32(10): 105003, http://iopscience.iop.org/0264-9381/32/10/105003/ [accessed 19 Jun. 2015].

DasGupta, S. (2007). Between stillness and story: lessons of children's illness narratives. *Pediatrics*, 119(6): e1384-e1391, http://pediatrics.aappublications.org/content/119/6/e1384.abstract [accessed 19 Jun. 2015].

Dobkin, P. (2009). Fostering healing through mindfulness in the context of medical practice. *Current Oncology*, 16(2): 4–6, www.ncbi.nlm.nih.gov/pmc/articles/PMC2669230/ [accessed 19 Jun. 2015].

Fortney, L. and Taylor, M. (2010). Meditation in medical practice: a review of the evidence and practice. *Primary Care: Clinics in Office Practice*, 37(1): 81–90, www.primarycare.theclinics.com/article/S0095-4543%2809%2900083-9/fulltext [accessed 19 Jun. 2015].

Gary Tatintsian Gallery (2015). Lee Ufan. Gary Tatintsian Gallery, www.tatintsian.com/artists/lee-ufan/works [accessed 19 Jun. 2015].

Gross, D. (2014). This is your brain on silence. *Nautilus*, issue 16: Nothingness, http://nautil.us/issue/16/nothingness/this-is-your-brain-on-silence [accessed 11 Jun. 2015].

Urazmetova, N. (2014). Some/art: James Turrell at Pace London [blog], http://www.someslashthings.com/online-magazine/2014/2/20/someart-james-turrell-at-pace-london [accessed Mar. 2016].

How does stilling act on our physiology? 4

> *Unnecessary noise, then, is the most cruel absence of care which can be inflicted either on sick or well.*
>
> Florence Nightingale

External stimulus for stillness and silence

Researchers initially used stillness and silence as a baseline to be able to study the effects of sound, music and noise on our physiology and brain function. They discovered that the impact of any kind of sound led to changes in carbon dioxide levels, blood pressure and circulation, especially in the brain. However, a study by Bernardi and colleagues showed not only that during almost all sorts of music there was a physiological change compatible with a condition of arousal, but also that only two minutes of silent pauses appeared to be far more relaxing than calming music or much longer phases of silence (Bernardi, Porta and Sleight, 2005). This makes sense, according to Wehr (2010), because 'the assumption that signalling of a sound's appearance and its subsequent disappearance are both handled by the same pathway' has been replaced by a theory that a separate set of synapses is responsible for each. 'It looks like there is a whole separate channel that goes all the way from the ear up to the brain that is specialised to process sound offsets (distortion or loss of audio volume).' These two channels finally merge together in the auditory cortex, which is situated in the temporal lobe. This suggests that we all possess two hearing faculties in each ear: one that responds to sound and one that responds to silence. So, why is the stimulus for stillness and silence so important to us?

Moran et al. (2013) discuss Raichle's view that there is a default mode network, a background activity taking place in the resting brain (situated in the prefrontal cortex), which is also enlisted in self-reflection. That is, in stillness and contemplative self-reflection, our brain is able to integrate information into a conscious workspace.

However, a different paper by Kirste and team in 2013, called 'Is silence golden?', led to completely unexpected results, highlighting further the possible magnitude and importance of stillness as a stimulus. Kirste states: 'We found that except for white noise, all stimuli, including silence, increased precursor cell proliferation ....' (Kirste et al., 2013). But far more important, says Kirste, is that 'after 7 days, only silence remained associated with increased numbers of BrdU-labeled cells [a synthetic nucleoside commonly used in the detection of proliferating cells in living tissues]'. She goes on: 'We saw that silence is really helping the new generated cells to differentiate into neurons, and integrate into the system' (Gross, 2014). In her 2013 paper, Kirste concludes that, 'In absolute terms, silence resulted in statistically increased levels of neurogenesis.' Additionally, Kirste found that two hours of silence per day prompted cell development in the hippocampus, the brain region related to the formation of memory and involving the senses. Gross (2014) commented: 'While Kirste emphasises that her findings are preliminary, she wonders if this effect could have unexpected applications.' According to Gross (2014), it is well known that pathologies such as depression and dementia have been associated with decreasing rates of neurogenesis in the hippocampus, which requires further research, but 'if a link between silence and neurogenesis could be established in humans, Kirste says, perhaps neurologists could find a therapeutic use for silence'.

But stimulus-stillness does not stop there. It focuses our attention to turn inwards. A study by Farb suggested 'that the neural networks of interoceptive attention may provide an inbuilt system separate from the thinking mind to help ourselves find calm' (Seppala, 2012). Seppala says Farb's study shows that 'we can't control our mind with our mind (or our prefrontal cortex with the prefrontal cortex), but with

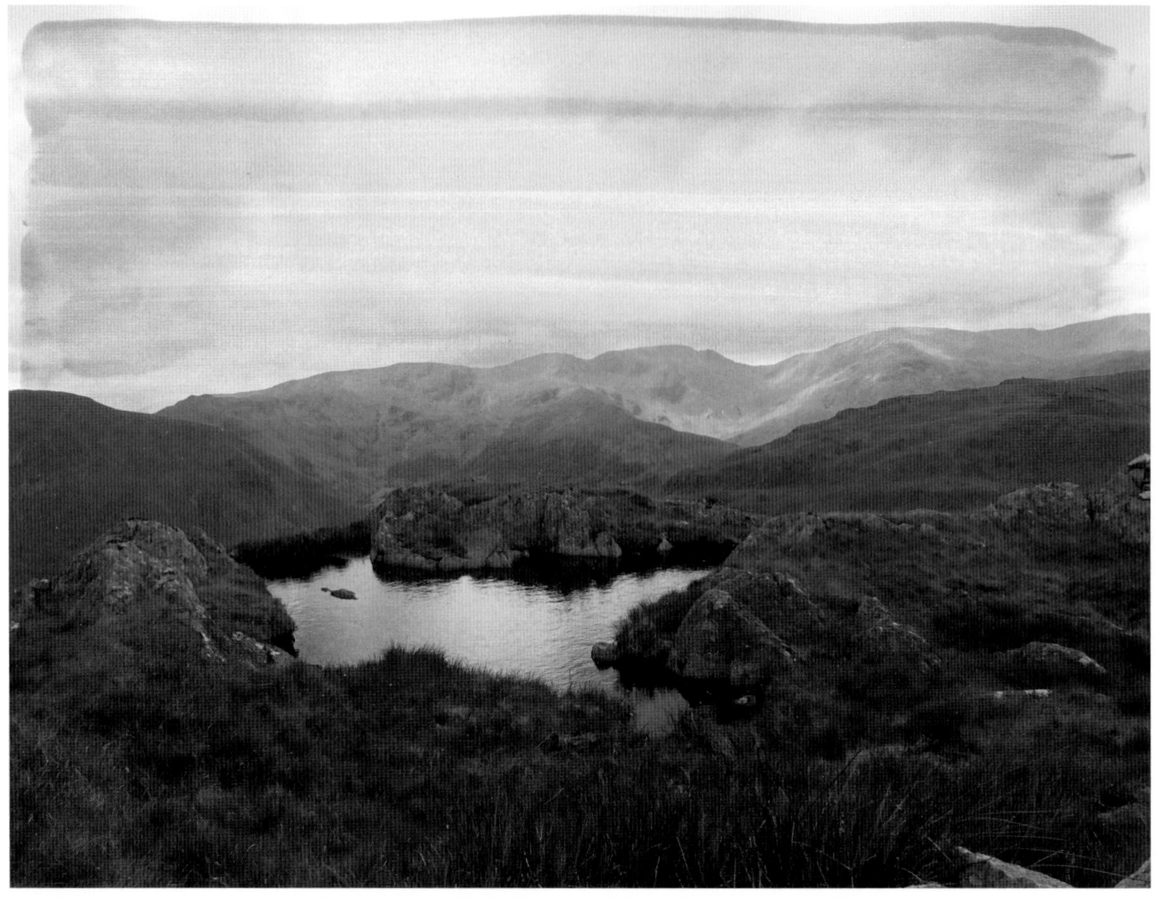

Figure 4.1

Space can be utilised as a therapeutic use for stillness and silence. Artwork Victoria Dokas; photography Alexander Filmer-Lorch

interoceptive awareness, we may be able to escape our racing thoughts'. Just imagine for a moment how this could benefit you, your work and your clients. In light of this question, learning how to access, strengthen and utilise this inbuilt system becomes very much worth pursuing.

The physiological benefits of stillness

- Focuses our attention inwards
- Increases grey matter
- Integrates information into a conscious workspace
- Leads to brain synchronicity
- Decreases mood disturbances
- Changes brainwave patterns

The following case studies from my own practice demonstrate the powerful impact of stillness and silence.

Case study 1

Miss D suffered from severe anxiety attacks. Like many people with anxiety, Miss D was not able to meditate. To my question 'What do you enjoy most?', she immediately answered, 'I love walks in nature.' So I asked her if she would like to participate in a little experiment, which required her on her daily walks to stay connected with the natural flow of her breath whilst keeping a soft gaze. After three to four months her anxiety attacks had dropped from three times a week to twice a month, and after a year they had stopped. She was then open to experiment with meditation practice, and this has now become a routine part of her life. Today she successfully teaches meditation to people struggling with stress and anxiety.

Case study 2

Mrs R suffered from chronic stress. As a senior manager, she identified with every difficult situation and conflict her staff had to deal with, which stayed with her even after work. She initially practised two simple exercises, the 'pause exercise' and the 'Da Vinci star' (see Part 5: The practitioner's toolkit). Within a couple of months she reported that she had stopped losing her own sense of self to that extent whilst dealing with difficult situations, and after a further four months of implementing regular stilling practice, she was able to completely separate work from private life.

Case study 3

Mrs H suffered from chronic pain in her neck and shoulders. After six months of weekly treatments she told me that she could never control her negative emotions and was struggling with it on a daily basis. She said that during each treatment she felt a soothing stillness coming through my hands, streaming into every cell of her body. Within this silent place she could witness the trigger points for her negative emotions, which were caused by her own unrealistic expectations of herself and others. I realised that we had never engaged in a dialogue throughout her treatments, and that I instinctively connected with the silent space within myself during the sessions. This demonstrates that the moment we have developed a certain depth of inner stillness ourselves, we might become an external stimulus of stillness for others. Today Mrs H does not suffer from negative emotions any more and her shoulder and neck problems have completely disappeared.

Brainwaves

Once our attention is turned inward, it is our very own brain that starts promoting an internal stillness-stimulus in the form of different brainwave patterns. According to Idris and colleagues (2014), 'A brainwave is a kind of traceable neurophysiological energy in a living brain.' Brainwaves are not visible to the human eye, but can be measured by using an electroencephalogram (EEG), and are created by different brain networks including the cortical-cortical, thalamo-cortical and extra-thalamic cortical networks. The limbic system, which receives information from both inside and outside of the body and distributes it throughout the whole brain, has a major influence on those networks. Brainwaves oscillate, creating wave-like patterns. The action potential of one single brain cell can create microscale oscillation, and the activity of different parts of the brain can spark macroscale oscillations. Interactions of different synapses play a major part in synchronising the information they have received from other neurons to pass them on to other regions in the brain. Similar wave-like patterns can be found in our breath cycle, our cardiovascular system and our digestive system, in the craniosacral rhythm, in sound and light waves, as well as at the level of atoms and neutrons. Even the increasing and decreasing depth of inner stillness, together with the expansion and diminishment of consciousness, oscillates.

Brainwaves and higher states of consciousness

Oscillations created by the stilling process, along with changes in oscillation created by sudden or gradual shifts in consciousness, manifest at a physiological level as different brainwave patterns, and can be said to be a result of what we are doing. There are five main brainwaves, which differ in frequency and amplitude, ranging from low to very high (0.4–200+ Hz). Frequencies are measured in hertz (HZ), which is a unit of frequency equalling one cycle per second, and their

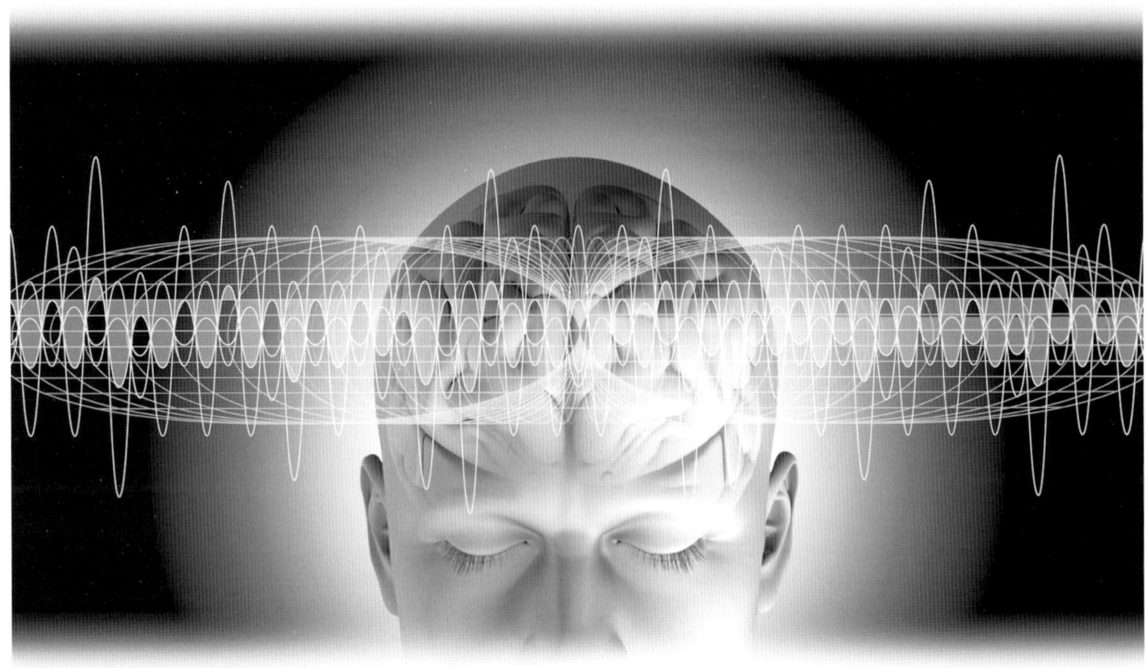

Figure 4.2

Brainwave patterns change throughout the stilling process

amplitude is measured in microvolt units (μV). We spend most of our waking time in beta wave activity (13–30 Hz), which oscillates out from the frontal and central regions of the brain. These brainwaves are associated with focused attention and conscious thinking. However, the moment we relax a bit more and find ourselves in a state of calm, we have shifted into slow alpha wave activity. Mu waves (8–13 Hz) are associated with intended movement, whilst kappa waves (10 Hz) are associated with our thinking processes. The powerful alpha wave activity (8–13 Hz) is known to be the most prominent rhythm. In this state of relaxed awareness, alpha waves are associated with absorption of knowledge, enhanced learning abilities, improved problem-solving, calming our emotions and enhanced creative thinking. Slow theta wave activity (4–8 Hz) originates from the thalamus. Theta brainwaves are associated with deeper meditation, long-term memory, periods of intuition and inspiration. Sleep spindle waves (7–14 Hz) arise during deep sleep and, according to Idris and team (2014), are generated in the reticular nucleus of the thalamus, and are related to brain synchronisation.

Delta waves (0.5–4 Hz) are active in deep, dreamless sleep in which we recuperate. In addition, they are associated with states of empathy and have been measured in a very deep state of meditation. Gamma wave oscillation (30–100 Hz) can be found in all parts of the brain and are linked with optimal brain function, above average integration of sensory information and high levels of brain organisation. They also are observed when subjects experience clarity of mind, enhance self-awareness and insight and are most predominant in highly experienced meditation practitioners. Furthermore, gamma waves are associated with compassion, empathy and feeling like one undivided 'self'. They are also known as the harmonising frequency, unifying all different kinds of information, and are involved in synchronising the brain, which is vital for maximum and more balanced brain function.

According to Thompson (2000) of the Centre for Neuroacoustic Research, hyper-gamma (100–199 Hz), lambda (200+ Hz) and epsilon (0.4 Hz) waves 'must be linked together in a circular relationship'. In other words, the very slow epsilon waves form the pivot point around which the super-fast hyper-gamma and lambda waves ride and circulate. They appear in stilling practice, the deepest states of meditation, highly creative states, the deepest levels of inner stillness and mystic transport, in which one's sense of time becomes extremely spacious and duality or multiplicity seamlessly transforms into unity.

Conclusion

Siegel mentions in his book *The Mindful Brain* (2007) that our personal experiences are shaping our neural structures. Hence, it is no coincidence that the key to our own inner development, and our possible inner evolution, can be found right here in our physiology. Inner stillness, silence, contemplative and meditative practice provide a form of experience that leads to neuroplasticity, and we now know that these specific neural modifications result in actual functional changes. It is no surprise, then, that much of the successful implementation of these functional changes lies in our own hands in the form of conscious effort. Exclusively working, treating and facilitating from conscious thinking and focused attention (predominantly beta wave activity) prevents us from working at our full potential. However, the repeated creation of stillness-memory will stimulate our brain to become active in ways that promote the continuous growth of fully functional and integrated neurons in the respective regions of the brain. This is of paramount importance from a philosophical point of view, because (according to Siegel) now we start seeing the notion that consciousness is utilising the brain to literally create and multiply itself.

Other insights from the scientific perspective and understanding of the body will be discussed in Part 2 by my co-writer, colleague and friend Caroline Barrow, who has always had a passion for blending science into this field in an accessible and thought-provoking way.

References

Bernardi, L., Porta, C. and Sleight, P. (2005). Cardiovascular, cerebrovascular, and respiratory changes induced by different types of music in musicians and non-musicians: the importance of silence. *Heart*, 92(4): 445–452, http://heart.bmj.com/content/92/4/445.full [accessed 11 Jun. 2015]. doi:10.1136/hrt.2005.064600.

Farb, N., Segal, Z. and Anderson, A. (2012). Attentional modulation of primary interoceptive and exteroceptive cortices. *Cerebral Cortex*, 23(1): 114–126. http://cercor.oxfordjournals.org/content/early/2012/01/19/cercor.bhr385.full.pdf+html [accessed 11 Jun. 2015].

Gross, D. (2014). This is your brain on silence. *Nautilus*, Issue 16: Nothingness. http://nautil.us/issue/16/nothingness/this-is-your-brain-on-silence [accessed 11 Jun. 2015].

Idris, Z., Muzaimi, M., Ghani, R., Idris, B., Kandasamy, R. and Abdullah, J. (2014). Principles, anatomical origin and applications of brainwaves: a review, our experience and hypothesis related to microgravity and the question on soul. *JBiSE*, 07(08): 435–445, www.scirp.org/journal/PaperInformation.aspx?PaperID=47331#.VXnPEUYsxKg [accessed 11 Jun. 2015].

Kirste, I., Nicola, Z., Kronenberg, G., Walker, T., Liu, R. and Kempermann, G. (2013). Is silence golden? Effects of auditory stimuli and their absence on adult hippocampal neurogenesis. *Brain Structure and Function*, 220(2): 1221–1228, http://link.springer.com/article/10.1007/s00429-013-0679-3/fulltext.html#Sec2 [accessed 11 Jun. 2015]. doi:10.1007/s00429-013-0679-3.

Moran, J., Kelley, W. and Heatherton, T. (2013). What can the organization of the brain's default mode network tell us about self-knowledge? *Frontiers in Human Neuroscience*, 7: 391, http://journal.frontiersin.org/article/10.3389/fnhum.2013.00391/full [accessed 11 Jun. 2015]. doi:10.3389/fnhum.2013.00391.

Raichle, M., MacLeod, A., Snyder, A., Powers, W., Gusnard, D. and Shulman, G. (2001). A default mode of brain function. *Proceedings of the National Academy of Sciences*, 98(2): 676–682, www.pnas.org/content/98/2/676.long [accessed 11 Jun. 2015].

Siegel, D. (2007). *The Mindful Brain*. New York: W.W. Norton.

Seppala, E. (2012). *Decoding the body watcher*. Scientificamerican.com, www.scientificamerican.com/article/decoding-body-watcher/ [accessed 11 Jun. 2015].

Thompson, J.D. (2000). *Sleeping / waking / awakening*, https://www.scientificsounds.com/index.php/center-for-nueroacoustic-research/articles/sleeping-waking-awakening.html [accessed 10 Mar. 2015].

Wehr, M. (2010). Sound of silence [video], http://uonews.uoregon.edu/archive/news-release/2010/2/researchers-find-how-brain-hears-sound-silence [accessed 17 Jun. 2015].

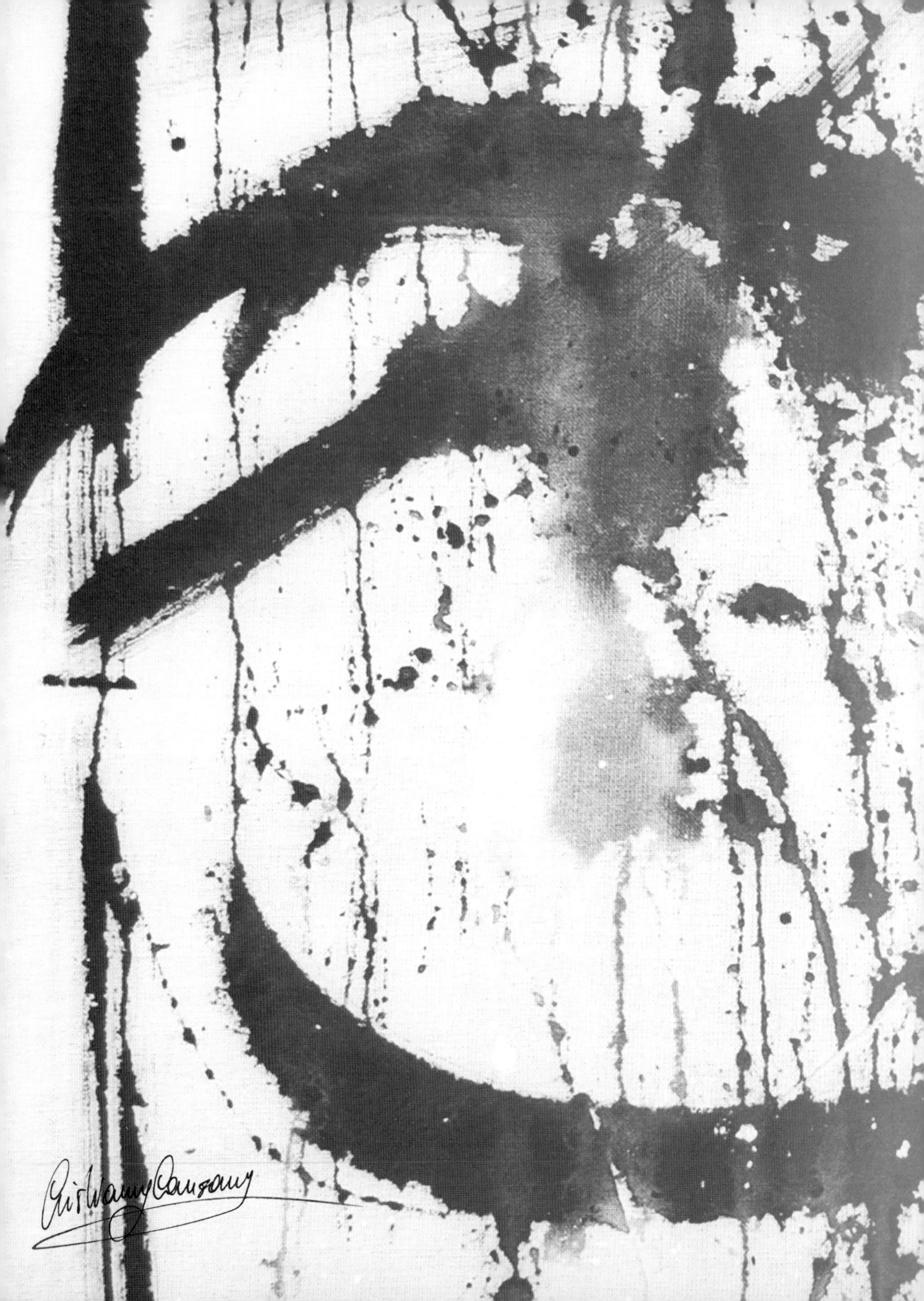

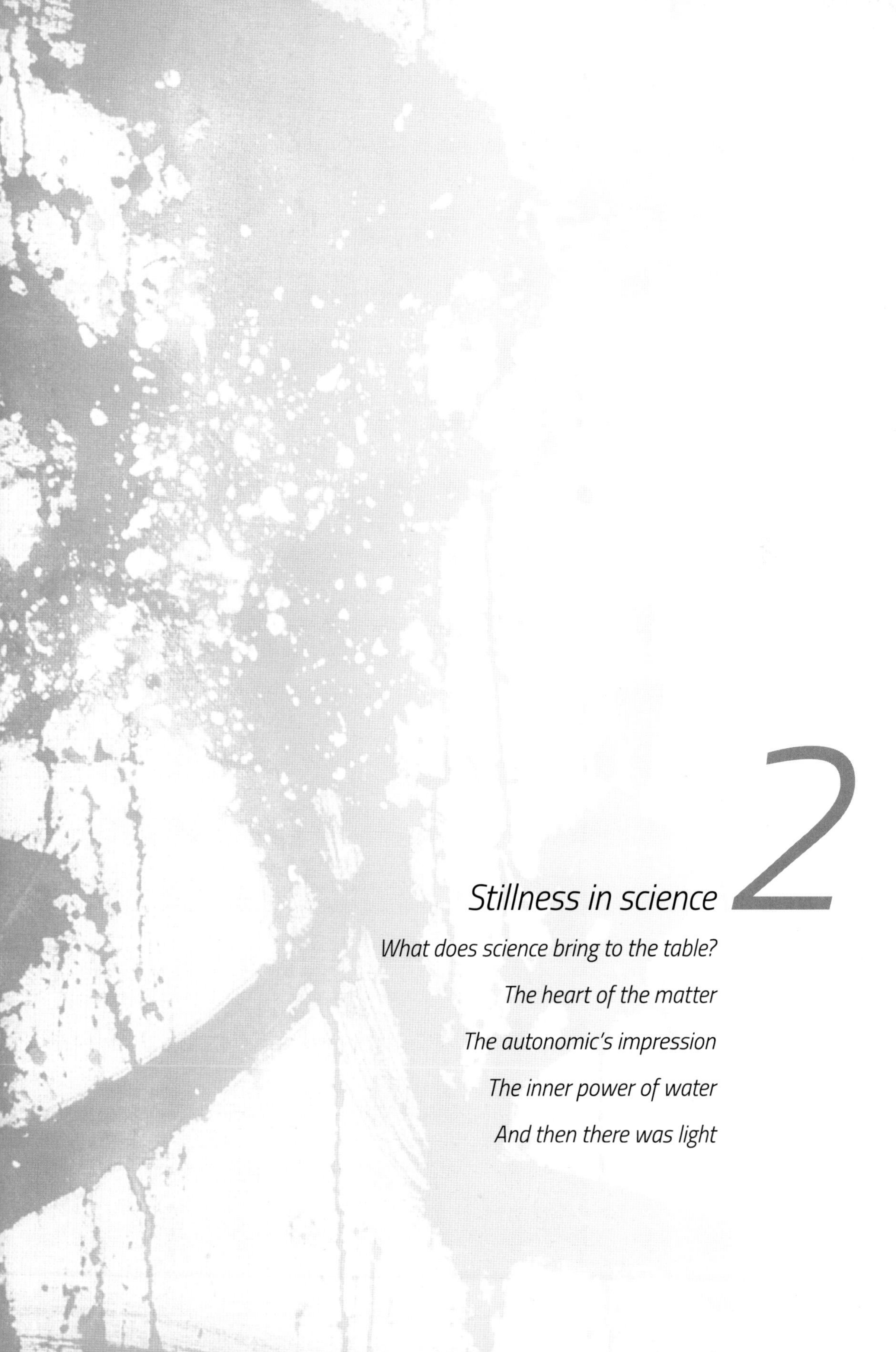

2 Stillness in science

What does science bring to the table?

The heart of the matter

The autonomic's impression

The inner power of water

And then there was light

What does science bring to the table? 5

> *If at first the idea is not absurd, then there is no hope for it.*
>
> Albert Einstein

Anyone who knows me will likely be amused by and perhaps even dubious about the concept of me contributing to a book on stillness. I am not really a still person, and when I work with this idea of stillness-memory it doesn't feel still. It feels *potent*, with qualities of depth and dynamism, filled with extraordinary possibilities, potential and opportunity. It is this place that I have found has helped me be more present as a therapist in sessions, hold the space as a CranioSacral Therapy teacher, keep my head as a parent amid emotional turmoil ... I love the idea of the scale of stillness too; that it is not one place to be reached when we are 'spiritual' enough or have meditated enough, but a moment-by-moment reflection of our coherence (as we discuss in the next chapters) – a subjective experience in the dance of awareness.

We talk a lot in the Upledger community, of which I am a part, of 'doing your own work' and taking your 'stuff' to the table, and I deeply believe it is through the myriad of different treatment sessions – some very physical, some very emotive, some going to intriguing places of my psyche – that I have been able to clear a path to the inner realms of who I am and 're-find' part of my inner self. It does not feel as if it is a new thing that we find but rather something that was there all along. So, the concept of stillness-memory resonates deeply, albeit in a dynamic and moving way!

I was honoured to be asked by Alexander to contribute to this book and incredibly moved by his story of what led him to his deep grasp of the importance that stillness had to play in his getting well. Naturally I agreed ... before really thinking through the unlikeliness of any straightforward answers to the question of what science can tell us of stillness-memory in the body (despite it being, as he shows, a state sought across countless generations).

Alexander touches on ways that stillness has been shown to affect our physiology, and this part will explore that in other ways. You could in fact subtitle the next four chapters 'Four (hopefully) compelling physiological reasons to keep us returning to our inner stillness'! My journey has taken me to the heart and its electromagnetic frequencies, and to the nervous system, particularly the autonomic nervous system and the depth of its integration with other systems. I have discovered where science is beginning to probe what more there might be to water and light and how these will become increasingly important areas for our understanding in the coming decades. What is shared here aims to be helpful in reference to what might be happening in our experience of stillness and what might support us in the way we work with others.

But before that we need to be clear about the *point* of looking at the scientific side. Why should this not simply be a philosophy book, applying Alexander's deep knowledge and practice of meditation? Whilst there can be a trend to try to marry philosophical ideas with scientific 'proofs', I actually do not think that is particularly important: what current science may confirm or not about our internal / meditative / spiritual experiences does not – and certainly should not – take anything away from them. What I do think important is that we reconnect to the very essence of science itself and be aware of what it does, and does not, bring to the table.

The changing boundaries of science

Peter Harrison, in his book *The Territories of Science and Religion* (2015), reflects that *scientia*, back in Plato's time, was the study of nature, with a philosophical slant that a good life was one lived in accordance with nature, and this was why some were drawn to understand more about the natural world. Harrison comments:

To make progress in science, then, was not to add to a body of systematic knowledge about the world, but was to become more adept at drawing 'scientific' conclusions from general premises. 'Science' thus understood was a mental habit that was gradually acquired through the rehearsal of logical demonstrations.

These ideas held strong for a long time. Harrison quotes William of Auvergne in the 13th century as feeling that this observational pastime could lead to both 'the exaltation of the creator and the perfection of our souls'. Harrison goes on to say that 'By 1700, *scientia* had shifted decisively away from being a habit that fostered human good towards a series of practices that generated knowledge and control over nature'. By the mid-19th century, collective material progress (rather than personal moral progress) became the justification for science.

It wasn't yet modern 'science' as we know it, but Harrison says it did acquire 'a special professional identity … the specification of a distinguishing set of methods … and … a traditional nomenclature'.

How interesting to think of science as a way to guide our progress towards 'a good life', to check on how in alignment with nature we are. Despite a few hundred years of arguably journeying away from this, are we not, paradoxically, slowly coming back to that way of thinking? As more people are awakening to the limitations of our industrial, technological and medical advancement in the bigger picture, are we not starting to demonstrate our desire to change, do things differently and align again with nature? We are moving towards understanding how to work *with* rather than conquer – think natural medicine, renewable energy, sustainable agriculture, biodiversity across the planet and so on. *To many of us this is our challenge right now, and one that surely has to start with ourselves and our inner journeys.*

In these contexts nature is still very much at the heart of science and generally scientific 'proof' is required to frame and guide the ways in which we proceed. Building the practice and methodology for science has been important and a big part of its guiding power – but we do need to remain mindful of potential vulnerabilities. What we are sometimes led to believe is cast-iron, authentic science may not be; because we cannot prove *how* something occurs does not mean it did not happen. Observations that can prove later to be vital (game-changers even) may be ignored, left behind or buried in the literature.

In essence, science observes the natural world. Scientists would agree that today our scientific method involves important steps. First, our observation of something happening may take us towards an attempt to explain it, or build a hypothesis for it. Karl Popper, a great philosopher of science, urged us to ensure that we create a falsifiable hypothesis, which can then be tested, ideally in a replicable manner, to try to disprove it – which is just as meaningful as offering proof for it. We then alter, expand or come up with a new hypothesis, continue to test, and may (or may not) reach the stage of developing a theory, which by then should be consistent with the data that we have collected, other available data and any other proven theories. Even better, we involve other scientists by publishing and inviting them to comment on our findings, or by replicating our work before or after publishing.

We try to stay abreast of the work others are doing so we can incorporate other evidence where appropriate, adjust hypotheses, research some more. Or, as Kandel (2006 p. 96–97) eloquently put it: 'Science proceeds by endless and ever refining cycles of conjecture and refutation. One scientist proposes a new idea about nature and then others work to find observations that support or refute this idea.'

Much excellent work has, of course, come from this approach over the past century and more, and from its revered seat at the top table, claims *The Economist* (2013), 'science still commands enormous … respect. But its privileged status is founded on the capacity to be right most of the time and to correct its mistakes when it gets things wrong'. This, the author claims, it is not doing adequately.

Has science gone 'to the darkness'?

Where is the wisdom we have lost in knowledge?
Where is the knowledge we have lost in information?

T.S. Eliot, *Choruses from the Rock* (1934)

Richard Horton (2015), editor of *The Lancet*, argues that there are some areas of science that have gone 'to the darkness'. He says:

> *The case against science is straightforward: much of the scientific literature, perhaps half, may simply be untrue. Afflicted by studies with small sample sizes, tiny effects, invalid exploratory analyses, and flagrant conflicts of interest, together with an obsession for pursuing fashionable trends of dubious importance, science has taken a turn towards darkness ... In their quest for telling a compelling story, scientists too often sculpt data to fit their preferred theory of the world.*

He is not specific about exactly where he is pointing his finger. But it is also suggested that of the 1.8 million articles that are published each year, in about 28,000 journals, about half are read only by the authors and journal editors (Eveleth, 2014). Further criticism includes that studies are not being replicated, peer review is not thorough enough, and competition over jobs and funding promotes publishing *something* over *not* publishing (with, it is suggested, a temptation to leave out the data not supporting the hypothesis). Our scientific model tells us we need to know what has been disproven too – not least so that others are saved the time of investigating. Yet such research tends not to get offered for publication, let alone accepted and printed these days. According to *The Economist* (2013), '"Negative results" now account for only 14% of published papers, down from 30% in 1990.'

How certain can we be?

Sometimes, ideas have been left behind so long ago that we have completed decades of research with some key pieces missing. There are many ideas in the literature that have never been disproven, gems that have been missed in the over one hundred years of papers, ideas lost in time for various reasons. If these avenues had not been left unexplored and their stones not left unturned, where might we be today? You will see a few of these tales in the upcoming chapters.

In a similar vein, what do we do with the 'good' things that we have evidence for but which are not followed up on, developed and applied for the benefit of all? For example, studies by Duke University exploring the possible benefits of prayer for people undergoing heart procedures showed that, whilst there was no statistical significance in primary outcomes of surgeries in those prayed for, there were significant improvements in secondary measures, including the reduction of emotional distress and rehospitalisation, and they noted that fewer patients died within the six-month follow-up period. If a drug offered that degree of improvement it would likely be seen as unethical *not* to prescribe it! Yet there has not been a mass move to integrate this as a regular part of care, despite the science offering good evidence that it has a positive effect. Krucoff, one of the surgeons involved in the study, acknowledges that it is not about replacing high-tech medicine, but he wonders if we have somehow 'missed the boat. Have we ignored the rest of the human being – the need for something more – that could make all the high-tech stuff work better?' (Lerche Davis, 2001).

This is especially challenging in the current world of medicine with the pull between very different approaches. Part of our medical system is so pharmaceutically based and biased by the potential for vast profits that ever more people suspect incidents of skewed science. The clinical trial that is supposed to be the pinnacle of evidence, assuring the public of both the efficacy and safety of existing and new drugs, is often, according to Marcia Angell, Harvard medical professor and author of *The Truth About the Drug Companies: how they deceive us and what to do about it,* biased through designs that are chosen to yield favourable results. She says, 'Perhaps most important, we do not know the results of the clinical trials they sponsor – only those they choose to make public ...' She is, in fact, far more damning of many of the arms of the 'machine' that has become this industry. There are certainly notably few papers that share doubts about the efficacy of the substances they are testing – or selling.

The complementary and alternative sides of healthcare, on the other hand, have struggled to respond to the call for the double-blind placebo-based trial as the gold standard of the scientific method, for a number of reasons (not least the financial support to make it possible). Some of the 'clinical trials' that have been done show a lack of efficacy. Offit (2012), commenting on money being spent on testing some of the many complementary approaches, concluded that

'Using rigorously controlled studies, none of these therapies have been shown to work better than placebo' but that such 'negative' results still did not lead to changes in behaviour. Should we dismiss therapies with a questionable biological basis and try to better understand the placebo effect? Then again, how certain are we really of our biological basis? The following chapters are going to give you some food for thought.

There are some things we don't know simply because no one has ever asked the question or looked closely enough. We assumed there were few white blood cells in the brain, but over the past decade or so Schwartz and her colleagues have blasted open our understanding about neuroimmunity, showing, for example, that the choroid plexus 'controls the access of immune cells to the brain tissue itself' (Schwartz et al., 2015 p. 41), and allows many immune cells across in times of damage. We believed there was no lymph drainage from the brain, yet Louveau and colleagues (2015) have demonstrated the presence of lymph vessels immediately lateral to the superior sagittal sinus, within the dura, through identifying endothelial cell types that match those in lymph vessels. We have learned that lymph vessels further afield are like open channels – Guimberteau's (2015) beautiful treatise on fascia suggests the distal vessels are more like sponges that soak up the interstitial fluid. These are just a few examples that show how much there still is to learn.

So what do we really know? I recall being told this old adage during my biomedical degree: half of what we are telling you now will be shown to be untrue in the next 50 years – the trouble is we just don't know which half! If the materialistic and reductionist efforts of most science up to now could answer all the questions generated by the things we experience then we would not need to peek past its boundaries, but many times it has not. This route has given us a strong way to proceed – but we must not be bound to a reductionist *perspective*, where we forget to remember the whole again or deny more complex observations because we cannot explain them.

Don't we need a bit of creativity and some crazy ideas to push us forward? Is this not an important aspect of our evolution as a species? Moments of inspiration and madcap wonder – at times these have moved us forward by leaps and bounds. I suspect we have lost many opportunities for radical shift through our fears of challenging the status quo (or being crushed by outright rejection when we have brought forth an unconventional challenge – or a challenge to the conventional). Some observers have captured something so outside of the current paradigm that it is rejected, sometimes out of hand, because it cannot be understood. This constitutes 'the common error in rejecting new scientific discoveries by using the absence of evidence as evidence for absence' (Roy et al., 2009).

Part of the paradigm is that scientists are 'supposed' to change their minds if additional evidence comes to light that suggests their theories are incorrect or their hypotheses need adjusting. But this can be hard to do. In the introduction to John Brockman's book *What Have You Changed Your Mind About?* Brian Eno says this is like all of a sudden 'a bit of the world we thought we'd secured is wild and mysterious again'. The very bedrock of a career might rest on an idea that had previously been accepted; if someone else questions it, it is simply human nature that 'proponents of a particular viewpoint, especially if their reputation is based on the accuracy of that viewpoint, cling to it like a shipwrecked man to flotsam' (Begley, 2009). On the other hand, 'it is important to avoid being seduced by theories that may be conceptually attractive but that in reality are inaccurate' (Guimberteau, 2015). How can we tell? We need to be able to spot the difference between something that has been *unproven* and something *disproven* – they are very different beasts. This is really how the scientific paradigm has evolved, as a continuous cycle of conjecture and refutation, ideally maintaining an open mind.

From knowledge to wisdom

One thing on our side is the technical advances that have been made. Science as observation occurs subject to the technical apparatus we have available to us. We have had the joy over the past 50 to 100 years of enabling many more details of nature to be 'observed' and thus more opportunities to explore testable hypotheses through the technology that we have created. As technology evolves we need to embrace the new vistas that open up to allow us to 're-view' some of our assumptions. Who knows where we will be in the next 50 to 100 years – the technology and instruments we have today, whilst amazing to us, will no doubt appear quaint and simplistic to future generations, whilst concepts that are discredited today may be accepted as absolute and vice versa.

So, science rightly has its place at our table. Just remember that it is an iterative process, always growing, changing, testing and clarifying. Some science is good, some jumps to incorrect conclusions and needs to alter its hypothesis, and some is not so good. As Buckberg (2002) beautifully puts it: 'Knowledge develops through analysis, differentiation, or taking things apart. Wisdom evolves by synthesis, integration, or by putting things together ...'

Do we need science to be able to prove what is happening when we experience a sense of inner stillness? Do we need to know the exact mechanisms by which our practice and repeated experiences (with, for example, the techniques in this book) take us forward and bring strength to our experience of everyday life? Probably not. People have been experiencing this for centuries without needing to know the ins and outs of neurological, immunological, energetic or other physiological coherences.

However, why it matters, I hope, is because by finding out more about what is actually going on we will help heal the rift that was created so many centuries ago by the separation of mind and body, and when physics, chemistry, biology and the other sciences divvied up the areas they would explore and created a somewhat artificial distinction between what are in fact overlapping strands of nature. As evidence amasses that encourages us to view ourselves as more holistic, and reductionist scientific paradigms change to reincorporate the pieces we haven't been looking at, we can be brave with our observations of our nature and also with our hypotheses about them. I hope to show the extent to which science is supporting the value in our efforts to connect with our stillness-memory and deepen our inner power of stillness.

To that end, in subsequent chapters I have explored the latest physiological and scientific information available to look at the possibilities that are opening up, challenging our paradigms and developing our understanding of what a wondrous thing it is to be alive and human. Some of the science may be regarded as being at the forefront, and it carries with it some establishment scepticism and a risk that it does not represent reality. It may turn out to be way off the mark, or in fact very close to it; only time and more research will tell. I hope that I have represented it respectfully and correctly and that you enjoy my interpretation of how it could fit with Alexander's experience and understanding of stillness and meditation.

References

Angell, M. (2004). *The truth about the drug companies.* The New York Review of Books, www.nybooks.com/articles/2004/07/15/the-truth-about-the-drug-companies/ [accessed 10 Mar. 2016].

Begley, S. (2009). Why scientists need to change their minds. *Newsweek.* http://europe.newsweek.com/begley-why-scientists-need-change-their-minds-78309 [accessed Jan. 2016].

Brockman, J. (2016). *What Have You Changed Your Mind About? Today's leading minds rethink everything.* Harper Perennial.

Buckberg, G.D. (2002). Basic science review: the helix and the heart. *Journal of Thoracic and Cardiovascular Surgery,* 124(5): 863–883.

***Economist, The* (2013)**. How science goes wrong [leader], www.economist.com/news/leaders/21588069-scientific-research-has-changed-world-now-it-needs-change-itself-how-science-goes-wrong [accessed 6 Jan. 2016].

Eveleth, R. (2014). *Academics write papers arguing over how many people read (and cite) their papers.* Smithsonian.com, www.smithsonianmag.com/ist/?next=/smart-news/half-academic-studies-are-never-read-more-three-people-180950222/ [accessed Jan. 2016].

Guimberteau, J. and Armstrong, C (2015). *Architecture of Human Living Fascia: the extracellular matrix and cells revealed through endoscopy.* Handspring Publishing.

Harrison, P. (2015). *The Territories of Science and Religion*. University of Chicago Press.

Horton, R. (2015). Offline: what is medicine's 5 sigma? *The Lancet*, 385: 1380, www.thelancet.com/pdfs/journals/lancet/PIIS0140-6736%2815%2960696-1.pdf [accessed 10 Mar. 2016].

Kandel, E.R. (2006). *In Search of Memory: the emergence of a new science of mind*. New York: W.W. Norton & Co.

Lerche Davis, J. (2001). *Can prayer heal?* WebMD, www.webmd.com/balance/features/can-prayer-heal?page=52 [accessed 10 Mar. 2016].

Louveau, A., Smirnov, I., Keyes, T., Eccles, J., Rouhani, S., Peske, J., Derecki, N., Castle, D., Mandell, J., Lee, K., Harris, T. and Kipnis, J. (2015). Structural and functional features of central nervous system lymphatic vessels. *Nature*, 523(7560): 337–341. doi:10.1038/nature14432.

Offit, P.A. (2012). Studying complementary and alternative therapies. *JAMA*, 307(17): 1803–1804, http://paul-offit.com/wp-content/uploads/2013/05/JAMA1.pdf [accessed 11 Mar. 2016].

Roy, R., Tiller, W.A., Bell, I. and Hoover, M.R. (2009). The structure of liquid water; novel insights from materials research; potential relevance to homeopathy. *Indian Journal of Research in Homeopathy*, vol. 3(2) April–June (revised from 2005 paper), http://ccrhindia.org/ijrh/3%282%29/1.pdf [accessed 11 Mar. 2016].

Schwartz, M., London, A. and Lindvall, O (2015). *Neuroimmunity: a new science that will revolutionize how we keep our brains healthy and young*. Yale University Press.

The heart of the matter 6

> *Go to your bosom; Knock there, and ask your heart what it doth know.*
>
> Shakespeare, *Measure for Measure*

It may seem odd, if we are contemplating stillness and the possible inherent memory of it, to begin by considering the heart, an organ that is always beating and is thus never still. But there are new understandings about its anatomy that lead us to reassess aspects of its physiology as well as its influence on other systems. Is it an energetic keystone for our attempts to find the stillness within ourselves?

Let's start where Alexander left off in Chapter 4 considering the effect of stillness on brainwaves. He highlighted evidence from the electromagnetic fields created from brain activity showing there are different patterns in the various states we experience such as waking, concentrating, meditating, sleeping and so on, and that these patterns weave together. Activity that generates brainwaves is not exclusive to the brain – an electromagnetic field is created anywhere there is oscillating movement of charged particles. We happen to have a lot of this going on within us; it's just that most fields are too small to measure. The other organ with a field large enough for measurement is the heart, and researchers are exploiting this to explore what is happening in various physical, emotional and psychological states. The heart emits an electric field about 60 times greater than the brain in its amplitude, whilst the magnetic component is 5,000 times stronger than the brain's – making it the strongest field in the body and one that can be measured from up to several metres away (McCraty and Zayas, 2014).

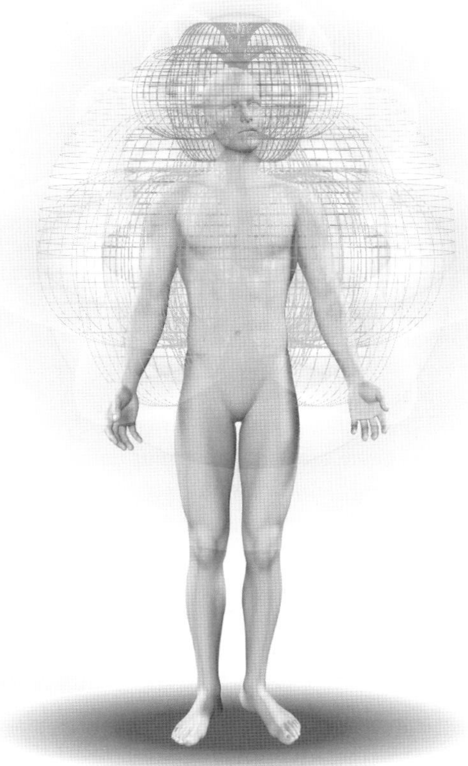

Figure 6.1

An illustration of the electromagnetic fields produced by the heart and the brain

Making use of this invisible physiology

One potent measure that can be extracted from an ECG (electrocardiogram) of our heart's beating is called *heart rate variability* (HRV). First noticed in 1965, it has been used since the 1980s as a window to the connection between the heart and brain, particularly via the autonomic nervous system (the heart's 'rhythm monitor'). The exact mechanisms of these relationships are complex and still debated, but it is an area rich in applications for improving health and monitoring pathology. It is important for us here because the work that has been done in this area suggests that we can positively affect our HRV when we work with the practice of stillness and therapeutic presence. Let me explain why.

Heart *rate* is controlled by the actions of the vagus nerve on the sinoatrial node of the heart, by its secretion of a neurotransmitter (acetylcholine) that prolongs the time to the next heartbeat, thus slowing the rate. HRV is a measure of the differences in the time *between* heartbeats, as opposed to heart rate itself (how many times it beats per minute), and thus of vagal activity, which we call vagal tone (more on that in the next chapter). From an ECG you can extrapolate these time intervals and plot them as a graph. A healthy heart is constantly changing this interval to adapt and respond quickly to the various demands placed upon it; this enables good resilience and homeostasis. It is generally seen as a good sign when, over a longer period, it looks spiky and a bit chaotic!

When measured, HRV should be reported alongside heart rate and the length of time over which the recording was made.

Normal fluctuations result from a combination of complex interactions within other systems. For example, there are slight rhythmic variations in the HRV in response to breathing: when we breathe in, the heart rate tends to speed up slightly (to make the most of the oxygen available); when we breathe out, the heart rate will slow slightly (as less oxygen is available). When our heart rate is higher then there will be less variability in the time between the beats (as there is less time for variability). There are changes from hormonal effects, and for some people from pathological conditions. HRV has been shown to reduce with age, is affected by dehydration (Carter et al., 2005) and by certain pathologies, to the extent that it has a strong ability to predict prognosis of some conditions such as heart or kidney failure, diabetes and after heart attack. A steady, non-changing heart rate over a period of time may be a sign of lowered adaptability (Malik et al., 1996). There may also be a genetic influence (Voss et al., 1996).

It is thought that the different factors that influence our heartbeat are also represented within this measurement. Imagine hearing a string quartet, then separating out the contribution from each instrument. Similarly (through clever maths) we can isolate different patterns from the overall rhythm: mediation by the vagus nerve; influence through the baroreceptor reflex (for control of blood pressure); fluctuations related to circadian rhythms (e.g. daily hormonal secretions); and the heart's own internal influence. However, there is still much work needed to identify the precise range and extent of the potential controlling factors.

How do we measure magnetic fields?

Researchers typically use a magnetometer dubbed a SQUID (superconducting quantum interference device), which is an accurate but very large, and very expensive, piece of kit that requires a very cold temperature of −267 °C to operate. It measures very subtle magnetic fields.

A new tool is currently being developed that is small enough to be held in the hand and does not need cold conditions. It has successfully measured alpha brainwaves and with some more enhancements could become as accurate as the SQUID. This may help the research effort in the future (Ost, 2012).

How do we measure electric fields?

Electrodes are placed on the body to measure voltage fluctuations, providing readings that some suggest can be 'mined' for more information (one example is heart rate variability). Advancing technology might in future enable us to analyse electroencephalogram (EEG) recordings more precisely to better understand cognitive and emotional processes and possibly use this information in feedback training methods.

Reviewing these in any more depth is beyond the scope here, but through showing the positive effect that our efforts to find stillness are likely to have on this measure, we hope you will be inspired to apply these practices, as appropriate, to support your patients and clients.

Towards 'self-sustaining upward spirals'

McCraty and Zayas (2014) from the HeartMath Institute have shown that our heart's rhythm and resulting electromagnetic field can change, affecting and being

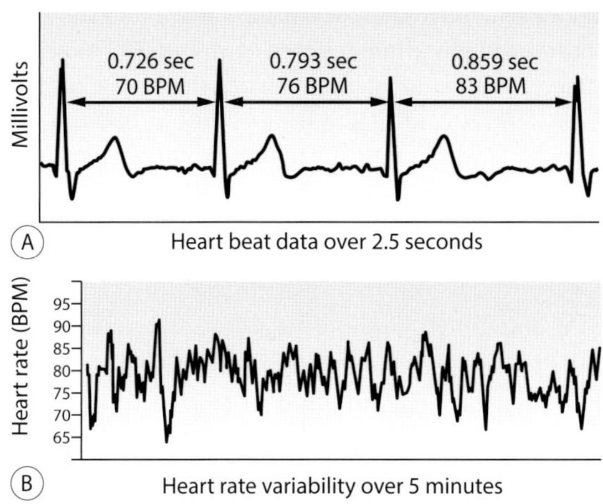

Figure 6.2

Examples of recordings from the heart: (A) the electrical activity of the heart over 2.5 seconds, measured in millivolts – the time between each beat can be extrapolated to equate to an overall beats per minute measure, which itself can be plotted as (B) heart rate variability (HRV), the graph of the time between each beat

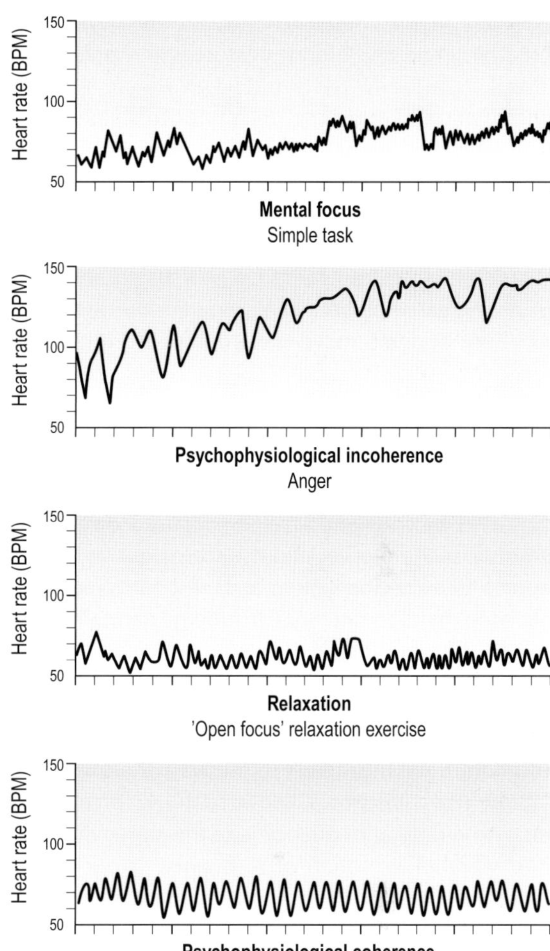

Figure 6.3

Patterns of HRV during certain emotions or mental tasks. The patterns shown are those that are typically observed during: concentration or mental focus, anger, relaxation and psychophysiological coherence

affected by our emotions and moment-to-moment experiences – it is a two-way street. They consistently observed that there are 'typical' patterns of HRV when we experience certain emotions or types of mental activity, such as anger, mental focus, relaxation and appreciation (see Fig. 6.3). In addition, HRV measures have been shown to predict how well we can self-regulate our emotional states.

Kok and colleagues (2013) demonstrated the links between the time we spend in a practice such as loving-kindness meditation, our experience of positive emotions, our perception of social connections and our vagal tone (noted using measurement of HRV). Subjects recording regularly for two months showed that an increase in positive emotions improved perception of social connections, increased parasympathetic tone and seemed to create a self-sustaining upward spiral that positively influenced health.

(I wonder if regular focus on our less 'positive' emotions also takes us in a self-sustaining spiral, just in the opposite direction?)

Physiological coherence – stillness in our system?

'Most people know what it feels like to be in harmonious state, the place where our hearts, minds and bodies are united in a feeling of wholeness', says McCraty (2014). He has coined the term 'physiological coherence' to express the patterns he observes, not only in the measurements of HRV but also in breathing rate and blood pressure when people are in this state. He suggests that when we are in coherence (which we suspect corresponds to stillness), the HRV becomes very stable. This can alter vagal innervation to the heart, stabilise the afferent vagal flow and in turn regulate sympathetic outflow. The heart synchronises with brain activity, which McCraty has shown enhances our cognitive processing and gives us an increased ability to self-regulate our emotions. As these systems move towards operating at their resonant frequencies, other subsystems do so too, so that other rhythms in the body become entrained.

McCraty's team found these rhythms reach coherence most thoroughly when the breathing cycle takes about 10 seconds and ideally is focused on positive emotion such as appreciation: 'Sincere positive feelings appear to excite the system at its resonant frequency, allowing the coherent mode to emerge naturally.'

The physicists amongst you may not be comfortable with the borrowing of terms you have clearly defined. However, for our use here they are taking the idea that resonant frequency refers to the way one object will vibrate when it is struck, and in so doing force another, whose natural frequency is of the same vibration, into vibrational motion or resonance. If our heart's system moves into its resonant frequency – perhaps the one at which it functions most efficiently, needing the least modulation to accommodate outside influences – then it will be the guide for the other systems of our body. It makes some sense that all our systems would function best at the same frequency, yet we are adept at accommodating other influences that bump us around in life. Do you have a memory or sense of a moment when you have functioned in physiological coherence? Our perception is that this state relates to moments of being in the stillness Alexander has been exploring and as have been portrayed through the ancient philosophy.

Using a biofeedback approach, where HRV is monitored alongside breathing rate, skin conductance and temperature, Gevirtz (2014) shows how we can learn to adjust our breathing to stabilise HRV. To understand what was possible he first worked with experienced meditators to map likely physiological changes as they reached their meditative or entrained state. He observed them attain a space of stable HRV in about three to four breaths. Interestingly, the breathing pattern used was consistent for each individual but not everyone's was identical. Those meditating explained that part of the shift for them included a transition to becoming a witness of the world, as opposed to a judge. (Sound familiar, anyone?)

Putting these findings together, the rate of the breath (rather than the depth), alongside generation of genuine positive emotion, gives a direct route, if you like, into this physiologically coherent state, affecting the heart, which in turn affects and is affected by the brain. With practice we can make the shift quite fast. Of course, meditators, yogis, martial artists and others have known this for centuries.

It is fascinating and exciting that there is research looking at our physiology in these states. Hopefully we will be able to measure our experiences of stillness at some point to determine how closely they are related to this other definition of coherence (or not). Future study will also enable researchers to follow up another prediction that, if breathing and blood pressure systems entrain, then 'low frequency brain rhythms, craniosacral rhythms, electrical potentials measured across the skin, and most likely, rhythms in the digestive system' would do likewise (McCraty, 2014).

Craniosacral rhythm?

Those who know me and my constant musings about the craniosacral rhythm will be well able to imagine my curiosity and excitement as I came across this. I was straight on the phone to Alexander to ask him what he had observed the craniosacral rhythm doing in meditation and periods of stillness.

For those of you who are not familiar with this rhythm, let me digress for a moment. The craniosacral rhythm is one that is created through movement of the cerebrospinal fluid within the meningeal system (the connective tissue layers that surround the brain and spinal cord) (see Fig. 6.4). We can palpate it, particularly on the head and sacrum, as it produces a subtle rhythm, feeling as if the fluid in the meningeal 'bag' empties a little, then gets topped up again. This

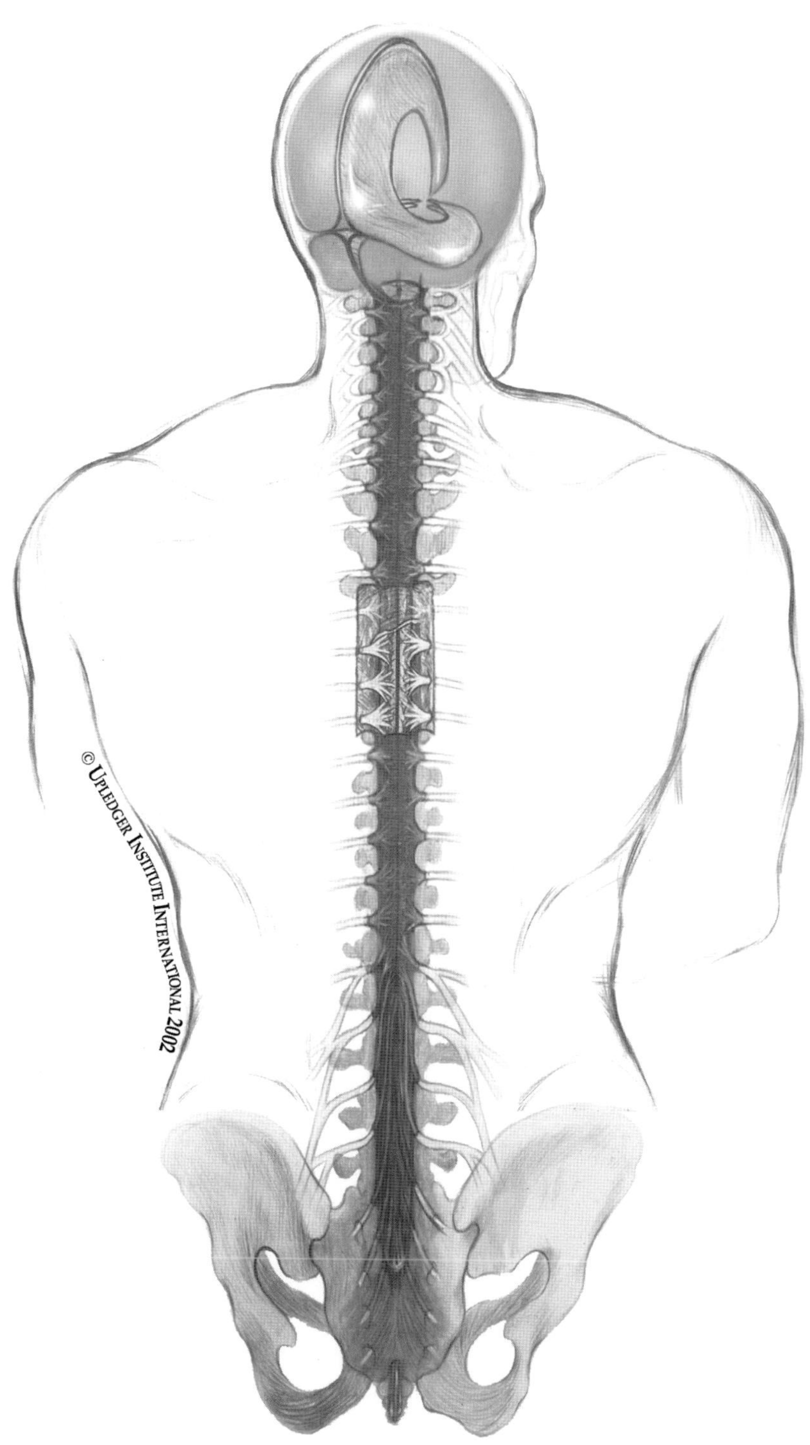

Figure 6.4

The craniosacral system: made up of the meninges, the bones to which they attach in the cranium and vertebral canal, and the cerebrospinal fluid within. A very subtle rhythm is produced from the way the cerebrospinal fluid is secreted and reabsorbed creates very slight movement on the bones these attach to (yes, I know, those bones are connected by supposed rigid sutures), which is what we can learn to feel. Whilst not yet an accepted feature in biomedical textbooks, those of us who work with CranioSacral Therapy, cranial osteopathy and similar bodywork methods have experienced palpating this rhythm for decades. Before you throw me into the pile of unscientific wackos, let me say that there will be some more science coming your way soon ...

However, if you are happy to let me proceed, according to Dr John Upledger (the developer of CranioSacral Therapy from cranial osteopathy), sometimes when we are working with a client, the rhythm will suddenly seem to 'stop'. (We don't think that it stops completely but that it reduces to the point that we can no longer palpate it.) He termed this the 'significance detector' because he repeatedly observed that, when this happened, something seemed to be occurring in the person's tissues that was 'significant' for them. Often, in practice, this results in an expression of emotion, a pathway to some self-realisation or a process that leads to a change in the tissue. Whatever occurs, it seems that the 'stop' in the rhythm signifies something important.

So, when I asked Alexander what happens to the rhythm in an experience of stillness, he unhesitatingly replied that it goes into significance detector and stops. Perhaps we would be more accurate to say it entrains, with the lowered breathing and heart rates and the steadying of HRV? We know that these systems are mediated by the autonomic nervous system, and so I wonder if this is also true of some part of the craniosacral rhythm's control system? Is the moment when the rhythm stops in a treatment session a time of physiological coherence that is supporting the body to take the opportunity to realign on some level and release energy or emotion from the tissues? It often seems as if there is a degree of clarity for people at these moments, perhaps similar to the enhancing of cognitive processing that McCraty noticed was possible in this state. Is this the space from which our 'aha' moments arise? Perhaps being in a still or coherent state also enables us to receive more from therapeutic interactions as a client and to assimilate things that change for us. This is in line with the way we work in CranioSacral Therapy, in the sense that our clients are always 'in the driving seat' of their process and we aim simply to facilitate.

Electromagnetic interplay between people?

The question of what communication may occur between people via these 'invisible' fields has often been contemplated, particularly by those in the therapy profession. Despite the fact that we know the heart emits an electromagnetic field, scientists have been doubtful that the neurology is in place to 'read' information from it. McCraty and colleagues have conducted many experiments to observe what happens in one individual's EEG recordings in response to the changes in another's ECG, for example when two people were seated opposite one another, and then again as they held hands. Prior to hand-holding there was no correlation of output, but during hand-holding one person's ECG pattern was detected in the other's EEG alpha wave output. In 30 per cent of cases the mirroring went both ways. They checked whether this occurred via skin conduction or through radiation and found there was 10 times less synchronisation when gloves were worn, but still some 'information' shared through radiation.

However, they noted the responses were greater when at least one subject was in a physiologically coherent state. The subjects became 'more sensitive to receiving information contained in the fields generated by others' and 'their electromagnetic field and internal systems were more stable and efficient'. McCraty wonders if this is the way in which the nervous system can act as an antenna. Subjects reported an increase in feelings of empathy at times of physiological coherence. The suggestion that this plays an important role in therapeutic interactions certainly mirrors our experience and supports part of the purpose of this book: that if we can access this state more efficiently, we can work with others in a different, perhaps more empathetic, way.

The 'heart brain'

A further piece of the evolving picture of our hearts comes from research pioneered by Canadian neurocardiologist J. Andrew Armour. He has demonstrated that there is a much more complicated set of neurons

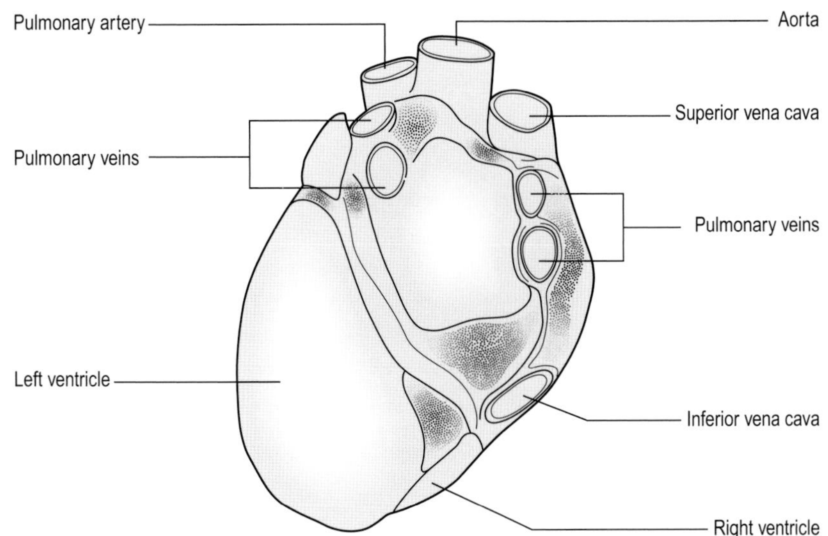

Figure 6.5

The intrinsic cardiac ganglia: posterior view of the heart showing the locations of some of the intrinsic ganglia identified so far (shaded areas). These areas have neurons within each plexus as well as others that connect the different plexi

within the heart itself, forming an internal communication network that has affectionately been dubbed the 'heart brain' or 'little brain'.

The cell bodies of many intrinsic cardiac nerves, spread throughout the heart, gather into groups or clusters, which are referred to as ganglia (see Fig. 6.5). Whilst it was thought that the heart responded only to messages from sympathetic and parasympathetic nerves at the sinoatrial (SA) and atrioventricular (AV) nodes, neurons within these ganglia have been shown to synapse with the extrinsic nerves, both efferent and afferent, via the vagus, sympathetic nerves and dorsal root nerves of C7–T4, and with neurons from other ganglia in the thorax, clearly sharing more information than previously appreciated.

In each of the ganglia (usually located within the epicardia of atria and ventricles) there are cell bodies of neurons that connect to the SA and AV nodes (and thus can modulate heart rate?), and others that make links between the different ganglia, creating a heart-wide network. In addition, there are many other 'interneurons' that never leave the ganglia. Many of these appear to fire in phase with the heartbeat; others distinctly not. Armour (2015) describes it as like having a 'computational capacity' within the heart of the heart, not dependent on external input. The full extent of the heart brain's regulatory capacity and other activity is still to be unravelled, but Armour (2011) urges us to 'appreciate not only the anatomy of all local neuronal elements but also the diversity of functional outcomes that such local elements are capable of initiating'.

To fully appreciate the heart, I want to finish this chapter by sharing an extraordinary recent discovery.

Unravelling the mystery of the heart

A Spanish cardiologist named Francisco Torrent-Guasp devoted his attention over 25 years to the structure of the heart. Early in his medical career he had not been happy with the idea that the heart was just a pump, passively waiting for venous return. His curiosity took him 2,300 years back in history to Erasistratus, a Greek anatomist, who believed suction occurred from within the heart to aid venous return. This view had held until the early 1600s, when it was superseded by the theory that the heart was part of one continuous circuit involving the lungs and functioning simply as a pump. Torrent-Guasp (re-)theorised that the heart should be sucking in diastole, as well as pumping in systole, and set about trying

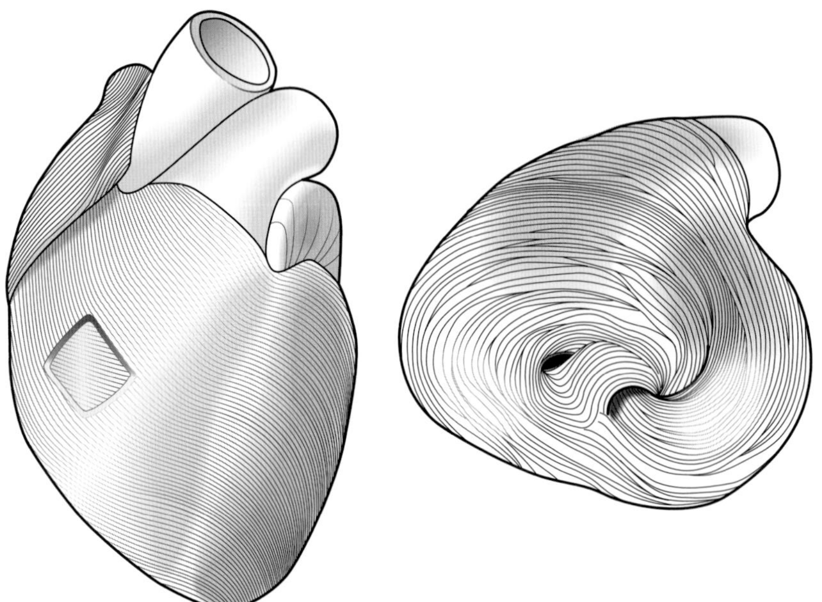

Figure 6.6

The spirals of the heart: demonstrating the clockwise and anticlockwise twists of the muscle fibres

to understand how that could occur. The complexity in the detail of the anatomical structure had remained confounding, but through comparing the evolutionary anatomy and function of many animals he eventually unravelled – literally – the heart's mystery.

If you look at the muscle fibres of the heart from under the apex (at the bottom, Fig. 6.6) you see them going in both clockwise and anticlockwise directions. This pattern is often seen as part of nature's secret code or sacred geometry, as it is common in flowers, shells and many other natural forms, as far afield as other galaxies: the repeating pattern of spirals within spirals. Another example we are familiar with is the double helix of our DNA, and it turns out that this has a similarity to the heart. What Torrent-Guasp discovered is that the heart also forms a double helix by a continuous band of muscle fibre that stretches from the start of the pulmonary artery (the inside of the right atrium) to the aorta (the exit of the left ventricle) with an inner and outer loop. This 'myocardial band' has twists within it like a rope, forming the shape of a Gordian knot in a figure of eight.

What then occurs is that the impulse travels along the band, starting at the pulmonary artery end. As systole begins, the outer band begins narrowing and twists the heart downwards, in an anticlockwise direction, swiftly followed by the inner cone portion, which also moves in a downward, narrowing, twisting helix, which will eject blood from the ventricles (think of wringing out a cloth) through the twist to the aorta.

In diastole, as the muscle relaxes, the heart then untwists, widens and lengthens, moving back upwards, the outer helix first, followed by the inner cone; importantly, as the muscle dilates, a vacuum is created that pulls the blood in by suction from the veins.

The apex of the heart therefore remains fixed but the upper tissue of the base is drawn up and down, which is what is observed from MRI scans of a beating heart but has never been adequately explained before. The heart is not simply pumping but also twisting and untwisting. It is the untwisting that opens the atria and ventricles, and most of their refilling is done in the first phase of this. Venous return then is not to do with pressure differences, as we have been taught for hundreds of years (other than in pathological conditions such as heart failure).

It has also been suggested that this pumping pattern sends out a pressure wave on each beat that travels through the arterial system faster than the blood,

Tying the knot

If you start with an open band at the aorta (1, aorta is on right), imagine twisting the band towards you all the way round (2) and then bringing that twisted section upwards and back on itself (3); you now have a twisted cone of muscle fibres (4). A further internal turn of the whole of the cone (5) then begins the formation of the outer layer of the structure, which wraps over the inner cone from behind and over, from the left side as we are looking at it (6), such that the pulmonary artery end point ends up in front and to the right of the aorta exit point.

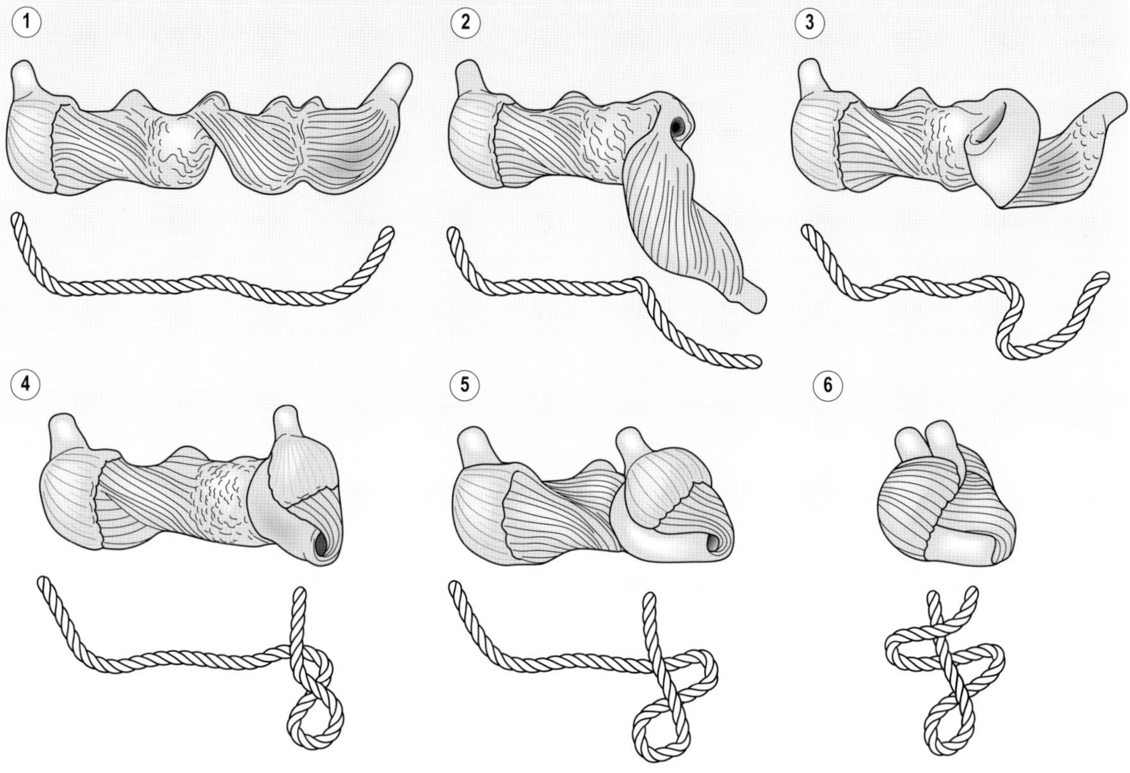

Figure 6.7

Tying the knot: compare the tying of a Gordian knot with the structure of the helical heart

which is part of what helps force oxygen and nutrients into interstitial fluids and gives a gentle rhythmic pressure to the cells around capillary beds, and may be helping create each individual cell's electrical activity, including those in the brain.

The spiral within the helical heart conforms to the Fibonacci sequence in that the different lengths of each section are in this 'harmonic proportion'. Does that make it one of nature's secrets? We have within us our own never-ending motion, reflecting movements that exist in a myriad other forms of life. Does the heart act as our own internal tuning fork to the vibration of nature? In our journey towards stillness, if we sit quietly in the midst of this gentle spiralling motion, might we hear the hum of the universe?

Summary: moving beyond the pump

Your heart is so much more than a muscular pump! We have seen that it:

- exhibits activity that generates a large magnetic field
- has patterns within the heartbeat (e.g. HRV) that have been shown to correlate with physiology, particularly vagal tone, and can measure our adaptability and resilience, reflect our emotional and cognitive processing, and predict prognosis of some pathologies
- has a large number of intrinsic cardiac nerves
- has many afferent autonomic nerve fibres taking information back to the brain from the heart (causing some to view it as a sensory organ)
- receives efferent fibres to more than just the SA and AV nodes
- responds to hormones circulating in the blood
- secretes hormones (and some have suggested that there may be an inherent encoding of information via rhythms in the timings of these secretions)
- has an exquisitely simple double helix structure within its anatomy (which should mean rewriting the textbooks!) where contraction along the myocardial band causes the heart to narrow and twist downwards in an anticlockwise direction to eject blood; relaxation causes the heart to widen, lengthen and move upwards, creating a vacuum that acts via suction.

Moreover, think about the fact that embryologically it is the first organ to develop functionally and starts to pump by about day 22, with its development by day 50 encompassing one billion years of evolution (Buckberg, 2002 p. 867).

Experiment

Reaching to the heart of the matter

Spend some time sitting with an image or sensation of your heart in your mind's eye. What do you see?

Whilst still in touch with your heart, allow yourself to feel what happens as you explore the ideas of:

- stillness
- coherence
- resonant frequency
- appreciation, gratitude
- allowing your breath to be.

How are these the same? How are they different?

References and further reading

Abboud, F.M. (2010). In search of autonomic balance: the good, the bad, and the ugly. *AJP: Regulatory, Integrative and Comparative Physiology,* 298(6): R1449–R1467.

Ardell, J.L. (2004). Intrathoracic neuronal regulation of cardiac function. In J.A. Armour and J.L. Ardell, *Basic and Clinical Neurocardiology.* Oxford University Press, 118–152.

Armour, J.A. (2008). Potential clinical relevance of the 'little brain' on the mammalian heart. *Experimental Physiology,* 93(2): 165–176.

Armour, J.A. (2011). Physiology of the intrinsic cardiac nervous system. *Heart Rhythm,* 8(5): 739.

Armour, J.A. (2015). The intrinsic cardiac nervous system: the cornerstone of cardiac neural control [video]. The Second UCLA Autonomic Nervous System Control of the Heart in Health and Disease Symposium, https://www.youtube.com/watch?v=_XBI70WUbAc [accessed Jan. 2016].

Brack, K.E. (2014). The heart's 'little brain' controlling cardiac function in the rabbit. *Experimental Physiology,* 100(4): 348–353.

Buckberg, G.D. (2002). Basic science review: the helix and the heart. *Journal of Thoracic and Cardiovascular Surgery*, 124(5): 863–883.

Carter, R., Cheuvront, S., Wray, D., Kolka, M., Stephenson, L. and Sawka, M. (2005). The influence of hydration status on heart rate variability after exercise heat stress. *Journal of Thermal Biology*, 30(7): 495–502.

Gevirtz, R. (2014). HRV training and its importance [video]. YouTube, 30 May, ThoughtTechnologyLtd, https://www.youtube.com/watch?v=9nwFUKuJSE0.

Kok, B., Coffey, K., Cohn, M., Catalino, L., Vacharkulksemsuk, T., Algoe, S., Brantley, M. and Fredrickson, B. (2013). How positive emotions build physical health: perceived positive social connections account for the upward spiral between positive emotions and vagal tone. *Psychological Science*, 24(7): 1123–1132.

Malik, M., Bigger, J., Camm, A., Kleiger, R., Malliani, A., Moss, A. and Schwartz, P. (1996). Heart rate variability: standards of measurement, physiological interpretation, and clinical use. *European Heart Journal*, 17(3): 354–381.

Mann, M. et al. (2013). Vitamin D levels are associated with cardiac autonomic activity in healthy humans. *Nutrients*, 5(6): 2114–2127.

McCraty, R. (2014). The energetic heart: bioelectromagnetic interactions within and between people. *The Neuropsychotherapist*, 6(1): 22–43.

McCraty, R. and Shaffer, F. (2015). Heart rate variability: new perspectives on physiological mechanisms, assessment of self-regulatory capacity, and health risk. *Global Advances in Health and Medicine*, 4(1): 46–61.

McCraty, R. and Zayas, M.A. (2014). Cardiac coherence, self-regulation, autonomic stability, and psychosocial well-being. *Frontiers in Psychology*, 5.

Oschman, J.L. (2015). Vortical structure of light and space: biological implications. *Journal of Vortex Science and Technology*, 02(01).

Ost, L. (2012). NIST mini-sensor measures magnetic activity in human brain. NIST *Tech Beat*, 19 April, www.nist.gov/pml/div688/brain-041912.cfm [accessed Jan. 2016].

Voss, A., Busjahn, A., Wessel, N., Schurath, R., Faulhaber, H., Luft, F. and Dietz, R. (1996). Familial and genetic influences on heart rate variability. *Journal of Electrocardiology*, 29: 154–160.

The autonomic's impression 7

> *The development of character is a progressive unfolding, splitting and antithesis of simple vegetative functions.*
>
> Wilhelm Reich
>
> *('Vegetative' is the old word for the autonomic system)*

Did you sit with your heart at the end of the last chapter? Were you able to get in touch with a sense of stillness or coherence? How did appreciation or gratitude resonate for you? The themes of the last chapter, including coherence and the ability to measure heart rate variability (HRV), are strongly connected, as we have mentioned briefly, to the autonomic nervous system and particularly the vagus nerve. We saw that the fastest way to even out our HRV and reach physiological coherence is via the breath and positive emotion. This is regulated by our autonomic nervous system. However, it turns out there is more to the neurophysiological part of the story than has long been thought (as you may have come across already).

You probably know that we use the term 'autonomic nervous system' (ANS) to refer to the peripheral part of our nervous system that controls our automatic functions – those that we think of as not being under conscious control. Autonomic also means to self-regulate. The ANS is made up of (a lot of!) *sensory* information that comes into the central nervous system (CNS) from our organs and other internal physiological reflexes (as opposed to the incoming information from our special senses or musculoskeletal proprioceptive afferents), and it has been shown that this input has connections from many areas of the brainstem to the hypothalamus for additional control of autonomic functions, as well as to the cortex via a variety of systems or assemblies of neurons. Porges (2011) refers to this as our 'sixth sense' and calls it interoception (in contrast to our exteroceptors, which receive information from outside of the body).

We also have different options for autonomic *motor* activity: the *sympathetic* system, which very quickly prepares us, if necessary, to fight or fly. These neurons innervate the heart and lungs to increase their activity, as well as reaching to distant areas of the body, piggybacking on the blood vessels, so that our muscles will have the blood they need for an upsurge in activity, to move us into action to protect or even express ourselves. Our *parasympathetic* pathways enable us to lower these arousal levels, bringing us back down and even inwards, helping us recover if necessary and, via neurons to various organs, especially the heart, lungs and digestive system, help us 'rest and digest'.

We learned in the last chapter that there are many neurons in the *intrinsic cardiac* system that are not part of the loop between organ and brain, and similarly there are very many nerves in our gut, known as the *enteric* nervous system (Gershon's 'second brain', 1998). Whilst some have communication to the CNS via the vagus, most actually get on with their jobs pretty self-sufficiently, without needing to follow commands from the CNS, so are not traditionally seen as part of the ANS.

This is the classic view, in which there has also been a tendency to think of high parasympathetic tone as 'good' and high sympathetic tone as 'bad', which is not entirely true of course. In fact, whilst it used to be thought that the two systems acted in opposition, sitting at either end of a see-saw, now it is reasonably well accepted that both divisions can be active and working at the same time. Porges' polyvagal theory was one of the first to contend that the conventional view was wrong.

It's not all a balancing act

Early in his career, working with HRV measures, Porges noticed that it tends to stabilise when we concentrate and that we have faster reaction times when it is more stable. Over time it was realised that these changes in HRV were due to changes in tone or activity of the vagus nerve.

Porges published a paper concluding that low cardiac vagal tone was a good clinical indication. His first clue that this general understanding had missed something came when a neonatologist, in response to this paper, stated that he had learned that the vagus – that we had come to think of as 'good' – could in fact be deadly. Sometimes babies born early or with difficulties experience bradycardia and apnoea that can be fatal for them – these are mediated from vagal nerve supply. Porges went back to the anatomy books and his search led him to realise that there are in fact (at least) two branches of the vagal nerve. One branch represents a highly conserved system of response to danger, and is the one we have retained from reptiles. These neurons have their cell bodies in the dorsal motor nucleus of the vagus (in the medulla, Fig. 7.1), many go to subdiaphragmatic areas and they are unmyelinated. Unmyelinated neurons are, Porges says, part of older, less efficient, less 'evolved' systems. This system, when firing, effectively allows an animal to 'play dead', hence the reduced heart and breathing rates; but as mammals have much higher metabolic needs than their reptilian ancestors, this response can sometimes lead to fatal bradycardia or apnoea.

The SNS and the vagal brake

Porges states that mammals have developed a higher level of defence, which enables us to do more than play dead – now we can pretty much instantly move to high alert, spring into action and either fight or fly. But this level of arousal also needs to be switched off again efficiently, and we need to ensure it is not activated too much of the time. For this we have evolved the 'newer' vagal branch. These neurons originate from

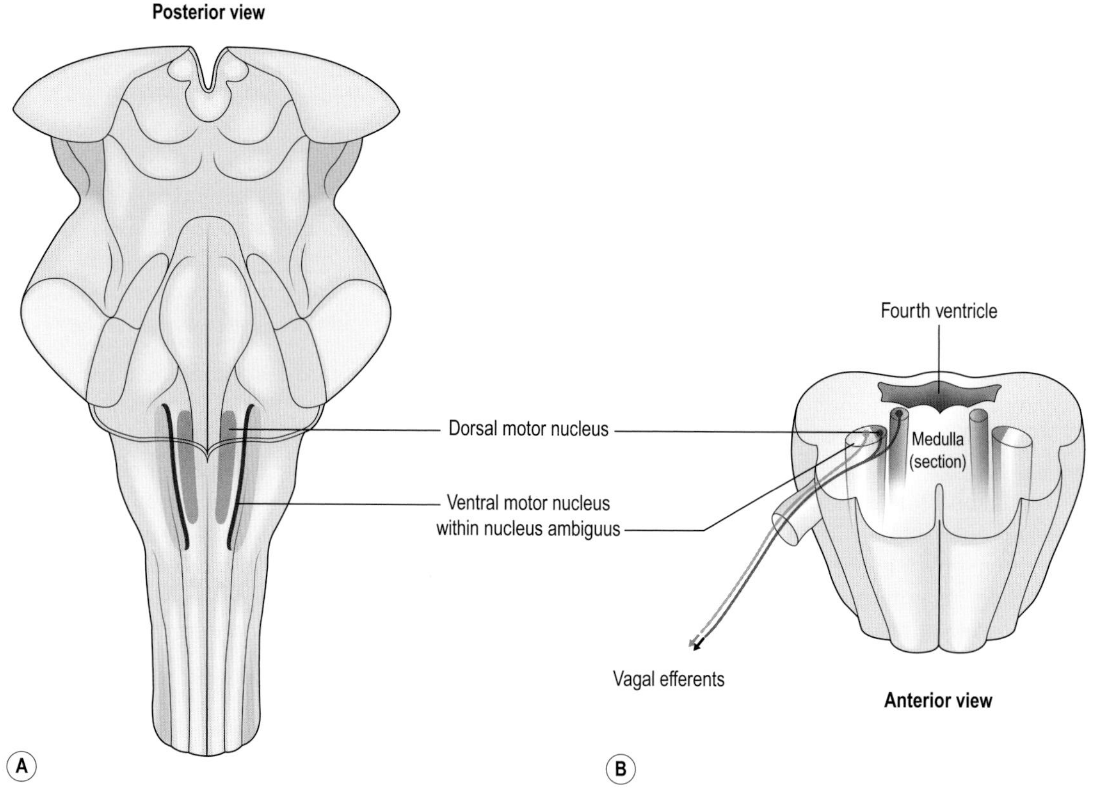

Figure 7.1 A and B

Locations of the vagal nuclei in the brainstem: dorsal motor nucleus (unmyelinated) and ventral motor nucleus within the nucleus ambiguus (myelinated) shown from posterior (A) view and in cross section (B)

the *nucleus ambiguus* on the ventral side of the medulla (Fig. 7.1); they are myelinated and one of their functions is to operate what Porges calls the 'vagal brake'. That is, their innervation to the heart and lungs overrides the sympathetic tendency to speed up activity – keeping the brakes on our (comparatively newly) evolved active defence mechanism. Other fibres project to other visceral organs and promote activity important for growth, repair and health. Any time that there is a perceived threat this vagal brake is removed and sympathetic activity and arousal can take over, allowing us to assess the situation and respond appropriately.

This deeper understanding of the neuroanatomy has helped explain the neonatologist's observations. The newer part of the vagal nerve does not function until at least 31 weeks and is not fully evolved until later in the first year (and needs communication with cortical areas that take time to develop during this first year), so for a stressed preterm baby the lesser-evolved defence mechanism can take over to move from tachycardia straight to shutdown mode, which in some instances could be fatal.

Indeed, there are still occasions when we may respond from our earlier defence mechanism – when we 'freeze'. We may experience weak muscle tone, lose control of our pelvic sphincters or pass out in the move towards shutdown. It was this part of Porges' theory that proved interesting for therapists working with people for whom this shutdown was a part of their response to trauma. It also explained why typical SNS markers such as high levels of cortisol were not always evident in trauma. Previously this had been hard to understand from seeing the nervous system as just having the 'good' parasympathetic or 'stressed' sympathetic response, without realising the third natural but ancient part of our nervous system response could account for the experience of shutdown mode.

Porges, therefore, sees the ANS as being about three systems (Fig. 7.2). Two are defensive – the older freeze response that is mediated by the unmyelinated vagal nerve and the newer sympathetic responses that permit us to fight or fly – whilst the third is the evolved vagus that can act as a brake on the SNS and help us to return from SNS activity to reapply the brake as appropriate and then be able to engage in and develop social interaction, which is a hugely important part of the evolved vagus's functioning. Why?

Because, in our development as a species, socialisation became more important to us and therefore we needed to communicate. This means connecting with others visually, expressing ourselves emotionally and through our facial expressions, using our voice and also being able to listen and respond. Much of the neurological foundation for these actions is connected to the evolved vagus (via its neural control of the throat, larynx and neck) and by nerves whose nuclei are adjacent or well connected in the brainstem (facial nerves, trigeminal, glossopharyngeal and accessory). Thus we have a basis for the face–heart connection that allows the step towards social engagement. As we grow and experience shapes us, the many pathways that connect into cortical areas let us give meaning and understanding to our lives (to put it very simply!).

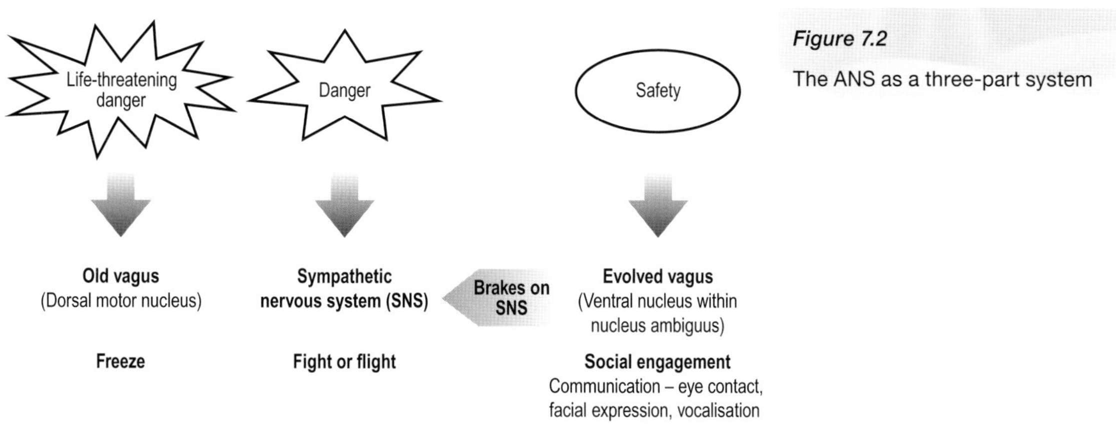

Figure 7.2

The ANS as a three-part system

Upwardly mobile information

Following these neurons into the brain takes us to a number of different brain areas (Fig. 7.3). It turns out that these afferent pathways feed into the nucleus tractus solitarius in the medulla, very close to input from the face, from taste and from the baroreceptors and chemoreceptors. These pass information on to the hypothalamus for hormonal communication; to the periaqueductal grey, which is a small area in the centre of the midbrain important for release of opioids in pain management; to the thalamus, from where information can be relayed to many places; and to the amygdala, so important for our emotional perceptions. It is also emerging that there may be a direct link from the nucleus tractus solitarius to the frontal cortex – might this more direct line of input give us a direct way of interpreting the perceptions from the heart and other viscera? ANS input, especially from the vagus, seems to give us more communication pathways between viscera and brain, and it is likely that these pathways are important for cognitive and emotional functioning as well as autonomic physical regulation.

Experiment

Take a moment to think about appreciation or gratitude, then allow yourself to feel it. Where do you feel it? Head? Heart? Neurons linking the areas in both directions give us another link to possible mechanisms of physiological coherence – from intention and cognition, working top-down, or from heart and emotion working bottom- (well, upper middle!) up.

How meditation affects vagal tone

Some studies that have explored what happens to the ANS during different phases of and different types of meditation give seemingly conflicting results. There are certainly changes in the ANS as measured by HRV, skin resistance, breath rate and other variables, but they are not always the same. Some studies have found that experiences of pure consciousness tend to correlate with breath suspension and reduced heart rate (Farrow and Hebert, 1982), whilst others have found that an even breathing rate is achieved in some forms of meditation more than others (Telles et al., 2013). Yet, since there are quite different states to be reached through

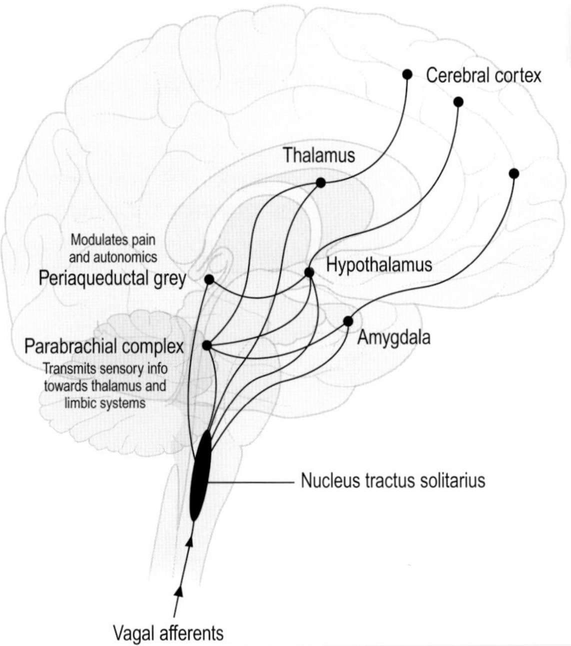

Figure 7.3

Diagrammatic representation of communications from the autonomic nervous system to the higher centres

the process of meditation, as Alexander shared in the second chapter of this book, is it a surprise that these would show up as different patterns of ANS functioning? Are we reaching different degrees of vagal tone?

In fact, is it possible that in moments of stillness we somehow go back to being regulated by the less-evolved vagal system? Would this account for the physiological responses? Perhaps this circuit is the one tapped into when yogis *really* slow their breathing and heart rate, and why, in deep meditation, our breathing rate stills and becomes imperceptible, the heart rate low and yet consciousness expanded. Is this the depth in our systems that we are drawn to when we let go of the SNS and upper PNS? If so, how would it correspond to the expanded sense of consciousness? My musings have led me to consider what the cognitive experience of lizards or reptiles, whose life is guided by the 'unevolved' vagal system, might be like. Without the activity of the SNS and additional vagal system, do they exist in the simple process of living, of being part of all that is? Do they live in the beauty of extended consciousness, which we usually experience only after years of practice?

I am also reminded of Jill Bolte Taylor's experience in her book *My Stroke of Insight*. Waking up one morning she knew something was not quite right, and being a neurologist she realised she was having a stroke. Her incredibly evocative story tells of her extraordinary experience, as her left brain shut down from the haemorrhage, of being at one with her body and of her feeling 'the composition of my being as a fluid rather than a solid. I was alone with nothing but the rhythmic pulse of my beating heart' (Taylor, 2008 p. 43). Was this right-brain functioning? Autonomic defence?

Thankfully, there are other ways that we can reach those moments of deep connection! In applying the ideas in this book we hope that you will be activating or reactivating your vagal brake and improving vagal tone, which will take you deeper into stillness. There are other benefits too: increasing vagal tone has been found to affect a number of other systems; another relatively recent discovery is its direct connection to the immune system.

Vagal regulation of the immune system

In the late 1990s Tracey (2002) stumbled across a neural circuit that directly reduced the inflammatory response. He noticed that vagal neurons heading into the brainstem could be activated by certain endotoxins that signal the presence of inflammation in

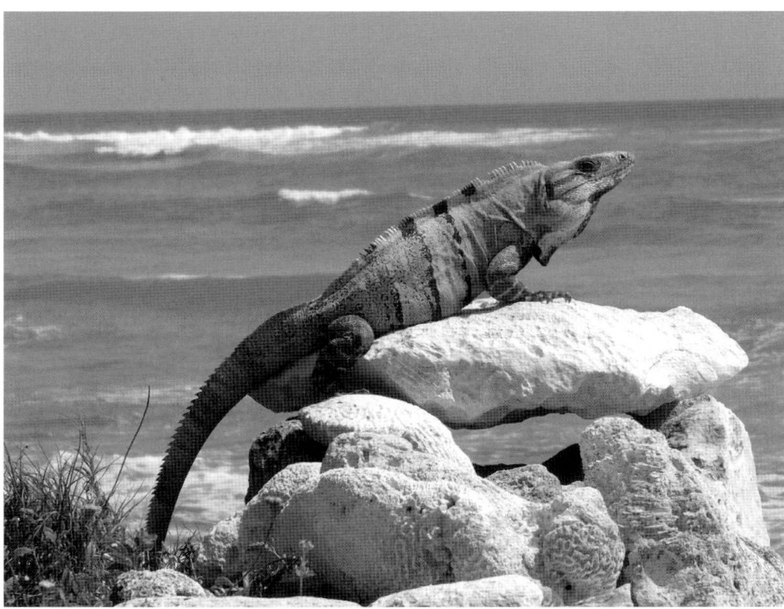

Figure 7.4

What is going on in the reptilian brain? (In this case a Mexican iguana.) Image courtesy of Alasdair Morrison

peripheral tissue. This generates a response via a branch of the vagal nerve heading directly to the spleen to limit production of cytokines – important pro-inflammatory molecules – from immune cells such as macrocytes. Other responses have since also been found to occur, such as down-regulation of neutrophil (another type of white blood cell) activation. Tracey termed this response the *inflammatory reflex.*

Tracey shows what a useful mechanism this is for controlling inflammatory responses as it works at top speed compared with the other mechanisms, which are far slower, such as waiting for blood cells to arrive to start the response, or routing the inflammatory mediators via the blood to the brainstem, which will cause a similar end response but just takes a bit longer. Also, responding so fast via the spleen enables greater control of circulating immune cells, therefore down-regulating immune responses further afield. Responses can also be modulated according to the amount of initial stimulation – a small amount of inflammatory endotoxins will cause a small response; more of them will amp up the overall response, initiating fever, for example (Huston and Tracey, 2010).

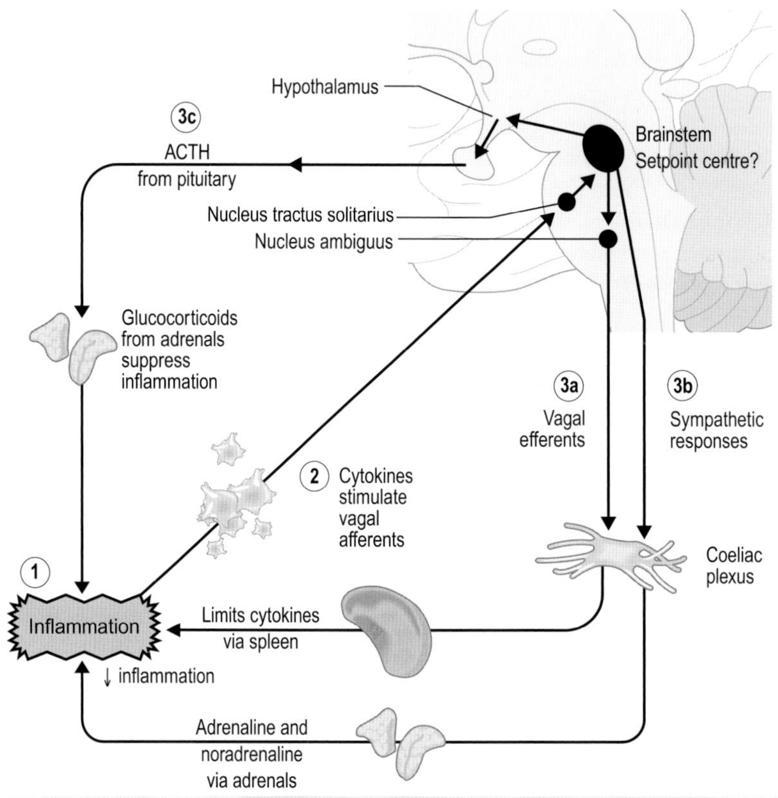

Figure 7.5

The inflammatory reflex: (1) inflammation in a tissue produces toxins such as cytokines which stimulate vagal neurons (2) taking the message to the brainstem (via the nucleus tractus solitarius or NTS). This then signals, possibly via some integrating and regulatory centre, (3a) vagal efferents (via nuclei in the nucleus ambiguus) and (3b) sympathetic neurons (that travel via the spinal cord); both synapse in the coeliac ganglion and the vagal signals cause the white blood cells in the spleen to help inhibit the inflammation, sympathetic neurons inhibit this via adrenaline and noradrenaline; (3c) messages reach the hypothalamus to cause the pituitary to secrete adrenocorticotrophic hormone (ACTH) that stimulates the adrenals to secrete glucocorticoids that also inhibit the inflammatory response

Application of this information

Much of the research in the past 20 years that links poor HRV (think vagal tone) with pathologies (such as heart disease, diabetes, heart failure, the autonomic dysfunction that can be part of multiple sclerosis, a poorer outcome after acute heart attack, to name a few) has also shown that people often have increased sympathetic tone *alongside* decreased vagal (parasympathetic) tone. It has repeatedly been found that the extent to which SNS activity is raised correlates with the severity of the problem. However, there has not been a clear understanding of the mechanism underlying the connection.

It seems the inflammatory reflex gives us at least part of the explanation. If vagal tone is low and is not giving its tonic influence to cytokine production then part of the inflammatory response may be over-responding, creating any number of inflammatory conditions – we know these are much on the rise and implicated in a number of conditions. Most often dietary changes and stress reduction are suggested for those who prefer to try a non-pharmaceutical route. This inflammatory reflex may also give us another, perhaps simpler, reason for the success of various stress reduction methods as well as some of our treatment approaches. If we are increasing vagal tone through touch and therapeutic presence then we may simply be supporting our clients' vagal tone to increase, bringing with that the range of benefits we have discussed.

We also know that the advantage of exercise is that it enables a rebalancing of SNS and PNS activity. A study by Lazzarotto Racatti and colleagues (2015) showed that electrical stimulation to leg muscles of animals with heart failure – mimicking light exercise – improved the heart modulation by the vagus and helped swing the sympathetic/vagal balance back towards normal, although the mechanisms for this are not entirely clear. This reinforces other evidence that exercise can increase vagal over sympathetic tone, and that even in patients whose condition is such that they are not able to exercise very much, electrical stimulation could be beneficial to their symptoms by improving the vagal tone.

There can be other metabolic reasons for ANS imbalances, such as vitamin D deficiency in cardiovascular disease and chronic kidney disease, because people are unable to synthesise this vitamin correctly, which precipitates 'exaggerated withdrawal of cardioprotective vagal tone' (Mann, 2013). We may see an oversupply of hormones such as adrenaline (epinephrine) and noradrenaline (norepinephrine) circulating in the blood, as can occur in heart failure when the body tries to raise these hormone levels in an attempt to increase blood pressure to get more oxygen to the cells. No doubt there are numerous other influences into these systems and other ways that imbalances arise.

Yet, whilst much of medicine's focus had been on considering how to reduce SNS activity, more recently it has been realised that a better approach is to increase vagal tone and allow the body to restore its own balance.

The research is increasing down this avenue to explore the range of benefits this might bring; not surprisingly it puts a strong case for lifestyle changes. Having improved access to your own inner power of stillness is surely one possibility ...

Is stillness hidden in our autonomic nervous system?

It does seem that some part of stillness can be found within the autonomic part of our nervous system, via the vagus nerve, and the basis of the polyvagal theory helps us understand a bit more about why.

I suspect that Alexander's instinct and ability to find the stillness when he was so ill correlated, at least in part, with activating his parasympathetic nervous system. This influenced his inflammatory reflex to find a way for his innate healing system to gain back control.

As a final thought, since it seems that exercise can have a positive and balancing effect on this system, and that stillness can also be experienced when athletes, sportspeople and performers are 'in the zone', as Alexander mentioned in Chapter 3, we wonder if vagal enhancement might contribute to these experiences? Is there a shift into physiological coherence that coalesces with physical action, enabling us to hold a still centre – or an autonomic impression – in the midst of motion?

Experiment

Next time you are exercising in your preferred fashion, experiment with applying your vagal brake through slower, regular breathing and positive intention in the midst of the movement ...

References

Farrow, J.T. and Hebert, R.J. (1982). Breath suspension during the transcendental meditation technique. *Psychosomatic Medicine*, 44(2): 133–153.

Gershon, M.D. (1998). *The Second Brain*. New York: HarperCollinsPublishers.

Huston, J. and Tracey, K. (2010). The pulse of inflammation: heart rate variability, the cholinergic anti-inflammatory pathway and implications for therapy. *Journal of Internal Medicine*, 269(1): 45–53.

Lazzarotto Rucatti, A., Boemo Jaenisch, R., Dalcin Rossato, D., Poletto Bonetto, J., Ferreira, J., Xavier, L., Sonza, A. and Lago, P. (2015). Skeletal muscle electrical stimulation improves baroreflex sensitivity and heart rate variability in heart failure rats. *Autonomic Neuroscience*, 193: 92–96.

Mann, M., Exner, D., Hemmelgarn, B., Sola, D., Turin, T., Ellis, L. and Ahmed, S. (2013). Vitamin D levels are associated with cardiac autonomic activity in healthy humans. *Nutrients*, 5(6): 2114–2127, www.mdpi.com/2072-6643/5/6/2114/htm [accessed Mar. 2016]. doi:10.3390/nu5062114.

Porges, S.W. (2011). *The Polyvagal Theory: neurophysiological foundations of emotions, attachment, communication, and self-regulation*. New York: W.W. Norton.

Taylor, J.B. (2008). *My Stroke of Insight*. New York: Viking.

Telles, S., Raghavendra, B., Naveen, K., Manjunath, N., Kumar, S. and Subramanya, P. (2013). Changes in autonomic variables following two meditative states described in yoga texts. *Journal of Alternative and Complementary Medicine*, 19(1): 35–42.

Tracey, K.J. (2002). The inflammatory reflex. *Nature*, 420(6917): 853–859.

The inner power of water 8

The weirdness of water

Water is weird. It has all sorts of strange properties that don't make sense: it freezes and melts at pretty high temperatures, it shrinks on melting, warm water freezes faster than cold water, water vapour forms into clouds, to name just a few.

Water is also one of the most important keys to life – it is 'the matrix of many processes' (Giudice, Spinetti and Tedeschi, 2010). We all know that it makes up 70–80 per cent of our bodies, the structure of plants and our planet's surface. If you were to count out individual molecules in our bodies, water molecules would account for 99 per cent of them (they are smaller than most of the others) (Pollack, 2013a). Understanding that water is made of an oxygen and two hydrogen molecules does not go too far towards explaining the joy and relief of drinking it when you are thirsty, the many aspects of the ocean or what exactly it is contributing to our biochemical inner workings. We know even less about what happens to it in our bodies during our search for stillness, so with ideas about coherence and vibration it seemed an interesting place to look. I got way more than I bargained for! Stay with me as there are some amazing secrets to be discovered. That will take us back to stillness shortly.

Many readers will be familiar with the photos produced by Masaru Emoto (Fig. 8.1) of the crystalline structure of water under different 'vibrational' influences. In many experiments, over many years, he flash-froze water samples taken from different sources or that had been exposed to music, emotions or thoughts, and then took pictures of their crystalline structure using a darkfield microscope.

He compared the images of water taken directly from a spring with that from Tokyo's water system. He had people hold different test tubes of water whilst praying. He placed a container of water between two speakers and played the classical music of different composers, and then compared these with the crystals that emerged after the water 'listened to' some heavy metal. He even taped different words onto the sides of the containers and left them overnight before taking pictures that showed quite different crystal formation from words such as 'love and appreciation' as opposed to 'I hate you'.

What is so remarkable is how different the crystalline forms are and, says Emoto, the visual clue they give us that water somehow has a structural response to vibration or a vibrational imprint. (I should point out that many in the scientific community give no credence to this interpretation.) For Emoto, the vibrational beauty hidden within these molecules represents part of the mystery of the universe, and a desire to uncover the universe's beauty is shared by us all, and throughout history. I wonder what the water crystals would look like after time spent with the words 'the inner power of stillness' taped to the side of its container …?

Not just an odourless, transparent and tasteless substance, especially in its liquid form, water has fascinating abilities that we are only really just starting to uncover. In fact, according to Rustum Roy (2009), materials scientist at Penn State for over 60 years, in the past 100 years we have missed a huge chunk of information, which is that the *structure* of water can be altered, unrelated to its *composition*.

That is, the way the H_2O molecules arrange themselves within a large or small body of water can vary, even though the building blocks have not changed. We have assumed that the only things that change structure are temperature and pressure, whereas we now know that the structure of some substances can also be changed by electric and magnetic fields, for example. The implications of this turn out to be huge.

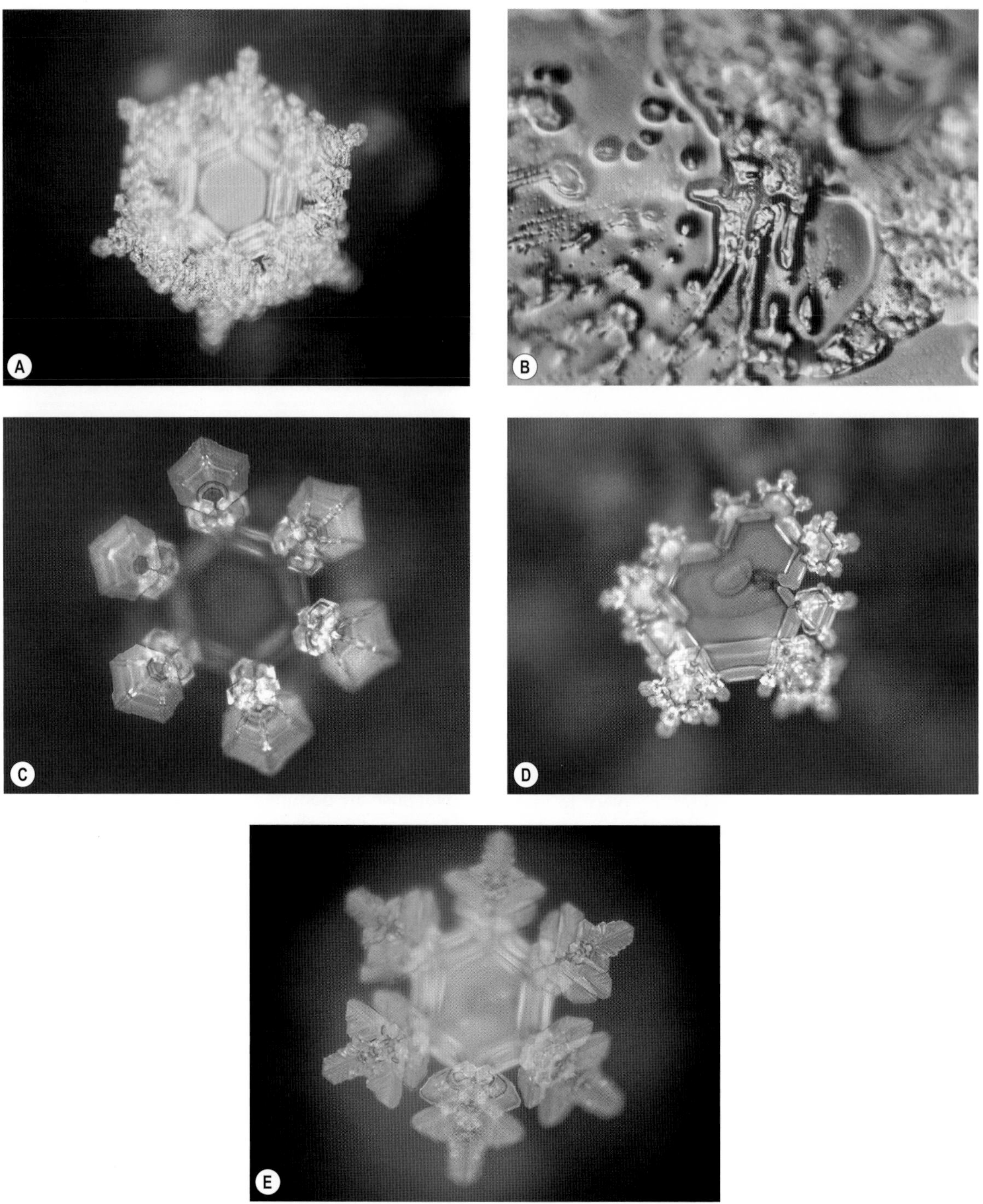

Figure 8.1

Images of crystalline structures of water: (A) water with words 'love and thanks', (B) water with words 'you make me sick I will kill you', (C) water from the source of the Honmyo river, (D) water from the end of the Honmyo river right before the bay, (E) water having had Vivaldi's *The Four Seasons*, Summer concerto played 'to it'

A whizz through the chemistry (if you need it)

Atoms

Atoms are made up of a centre of protons, which carry a positive charge, and neutrons, which are neutral. Both have mass. Organised in layers around this centre (sort of like the planets around the sun except they move a lot faster!) are electrons, which have a negative charge. The number of electrons will be equal to the number of protons, so that a single atom is overall neutral or has no dominant charge. These electrons are not arranged randomly but move about in 'shells', each shell further from the centre. The inner shell will hold only two electrons, then after this the next shell will hold up to eight, and the same for the one further out than that. (Beyond that it is a bit more complicated but unnecessary for the points made here.)

Adding a proton, neutron and electron to each atom successively roughly moves us through the periodic table. Each type of atom therefore has a unique number of protons, neutrons and electrons; protons and electrons are always equal in number so the atom is overall neutrally charged (usually the same number of neutrons too). A few are shown in Fig. 8.2 but consult a periodic table to see them all.

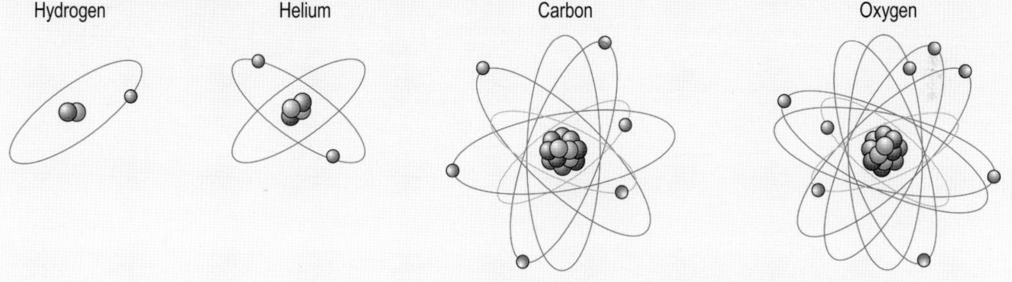

Figure 8.2

Basic structure of atoms with protons (p) and neutrons (n) in the centre and electrons (e) on the outside in shells at different distances: hydrogen (1p, 1n, 1e), helium (2p, 2n, 2e), carbon (6p, 6n, 6e) and oxygen (8p, 8n, 8e) are shown

Forming bonds

What changes the game the most is the arrangement of the electrons in the shells – the number of electrons in the shell will offer the atom its options for ways it can react with other atoms. There are three choices:

1. It can be given or donated an electron/s to fill its outer electron shell. In that case it will have an extra electron/s and this will give it an overall negative charge, for example chlorine (Cl^-).
2. It can give away the electron/s to another atom that has a space for one in its unfilled outer shell; then it would have one extra proton and so have an overall positive charge, for example sodium (Na^+).

When this has occurred the resulting attraction between these two ions (now called ions as they have charge) is called an *ionic bond* (Fig. 8.3A).

3. Or two atoms could share electrons, so that there is an overlapping bond between the atoms, and they both contribute an electron to assist in the stability of the outer shell. This is what happens for many structures, and shells can be filled with such contributions from more than one other atom.

These are called *covalent bonds* (Fig. 8.3B).

Figure 8.3

Ionic and covalent bonds:

(A) Ionic: sodium gives away the single electron in its outer shell, and this leaves it with a +ve charge from the one extra proton. Chlorine receives the electron to fill the one empty electron space in its outer shell, and this gives it a –ve charge. These two charged particles are then attracted to each other and can form a stable structure. This is known as an ionic bond.

(B) Covalent: the structure of an oxygen molecule O_2 where both share two electrons to make a full outer shell; and a water molecule showing the covalent bonds when each hydrogen atom shares one electron with the oxygen atom, which shares one too.

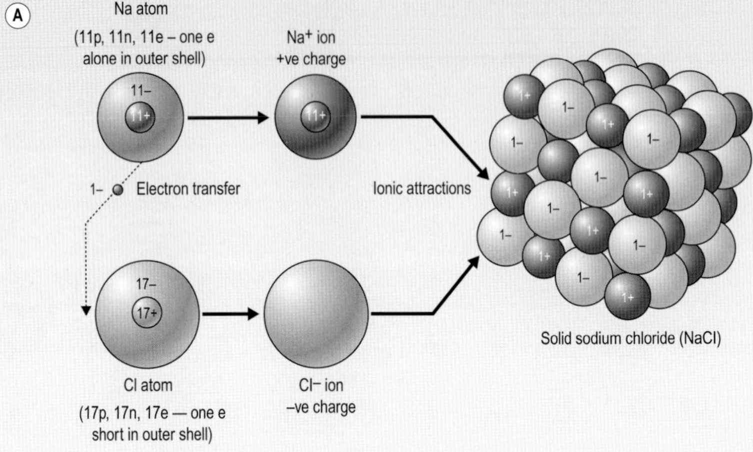

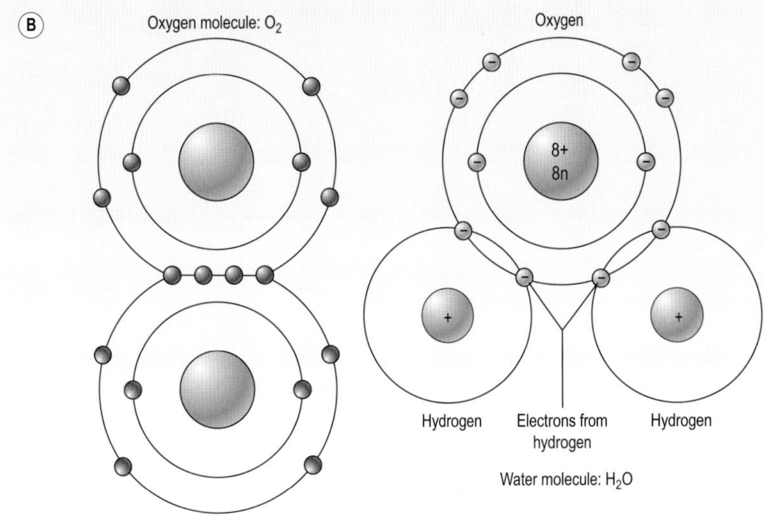

Oxygen and hydrogen → water

Oxygen has eight protons in its centre – two electrons in its inner shell, therefore six in the outer shell. This leaves it open to either receiving two or sharing two of its electrons with other atoms that can share two in return. In hydrogen's case each atom can share one, hence the build of H_2O – two hydrogen atoms bonding with one oxygen.

Hydrogen, the first element in the periodic table, has one proton in its centre and one electron in its first electron shell. Since the first shell around an electron prefers to be full (or in this case empty), it can actually be either H^+ or sometimes to fill it H^-.

Hydrogen bonds

Now, what is interesting is what happens next... Because there are four electrons in the oxygen atom not sharing they tend to give that side of the molecule a slight negative charge. The hydrogen atoms, on the other hand, have their electrons pulled towards those of the oxygen, as it has more positive protons, and hydrogen thus has a slightly positive charge on the 'outer' edge.

What this initiates is an attraction between the positive areas of the hydrogen and the negative areas of the oxygen (Fig. 8.4). These can form what are called hydrogen bonds, which are nowhere near as strong as the covalent, electron-sharing bonds, but are certainly implicated in water's 'weirdness'.

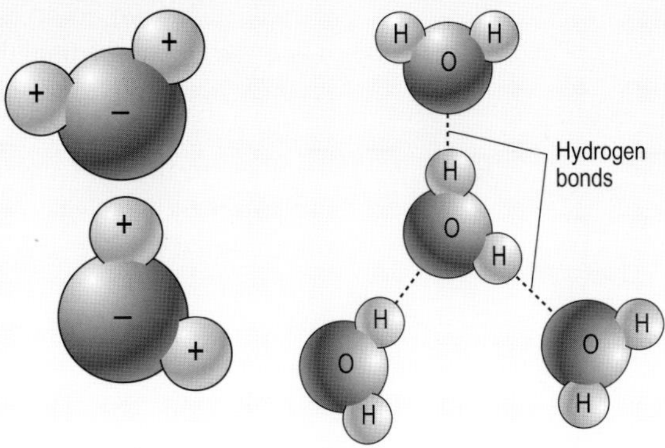

Figure 8.4

Hydrogen bonds: see how the unbonded side of the oxygen atom with its four electrons will have a slight negative charge, whilst the open side of the hydrogen atom will have a slight positive charge from the proton within the nucleus, as its electron is sharing with the oxygen atom. It is these two areas that have attractions we call hydrogen bonds

We are familiar with this idea if we consider the ways carbon bonds with itself. Diamond is the hardest material we know of. This is because the carbon atoms are arranged so that every bond has the same length (Fig. 8.5A). Graphite (Fig. 8.5B), on the other hand, is one of the softest materials we know: it has two ways that carbon bonds within its structure. Sheets of carbon molecules have short, strong bonds (even stronger than diamond's), but bonds between the sheets are longer and weaker, enabling the pencil! These differences in structure give the huge differences in properties. Same atoms, same composition, but different structure, different properties. It turns out that not only is water similar but that the variations in structure offer some extraordinary properties.

At the water's edge

If you were to place some very small particles (microspheres) in water, then put this water in a small dish next to a solid edge (say a gel) and watch what happened under the microscope, you would see a sur-

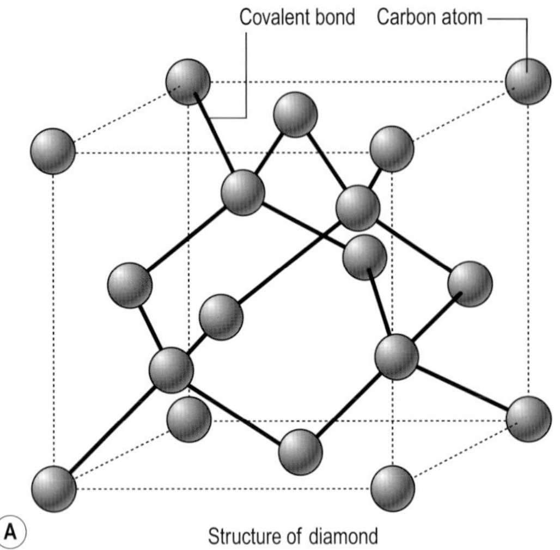

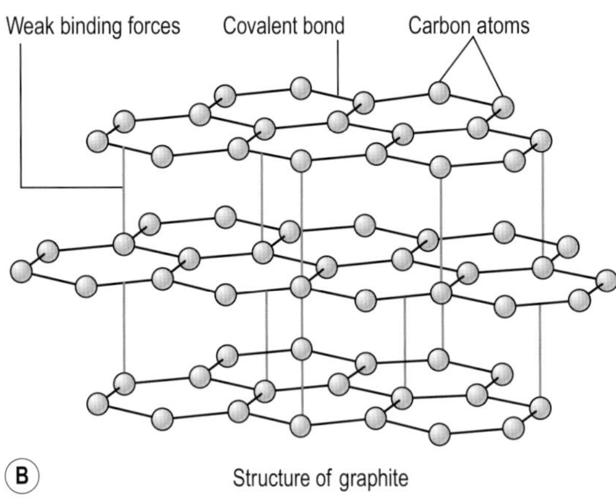

Figure 8.5

Differences between carbon and graphite. (A) Carbon: all the bonds are of equal length. (B) Graphite: bonds between carbons in layers are shorter and strong; bonds between layers are longer and weaker. The scientific term for a substance that has unequal bonds is anisodesmicity (for those of you who like words)

prising thing: the bulk of the water with the particles dissolved within it would move quickly away from the edge of the gel solid, until there was a distance of a hair's breadth – not seemingly so big to us but huge for the comparative size of water molecules. This newly formed area, if you could see the arrangement of the tiny water molecules, would consist of lattices of a honeycomb-type structure that quickly form from the surface inwards towards the rest of the water, pushing back the edge of the bulk water along with the microspheres within it (Fig. 8.6).

This is exciting new stuff from a researcher called Gerald Pollack, who is daring to push the boundaries and explore this science, despite having seen that 'immersing oneself in water science has become as perilous as immersing oneself in corrosive acid' (as we will see as we go on) (Pollack, 2013a). Aware that it is a tempestuous field, but one that still has many unanswered questions, Pollack decided to start back at the basics, unravelling any previous assumptions ... or so he thought until he discovered a 100-year-old paper by Sir William Hardy, who was the first to propose that water might have a fourth phase beyond its solid, liquid and gas states, the 60-year-old review that gave evidence for the long-range depth of structure on the surface zones of liquids (Henniker, 1949) and the 1969 paper that proposed the same structural model for water that Pollack ended up coming to, to name just a few. Two other key influences whose forward-thinking ideas have deeply contributed to this research are Albert Szent-Györgyi and Gilbert Ling. Have all these ideas been ignored and buried because they demanded too much of a rethink of accepted convention?

Whilst a layer or two of water molecules, and nothing else, at an edge had been thought likely, it was not supposed to be anywhere near as large as this – think 'a lineup of marbles extending over several dozen

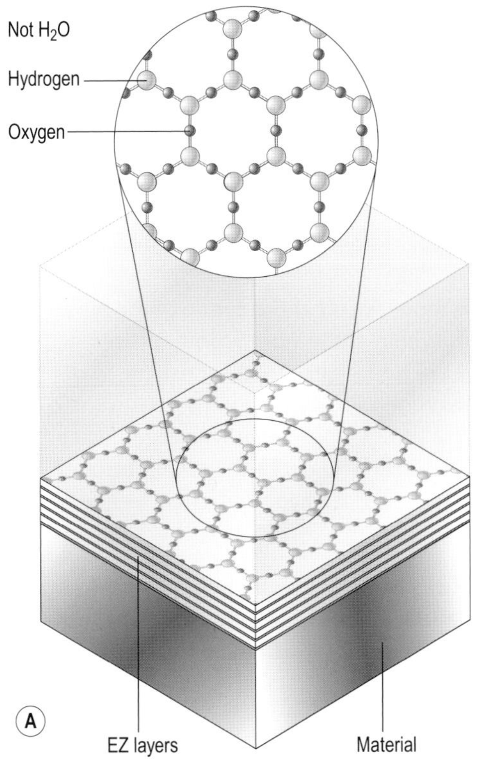

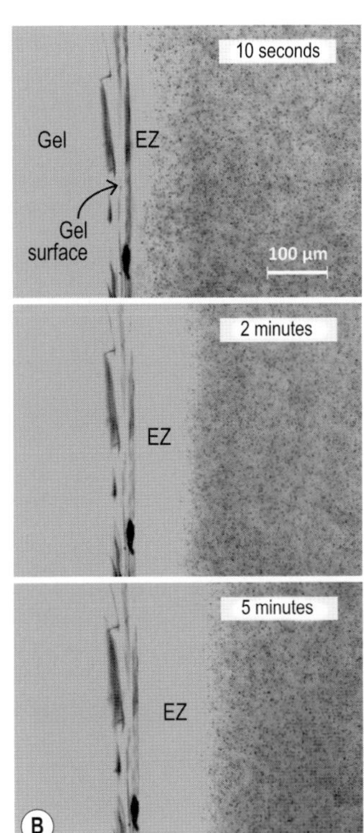

Figure 8.6

What you would see at the exclusion zone: (A) the honeycomb lattice of structured water molecules. (B) The build-up of the exclusion zone takes about five minutes. From *The Fourth Phase of Water: Beyond Solid, Liquid, and Vapor* by Gerald Pollack published by Ebner and Sons (2014). Illustration by Ethan Pollack

US football fields', says Pollack. A colleague playfully called this area the 'exclusion zone' or 'EZ' water as it 'excluded' anything other than itself, and the name has stuck despite the later thought that liquid crystalline or semi-liquid phase might have been better! They tested many dissolved substances for proof that they were excluded from this area and present only in the bulk water and the list was long. What is happening in the exclusion zone?

When is water ***not*** water ...?

Many experiments led Pollack to conclude that the water that forms in this zone is made up of highly ordered molecules, giving it a liquid crystalline structure that is more stable and viscous than liquid water. Liquid crystals are substances that have properties of liquids and solids. They are highly ordered on a molecular level, yet retain flexibility and responsiveness. This is the fourth phase of water, different from ice, liquid water or water vapour as a gas.

Pollack's team tested the plausibility of different models for this structure. The one that holds for the properties they observed in EZ water is 'sheets' of hexagonally arranged molecules aligned in planes that are offset against one another – similar to the structure of graphite shown in Fig. 8.5. There are a few different ways they can offset that will still allow the bonds between the sheets to attract, one of which, interestingly, appears to create a helix formation with the hexagonal structures (Fig. 8.7). Might this turn out to be relevant biologically when this layer needs to work with helically wound proteins and even DNA?

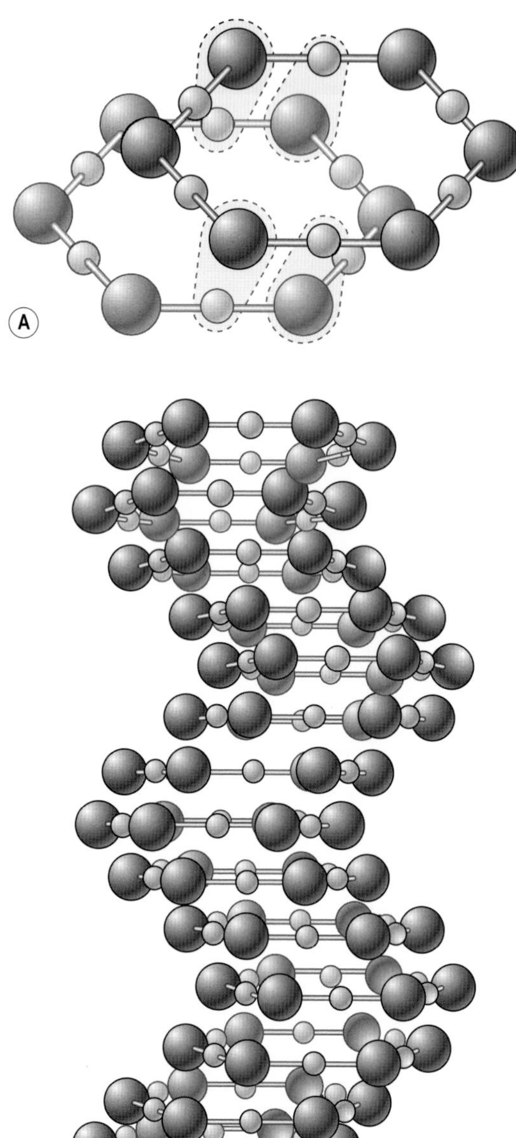

Figure 8.7

Possible alignments of hexagonal planes: (A) offset and (B) forming a helical structure. From *The Fourth Phase of Water: Beyond Solid, Liquid, and Vapor* by Gerald Pollack published by Ebner and Sons (2014). Illustration by Ethan Pollack

In searching for the structure within the EZ, Pollack's team also stumbled upon the discovery that the EZ is very negatively charged, which they were not expecting since water has an inherently neutral charge. Having found that, they knew there must be a positive charge somewhere too. They found it in the water just beyond the EZ. What was going on?

… when it's H_3O_2 in the EZ!

If we look more closely at the set-up of the hexagonal structures within these honeycomb lattices, we see that they are no longer, strictly speaking, water. The *ratio* of hydrogen to oxygen atoms goes from 2:1 (in H_2O) to 3:2 (H_3O_2) – not as individual molecules but because to form a joined hexagonal structure you effectively have to lose hydrogens (feel free to count!) (Fig. 8.8A).

Those kicked-out hydrogens migrate to the edge of the bulk water and join with another water molecule to form what are called hydronium ions (H_3O+), with a positive charge.

Thus, the bulk water just beyond the EZ is positively charged, to the same extent as the EZ is negatively charged (Fig. 8.8B).

Why do they form in the first place?

Pollack and his colleagues noticed that exclusion zones only form from water next to a hydrophilic surface, and the extent to which the surface is hydrophilic determines how large the EZ becomes. Quite why the first layer forms is not 100 per cent clear, but a hydrophilic surface typically has lots of oxygen atoms that, Pollack theorises, might form a template. (Of course, different surfaces will have different set-ups, which is shown by different depths of zones.)

Most interestingly, they found (again quite by accident – when one of the lab students was moving a lamp) that in the presence of *light* there would be more liquid crystalline build-up. Carrying out further experiments showed that all wavelengths will build this zone, with the near-infrared doing so the most. Water can absorb infrared from the environment (which is being emitted from things all the time – think of how much you still see in the dark looking through infrared

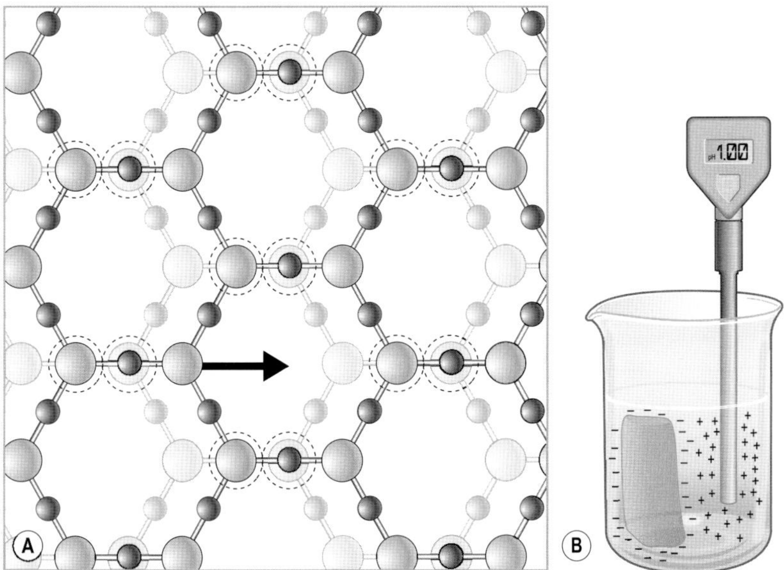

Figure 8.8

(A) Structure in the EZ: since hydrogen has a positive charge of 1 but oxygen has a negative charge of 2, rather than the neutral H_2O ($2H^+ + O^{2-}$), we now have three positive hydrogen charges but four negatives from two oxygen atoms ($3H^+ + 2O^{2-}$), leaving an overall negative charge to the structure.
(B) The negative charge in the EZ and the positive charge at the edge of the bulk water.

From *The Fourth Phase of Water: Beyond Solid, Liquid, and Vapor* by Gerald Pollack published by Ebner and Sons (2014). Illustration by Ethan Pollack

night goggles). Ultimately, Pollack ended up concluding that the energy for building this zone comes from the sun and the build-up is spontaneous.

Pollack relates some extraordinary experiments showing that the amount of light water absorbs changes during the day and according to the time of year. For example, an Italian scientist, Piccardi, conducted experiments every day for 12 years and noted the time that chemical reactions took. They varied by a few seconds from day to day. To explore why that might be his team carried out experiments in twos – one within an electromagnetically shielded beaker, the other identical but not shielded. The latter was the one that varied. Piccardi concluded that the only variable was the external environment and that the only substance common to all the experiments was water, therefore the water must have absorbed some kind of electromagnetic energy from the environment. We know that there are tiny changes from the sun's energy.

We therefore have water against a hydrophilic surface absorbing energy from the electromagnetic spectrum, spontaneously creating a liquid crystalline structure that has charge, with corresponding opposite charge in the adjacent area of bulk water. This also gives us two forms of potential energy – one from within the order or structure of the lattice, the other in the charge separation between the EZ and edge of bulk water. Or, in other words, the possibility of a battery! There are many ways this could be exploited – from the photosynthesis in plants to reactions in our cells. As Pollack (2013a) says, our 'EZ offers a ready source of electrons that could drive any of numerous biological reactions. The complementary hydronium ions may play an equally vital role.'

Like likes like

There is one other piece to this that is relevant. If you put two negatively charged particles in a beaker of water, not too far apart, what will happen when they get a sense of each other's charge – will they pull together or push apart? The unexpected observation is that they actually pull together, not so they are touching but close enough. Ise, a Japanese researcher, looked into this first and observed that charged particles 'hanging out' in solution would arrange themselves into ordered lattices. Conventional physical chemists have not liked this. However, Pollack and his team showed that these 'like-likes-like' attractions are in fact drawn together because of the unlike charges in between – but only if you consider the exclusion zone!

As long as the particle has a hydrophilic surface an EZ will build around it from radiant energy, as explained above. The EZ will be negatively charged and there will be a matching positive charge in the bulk water just beyond. When there are two particles in the same vicinity there will be more positive charge in the area between them, compared with the wider area around them. The negatively charged EZ will therefore be attracted to this area of greater positivity, thus moving together (Fig. 8.9).

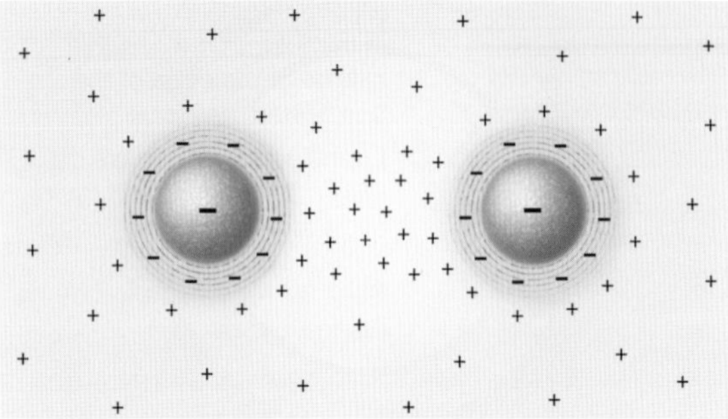

Figure 8.9

Like likes like. From *The Fourth Phase of Water: Beyond Solid, Liquid, and Vapor* by Gerald Pollack published by Ebner and Sons (2014). Illustration by Ethan Pollack

Does this have a role in holding us all together? I have included these ideas here because it seems really important to understand in reference to our bodies and cells. Recall how much of our structure is made up of water, and yet how little attention modern biology gives to its influence in our cellular processes. But this research shows that in fact a liquid crystalline structure might be what envelops every molecule, enzyme, macromolecule and organelle in our cells (Fig. 8.10). Could these liquid crystalline structures account for a signalling mechanism that is much faster than blood transfer of messengers? Even more intriguingly, since infrared or other electromagnetic energy is involved in the creation of and will affect the depth of the zone, and if the charge separation is important for supplying the energy for some chemical reactions, could there be a radically different way that our cells are powered, unlike the one we have conventionally learned?

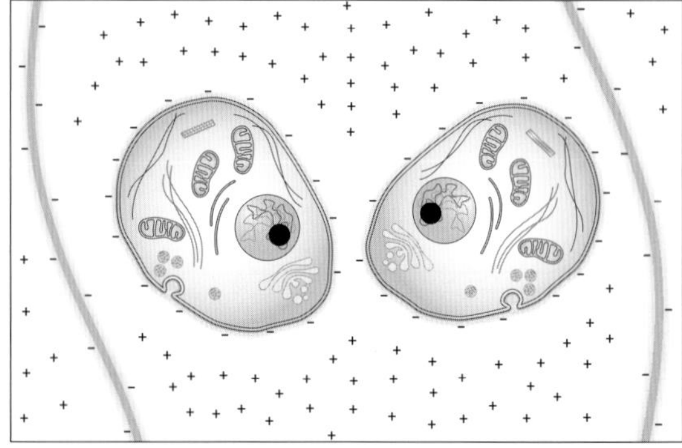

Figure 8.10

What if all of our cells, and everything inside and outside of them, were surrounded by an exclusion zone?

At the water's edge summary

- Water molecules spontaneously form an exclusion zone against any hydrophilic surface, making a liquid crystalline, fourth phase of water.
- They do this from light energy (especially infrared wavelengths).
- These molecules arrange themselves in slightly offset hexagonal planes.
- This arrangement leaves a negative charge in the exclusion zone; a positive charge is then found at the edge of the bulk water.
- This gives an inherent energetic set-up – a potential 'battery'.
- It also gives like-likes-like attractions between molecules of hydrophilic surfaces as the high level of positive charge between adjacent molecules attracts the negative charge of the exclusion zone.

Beyond the water's edge

What about the rest of the water in our bodies? Korean scientist Mu Shik Jhon suggests that around 60 per cent of our body's water is intracellular and 40 per cent of it extracellular, with 10 per cent running in the blood (Jhon and Pangman, 2004). The EZ properties exist up against any hydrophilic surfaces (which will include many of the structures within our bodies), but there will also be areas of bulk water, although we do not yet know how much of the other areas will contain bulk water, since the like-likes-like attractions will also pull much of our structure together. Is it likely that there is more to water's structure in other areas?

Ideas that water holds structure are not new. As mentioned above there are articles reaching back over many decades suggesting that this is the case.

A study from the Lawrence Berkeley National Laboratory materials Science Division (Velasco-Velez et al., 2014) using x-ray absorption spectroscopy (which essentially measures photons produced by excited atoms) showed that the water up against a gold electrode surface had a different arrangement to the bulk water beyond and that the depth of this would change with voltage. The team also showed that a negative or positive charge emitted by the electrode would alter the direction of alignment of the water's structure. This is interesting as it is such a similar finding but from a different field of research.

Jhon has published over 250 papers that point to the evidence that water exists in hexagonal structures, and he also talks about water surrounding ions in layers, which he calls hydration layers. He sees the first layer being the one held tighter as the molecules will have direct attraction to the ion; beyond this they will hold structure, and beyond that will be bulk water (similar to the exclusion zone above).

This idea of water structuring around surfaces includes larger molecules such as proteins and our DNA. Jhon suggests that the water structures support the bends and folds of a protein's structure – which is even more important in the larger DNA molecules to help maintain and stabilise its helical form. Jhon's team discovered that distortions in DNA structure are accompanied by fewer water molecules in place around its helix. They have also shown that 'cancerous and non-cancerous cells exhibit a similar hydration phenomenon'; that is, there is less structured water around them. Which comes first: disruption of the water's structure or disruption of the activity of the other molecules or cells?

Water clusters – in divine proportion?

The ancient Greek philosophers saw water as one of the vital elements, along with earth, fire and air, with water being the one most important for life.

Plato talked of each of these elements as being represented by a certain geometric structure: fire by a tetrahedron as it would be the lightest, earth by a cube because it would be the most stable, air by an octahedron, and water by an icosahedron. The universe or cosmos would be represented by a dodecahedron. All of these have similarly shaped surfaces and fit within a sphere; geometrically they are also 'all related to the Divine Proportion' (Fig. 8.11) (Hemenway, 2008).

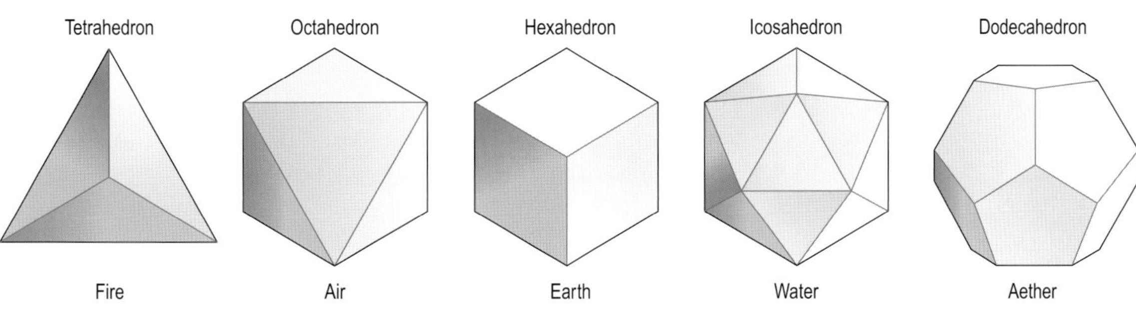

Figure 8.11

Martin Chaplin, Emeritus Professor of Applied Science at London South Bank University, has been studying the structure of water and the shapes that *could* form from the given molecular building blocks. He puts forward a detailed and elegant theory that many different *water clusters* will be present in a body of water. Intriguingly, for those of us who enjoy the conservation of ideas over millennia, he posits that some could indeed form the shape described by Plato.

The box 'A whizz through the chemistry' earlier in this chapter showed why hydrogen bonds exist in water; be aware too that as more molecules unite, bonds also form under the repelling influence of any two positive or two negative areas. Thus, water molecules can combine and arrange themselves to form a variety of shapes, for example those shown in Fig. 8.12.

Each of these possible clusters is fairly stable. The smaller ones can also build up into a tetrahedron, and

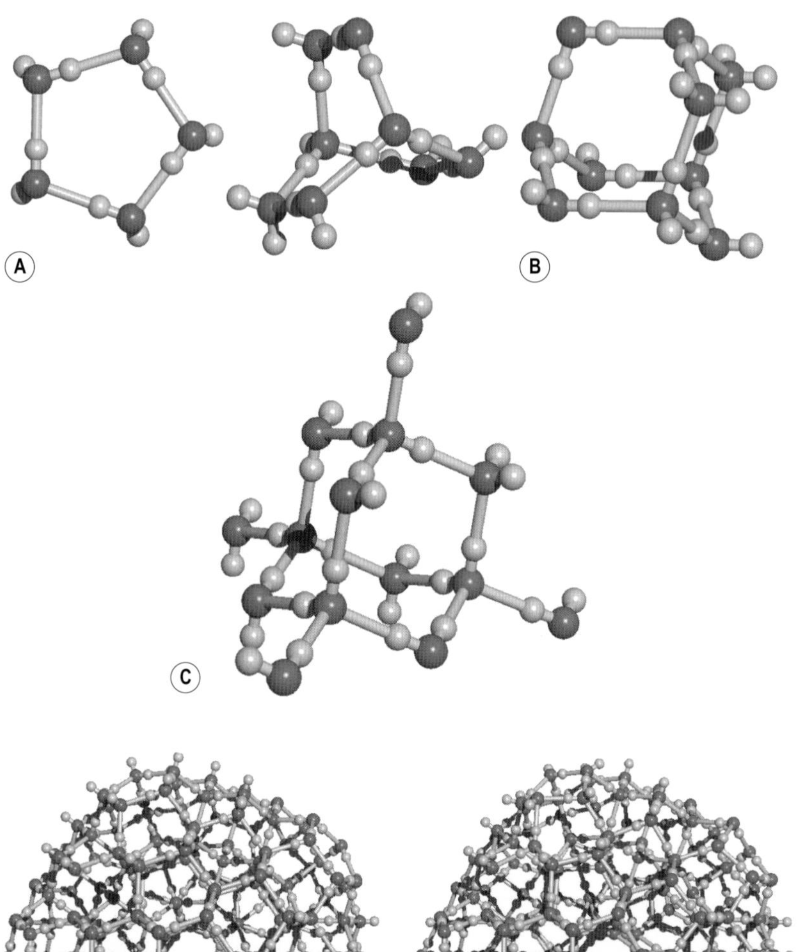

Figure 8.12

Examples of stable water clusters: (A) the five-sided shape or pentamer, (B) the bicyclo- or tricyclo-octamers (you don't need to remember the names!), (C) tetrahedra, (D) icosahedron, made up of 280 H_2O molecules, each molecule participating in four hydrogen bonds; it may also exist in both a more open and more condensed structure. Images courtesy of Martin Chaplin, Emeritus Professor of Applied Science, London South Bank University

14 tetrahedra can form an icosahedron – Plato's solid. Despite there being the possibility of 'small differences in geometry' of the larger structure compared with the 14 tetrahedra within it, on his website Chaplin notes that these 'may be taken up by the flexibility of the hydrogen bonding', since it is known that hydrogen bonds can bend slightly.

Chaplin goes on to geometrically extrapolate other superclusters that could occur – from 13 icosahedra creating super-icosahedra, to how they may also create other spherical structures or exist as strands, linked together in a more linear or elongated pattern. Chaplin is far from alone in having these ideas. Others have agreed that there are likely superstructures within bodies of water, even up to many millions of molecules. What he says is important to understand is that water's electrons and protons are not irrevocably tied to any individual molecule.

Therefore, he does not presume that these larger water clusters are stable and constant. They may not always be perfectly formed and can be affected by external influences, from temperature and pressure to solvents within, and even electromagnetic forces, we are now realising. Molecules are constantly moving and each hydrogen bond lasts only a very short time (picoseconds). The tendency is for the clusters to be continually changing and reforming as different individual molecules join and leave, or the centrepoint of the structure changes, prompting other molecules to recluster around the new centre. The fact that the behaviour of large bodies of water remains consistent, even though the individual molecules are constantly moving, may be due to this consistency of patterning of the clusters.

New theories for water's properties

Why are the molecules constantly moving about? Whilst it is typically accepted that the molecules within water move about due to the thermal energy, Pollack has questioned this, arguing that the theory simply doesn't hold for all that is observed. Citing a range of different experiments and observations, he offers instead evidence for radiant energy from the electromagnetic spectrum being a more likely candidate than temperature in instigating the ongoing Brownian motion. (Incidentally, researchers before Einstein had put this forward as a theory and others had argued against his initial temperature ideas, but the idea took hold anyway for the observations it did explain.) Is it possible that it could be both?

Does this geometric theory explain the beauty of structure of some of Emoto's images? By flash-freezing drops of water to −25 degrees and photographing the crystals at −5 degrees, where the hydrogen bonds have stabilised, was he capturing crystals formed from different arrangements of water clusters? Are we simply seeing more or less well-ordered geometric structures under the microscope? If so, does it suggest that vibration is an important part of forming more aligned structures? This is why it is relevant to us here: is it possible that when we practise finding our places of stillness we are affecting our vibration and therefore the actual build-up of our water clusters?

Which brings us back to Roy's work. Originally a materials scientist, he brought together 60 years of scientific endeavour to conclude that, at a temperature of 25°C and normal atmospheric pressure, water would be 'a highly mobile assemblage of interactive clusters' (Roy et al., 2009) that would consist of a variety of these larger and smaller geometric structures held together by hydrogen bonds, albeit with different molecules moving in and out of individual clusters. In addition, there are even weaker bonds possible (created from the constant moving of electrons within their shells creating temporary 'dipoles' or areas of charge) that can influence the structures. But, importantly, he is clear that these variations are endless and that the differences in the structural alignments will give water *subtly different properties*.

Additionally, Roy contends that because of the weakness of the bonds, water can be changed by weak vectors, such as light photons or magnetic waves, including the electric field around the body (Fig. 8.13). Bear in mind that these ideas move out of what conventional science is teaching into the realm of sometimes controversial evidence, alongside hypotheses that have not yet been fully proven – but not disproven – so maintaining an open mind is paramount.

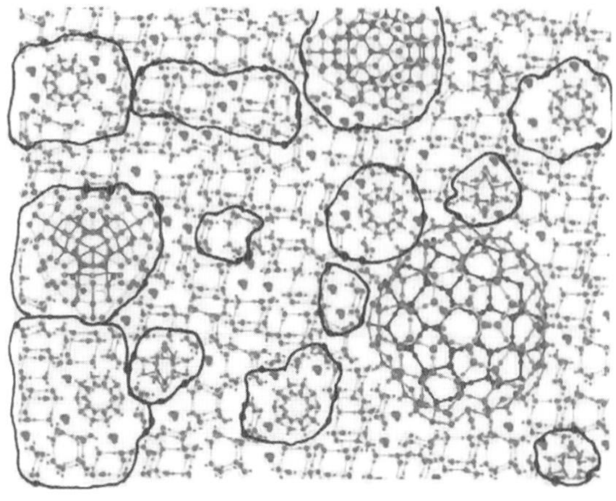

Figure 8.13

A cartoon image of the possible structures in bulk water and the forces that might alter the structures

McTaggart (2008, 2011) has been carrying out a variety of experiments exploring the effect that intention may have on the structural arrangement of water. Working with Roy, using Raman spectroscopy, and a Russian researcher named Korotov, who uses a technique called gas discharge visualisation (GDV) (Korotov, Williams and Wisneski, 2004), which essentially measure photons produced from substances (more on that in the next chapter), they have shown interesting indications that intention and healing energy can make changes to water. Their results have not always shown statistical significance, but it does seem that the more experienced a healer or intender you are the more change is made. Additionally, they have shown small effects from people 'sending' energy from all over the world, which also suggests that we do not have to be in situ to have far-reaching effects.

Is stillness-memory in water?

To what extent is this important within our bodies? Is it plausible that the various forms of electromagnetic radiation around us affect our vibration and the very arrangement of the molecules of water within us? If many shapes are possible, do some have different effects on the biochemical reactions going on within our cells? If so, what additional layers of vibrational information might be contained within the cytoplasm of each cell, the blood traversing each capillary bed, the cerebrospinal fluid circling the perimeter of our central nervous system?

Also, since we are ourselves electromagnetic generators, as we saw in Chapter 6, is it not conceivable that the 'health' of our EZs, as well as any other water clusters, will be affected by our own electromagnetic coherence, our vibration, our ability to hold stillness?

If we come back and think about our idea of an inherent memory of stillness, could one (or more) of the myriad possible arrangements of the water within our bodies hold a pattern of vibration that we might refer to as stillness? Might there simply be one or more 'natural' alignments of molecules that occur in response to the vibration we are calling stillness that somehow allow for an optimum experience of (universal) connection?

(Might the brevity of the hydrogen bonds be why we can only hold onto the sense of stillness for short moments initially? Perhaps this is why my experience of stillness feels dynamic and has an inner sense of dynamism to it – it *is* changing every picosecond! I am not really serious about this one!)

Is this a place for our stillness-memory? Is there such a thing as water-memory? (Of course, I am not referring to conventional memory but more a vibrational encoding of the moment.) This makes me intrigued enough to venture (stumble?) further into a very controversial area – the work of a scientist called Benveniste. Some may recognise the story ...

Beyond the water's edge summary

- Roy says we have missed a vital piece of information: that the structure of water can change even though its composition is the same.
- Jhon suggests water arranges in hexagonal forms and that ions have a hydration layer (similar to the EZ layer above though not as large).
- Chaplin theorises (and Roy agrees) that bulk water will contain a huge variety of water clusters because of the extent of hydrogen bonding.
- Even though these bonds are short-lived (picoseconds) they will continually reform.
- Roy adds that these bonds can be influenced by much weaker forces than temperature and pressure, including photons and magnetic waves – and possibly even intention.
- We put forth the idea that if all these water molecules within our body are subject to vibration, including our thoughts and intentions (as also suggested by Emoto's images), then a greater ability to hold stillness, which we suggested in Chapter 6 may create more physiological coherence, would be likely to be a positive influence on the way our water molecules arrange themselves.

A tale of controversy

In 1988 French doctor and researcher Jacques Benveniste, well recognised for his decades of work on mechanisms of allergies and inflammation, published an article in *Nature* that in the long run led to a downturn of his previously successful career.

He was head of ISSEM (Institute of Health and Medical Research) in France and had published many papers over many years, in particular looking at the effects of allergens on basophils. A basophil is a type of white blood cell that contains many histamine granules. It has antibodies on its surface that, when exposed to certain allergens, will react, effectively spitting its histamine granules into the surrounding tissue – a process known as 'degranulation'.

One of his team was a homeopath and asked if he could do some research. He wanted to run Benveniste's basophil degranulation test on some high-dilution solutions to see if the basophils would respond in the same way as they would with undiluted allergen. Despite his initial scepticism, and a certainty that they would have nothing but non-degranulating, plain water after the high dilution, Benveniste permitted his colleague to try.

To his extraordinary surprise the high-dilution solutions *were* precipitating degranulation of the basophils. They repeated the research time and again over five years, called in others to replicate their results and published their first two papers. In 1988 Benveniste sent a paper to *Nature*, who at first refused to publish, apparently as they couldn't believe the results, despite the fact that they could not fault the scientific procedure. Eventually they agreed to publish on the condition that they could bring a team to the lab to see the experiments performed (Poitevin, Davenas and Benveniste, 1988). Benveniste willing agreed.

Curiously, the *Nature* editor did not bring other scientists with him but an ex-magician-turned-pseudo-science-debunker and an unofficial fraud expert. After attempting to reproduce the experiments they could not replicate the previous results. They published an article in *Nature* themselves, denouncing Benveniste's previous paper.

What I find fascinating about this story is that Benveniste was an experienced and recognised scientist. He was quite willing to have those who wanted to repeat and replicate his experiments visit his lab. Four other labs had already tried and three had found the same results. As such, he was surprised to be treated as a fraudster rather than a scientist who had some extremely unusual results that could not yet be explained. He commented that his 'trial' became a 'pantomime' rather than an honest attempt to explore the controversy.

The way that Benveniste's team conducted the science has had overall approval. Since then other teams of researchers in many laboratories have repeated the studies and some have found similar results, whilst others have not been able to replicate them. There

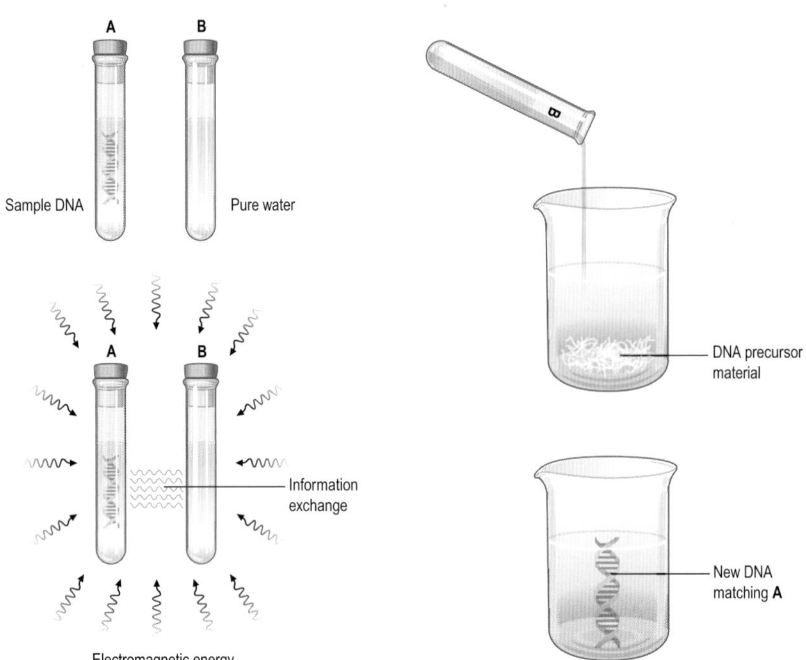

Figure 8.14

DNA information passed through water and electromagnetic waves

have also been a string of other papers that show something still happens with substances under high dilution (albeit not published in *Nature*!). It has also been noted, but not explored further, that some researchers consistently get results, whilst others do not.

It is a curious standoff that continues to this day. Our current general understanding of science cannot explain these findings – or why they don't occur every time. Did Benveniste simply make it all up? If you look closely at all the papers, and consider his experience as a scientist, that seems highly unlikely. Why was it only reproducible sometimes? Does that negate the times when there *was* a degranulating reaction?

Emoto found that the crystal structures of tap water in built-up areas were utterly different from those in cleaner areas or natural springs – is there a difference in the inherent crystalline structure of the water in different labs that could explain the difference in water's ability to retain 'information' under high dilutions? I wonder what images of the flash-frozen samples of the different waters would look like? Would water flash-frozen and then photographed before and after the high-dilution process have similar or different crystalline structures? If the premise was correct, what happened when the experiment was repeated under different circumstances? Think about cross-referencing Emoto's studies of how water seems to reflect vibration: if you add in the possibility that intention could alter water's structure, where would that leave us?

This is such an interesting edge of science where there are two directions available: to be open to possibilities far beyond what our current materialistic focus and patterns of scientific belief have space for, or to denounce the results because we cannot explain them in a scientifically reassuring and validating way.

But remember the essence of science: it is observation of what happens in the world, then we build hypotheses to account for what we have observed and then test and refine these hypotheses. I wonder if this process was cut short on this occasion? Certainly, Benveniste went further into the edges of science that many could not fathom and never regained the respect of the establishment before his death in 2004. I wonder what he would make of the hypotheses currently being put forward if he were still with us?

Now, he is not alone out on his proverbial limb. There are an increasing number of other researchers noting odd things that are really hard to explain. In 2011 another established and previously respected researcher named Luc Montagnier, receiver of the 2008 Nobel Prize for discovery of HIV, came to attention. He was reporting on what happened when he placed an aqueous suspension of sample DNA in a sealed test tube, then placed another test tube with plain water next to it and exposed both to electromagnetic energy for 18 hours. He reported that when the plain water was subsequently mixed with the constituent building blocks of DNA, the same structural sequence of DNA as had been present in the original sample had formed, with 98 per cent accuracy (Fig. 8.14) (Montagnier et al., 2011). The group's 2015 paper adds that 'this experiment has been repeated many times in our laboratory, with extraordinary precautions taken to avoid contamination ... and many controls were always done' (Montagnier at al., 2015).

I will give you one guess as to the general response of the scientific community. Such a similar story to Benveniste. Another highly skilled and weathered scientist who discovers something that cannot be explained by the current belief that 'visible' active molecules must be present to explain all of biochemistry's happenings ... But what if this premise is wrong (gasp!)? What if there is something else going on?

Most research to date has taken little of the eccentricities of water's behaviour into account, elements of which, as we have highlighted here, are just beginning to be understood. The information in the next chapter on light is also a key part of these new ideas and perspectives, which are closely linked. Thankfully, time is bringing forward more researchers to continue exploring logical explanations for these seemingly extraordinary things that occur. A whole issue of the journal *Electromagnetic Biology and Medicine* (2015) was devoted to research on water, honouring particularly the contribution of Del Giudice (1940–2014) who worked with Montagnier's team and who pioneered the application of quantum field theory to water. According to Ho (2011), Del Giudice's work shows that 'quantum coherence of water is really what makes life possible' and suggests how little we currently understand; nor will we until we incorporate the quantum paradigm into our framework, which may well need to blend with artistry. At the ISIS Colours of Water festival in 2013 Giudice said: 'Artistic experiences are resonances in the framework of our quantum field paradigm. Their relevance for the self-organisation of matter has been recognised by artists and humanists long before the scientists' (ISIS, 2014).

(Is it possible that we are up against the need for a paradigm change on a par with realising the earth is not flat?)

The tales here hopefully lead us to ponder whether the way water is organised and aligned in our bodies is actually part of a liquid crystalline communication system. And, if so, that it may even hold information from vibrational inputs that affect our health, vitality and even how the ageing process proceeds within our bodies. If the way that water is structured is important for our cells and the fluid spaces in our bodies, and if its structure can alter at the molecular level, surely the vibrational input of stillness and the coherence it brings are going to affect this level of our being as well?

As we ponder the effect that creating the inner vibration of stillness may have on our water molecules, let us also consider the effect our outer lives might be having: does our bustle and busyness affect the patterns that 'should' be held inside for biochemical reactions to happen effectively and efficiently? Are we creating or adding to health problems by disrupting these arrangements in an invisible way, subtly changing our inherent stillness or coherence? If we think of all the things that might affect the formation of the EZ layer, and thus the possible 'battery' within and between our cells, and the structure of bulk water anywhere else – from the food we eat, to the light we shine on us (indoor light vs the sun), to the thoughts we think and the impact from those around us, family, society, culture – maybe some of the health challenges we face could be helped by attention to our water within. We posit that the practice of connecting to and deepening our inner stillness could improve our vibrational imprint and the alignment of water and energy within our bodies.

You may have read the experiences of Dr Batmanghelidj (1992), who learned, from his experience of assisting a fellow political prisoner in Iran in 1979, that people who were experiencing illness could sometimes be greatly helped by simply increasing their water intake. 'You're not sick; you're thirsty' became his strapline and he encouraged us all to drink more water. However, if we are now beginning to appreciate that not all water is the same, it is also important what water we drink. Jhon emphasised that the best water is water that has been moving; turbulence leaves it oxygenated and highly energised, unlike water which has been stationary in reservoirs or has travelled in straight, confined pipes. This was also shown by Emoto's images. Perhaps this gives us another reason to keep our bodies, and the water inside them, moving and active!

Pollack ended a Ted Talk (2013b) with the comment 'What we like most is understanding the gentle beauty of nature', an echo of the feelings of Emoto with whom we started this chapter and the early scientists who observed nature to help them live a good life. Even if we don't yet fully understand this gentle beauty, we at least have the joy of the journey.

Experiment

Feel it in your water

Ponder a moment the water in your body: within and between each cell, travelling through the circulatory, lymphatic and cerebrospinal fluid systems; think too that our plasma is one of the few substances that can pass through the blood–brain barrier. If the inherent structure of water is subject to change – not just from temperature and pressure, but from all the different wave forms that have an impact upon us, including the electromagnetic fields of our environment and of others – we can see another, possibly literal, way that finding stillness and neutrality for ourselves may be affecting our clients.

We do not yet know what water's 'optimum' structure is for our internal biological processes to occur, be it large EZs, hexagonal structures, super-repeating clusters of icosahedra or other helical patterns. I invite you to explore it in your meditations or dialogues with your inner wisdoms (or whichever way you like to connect with your self) and to keep me posted on any insights you get whilst we wait for the science to show us some more.

References

Batmanghelidj, F. (1995). *Your Body's Many Cries for Water.* Falls Church, VA: Global Health Solutions.

Chaplin, M. [website] www1.lsbu.ac.uk/water/martin_chaplin.html [accessed Jan. 2016].

Electromagnetic Biology and Medicine (2015). Special issue: Emilio Del Giudice and the science of water, 34(2): 105–169.

Giudice, E.D., Spinetti, P.R. and Tedeschi, A. (2010). Water dynamics at the root of metamorphosis in living organisms. *Water,* 2(3): 566–586.

Hemenway, P. (2008). *The Secret Code.* Evergreen.

Henniker, J.C. (1949). The depth of the surface zone of a liquid. *Reviews of Modern Physics,* 21(2): 322–341.

Ho, M-W. (2011). *Quantum coherent water and life.* ISIS report 25/07/11, www.i-sis.org.uk/Quantum_Coherent_Water_Life.php [accessed Mar. 2016].

Institute of Science in Society (ISIS) (2014). *Emilio Del Giudice: illuminating water and life*. ISIS report 1/10/14, www.i-sis.org.uk/Emilio_Del_Giudice_Illuminating_Water_and_Life.php [accessed Mar. 2016].

Jhon, M.S. and Pangman, M.J. (2004). *The Water Puzzle and the Hexagonal Key*. Uplifting Press.

Korotkov, K., Williams, B. and Wisneski, L. (2004). Assessing biophysical energy transfer mechanisms in living systems: the basis of life processes. *Journal of Alternative and Complementary Medicine*, 10(1): 49–57.

McTaggart, L. (2008)., *The Intention Experiment*. London: HarperElement.

McTaggart, L. (2011). The Intention Experiment [website], http://theintentionexperiment.com/the-experiments [accessed Mar. 2016].

Montagnier, L., Aissa, J., Giudice, E.D., Lavallee, C., Tedeschi, A. and Vitiello, G. (2011). DNA waves and water. *Journal of Physics Conference Series*, 306: 012007.

Montagnier, L., Del Giudice, E., Aïssa, J., Lavallee, C., Motschwiller, S., Capolupo, A., Polcari, A., Romano, P., Tedeschi, A. and Vitiello, G. (2015). Transduction of DNA information through water and electromagnetic waves. *Electromagnetic Biology and Medicine*, 34(2): 106–112.

Poitevin, B., Davenas, E. and Benveniste, J. (1988). In vitro immunological degranulation of human basophils is modulated by lung histamine and Apis mellifica. *British Journal of Clinical Pharmacology*, 25(4): 439–444.

Pollack, G.H. (2013a). *The Fourth Phase of Water*. Seattle, WA: Ebner & Sons.

Pollack G.H. (2013b). *The fourth phase of water: Dr. Gerald Pollack at TEDxGuelphU* [video]. YouTube, 6 September, https://www.youtube.com/watch?v=i-T7tCMUDXU [accessed Mar. 2016].

Roy, R. (2009). *Water, water everywhere; and so little understood* [video]. YouTube, 5 April, https://www.youtube.com/watch?v=c8ajf_a9MRw [accessed Mar. 2016].

Roy, R., Tiller, W.A., Bell, I. and Hoover, M.R. (2009). The structure of liquid water: novel insight from materials research; potential relevance to homeopathy. *Indian Journal of Research in Homeopathy*, 3(2), http://ccrhindia.org/ijrh/3%282%29/1.pdf [accessed Mar. 2016].

Velasco-Velez, J., Wu, C., Pascal, T., Wan, L., Guo, J., Prendergast, D. and Salmeron, M. (2014). The structure of interfacial water on gold electrodes studied by x-ray absorption spectroscopy. *Science*, 346(6211): 831–834.

And then there was light 9

Walking on hot coals

A number of years ago I had the opportunity to do a fire walk. In preparation for it the people leading the course talked a lot about believing anything was possible, getting us into a space of focus and attention so that we could be in 'the zone'. However, when I reached the front of the queue my scientific brain took over and asked (very loudly inside my head) how is it possible that my feet will not be burned by these exceedingly hot coals? (We had been assured how hot they were.) The person in charge of letting us walk or not looked into my eyes and asked if I was ready – he and I knew instantly that I was not. I turned, ran and burst into stressed-out tears ... which gave me time to look around. People were walking over these coals. It obviously was possible. How? I did not know. But I knew I wanted to do it and I knew that I had to find a way. As I re-approached the coals I went back to the experiences I had had from my shiatsu training and from some years practising martial arts. I dropped my energy into my hara, the area below the belly button, turned to the guy in charge and he nodded. Something had changed in my eyes and I walked.

To this day I ponder what happened. How did we all do that? How can we change the 'expected' result of two surfaces connecting by doing something so fast within us? Did our physiological systems entrain and come into some sense of coherence (as we considered in Chapter 6)? If so, how did it happen so quickly?

In this chapter we are pushing the boat right out and looking at some of the possibilities that attempt to bring the quantum paradigm into our understanding of biological processes. In particular, we are going to consider the biophoton and the possibility that our biological processes are in fact controlled at the speed of light.

Think about the systems of the body made up of all our cells – that's roughly 10 billion cells (give or take) that have an estimated 100,000 reactions going on every second. Plus approximately 10 million cells dying every second and 10 million replacing them. Timing is crucial. How can all of this be coordinated? By molecules travelling around in the blood? By neural control? That's too little, too slow and not the whole picture, think an increasing number of researchers, as these processes only take into account the Newtonian approach to the body. This sees the variety of molecules and their reactions as the only things making up our biological action, which is missing the essence of the quantum view: that the universe (us included) is in fact made up of oscillating and vibrating particles, where 'each atom is like a wobbly spinning top that radiates energy' (Lipton, 2005). Each and every atom then has its own unique energy, and the energy from groups of them, so to speak, will become entangled, creating a mesh of interactions. Thus, the flow of information from the quantum perspective is complex, holistic and ultimately energetic.

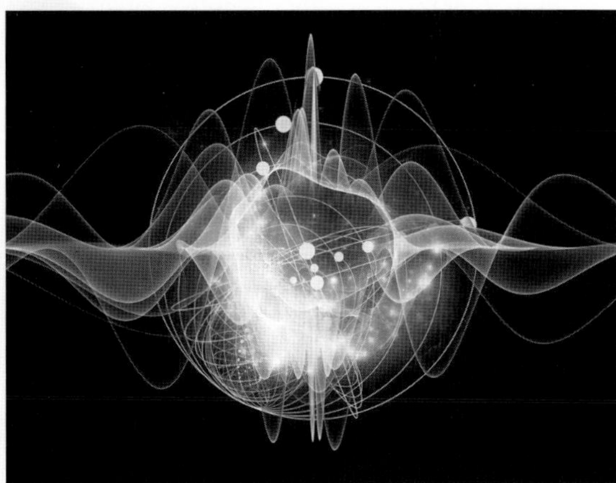

Figure 9.1

A quantum atom vibrating

What does this mean to us? It means that there could be a level of communication occurring that takes account of this energy perspective. Oschman (2015) argues that accepted biological theories, such as the lock and key model of cell receptors for hormones and other travelling molecules, simply do not account for enough. He suggests that chemicals journeying through the fluid pathways of the body 'chancing' a meeting with a specific cell that has a specific receptor 'is seriously deficient and outdated'; the mechanism is too slow to explain the speed with which organisms can adjust many aspects of their functioning.

But we can start to add to our knowledge of molecules and chemical reactions an understanding of an exciting, newer, evolving paradigm. Some of the introduction to this story is (coming up to a 100 years) old news, but it is not that well known so I would like to include it here.

The idea that all living cells emit weak light was discovered by Alexander Gurwitsch, back in 1926 or so, who observed that placing the tip of an onion root (with dividing cells) up against the side of another onion root would increase the amount of mitotic cell division at that specific point on the second root. That in itself is quite interesting but then he also found that putting normal glass between the two roots blocked the effect, whereas quartz glass did not. Working out that the latter allows UV light through whilst the former does not, he concluded that 'mitogenetic radiation' – or UV emitted from the first onion root – was responsible for the change in cellular activity in the second root. However, back then there were no instruments able to measure the light that was being emitted and the field of research, at the time up against the new genetics and molecular biology, got left behind.

In the 1950s a much more sensitive 'photomultiplier' was invented – actually by astronomers to look at distant stars; turned closer to home it also showed that plants and their cells did emit weak light, but after a bit of a hubbub from biologists of the time the research, again, got left behind.

That is until the 1970s, when a young Fritz Popp, in a doctoral thesis, wanted to explore why a substance called 3,4-benzopyrene (think cigarette smoke and coal tar) is carcinogenic whereas its very similar cousin 1,2-benzopyrene is not. The first 3,4 version, he discovered, has the unusual property of absorbing light in the UV part of the spectrum. He wondered if this was the property causing its carcinogenic nature rather than any molecular activity. Amusingly (in retrospect) he was funded to prove that there was no light emitted from cells, not to explore the idea that there might be. So, he failed (or succeeded, depending on which way you look at it) as, after building a more sensitive photomultiplier, he proved that light is indeed emitted from all living cells. The light emitted is in the UV range – which is why we cannot see it. The quantity of biophotons that are emitted can change over time and, he also noted, will 'spike' when cells receive radiation from an external source.

That's two game-changing discoveries – or re-discoveries:

- living cells emit light, and
- cells emit more when they have received some light themselves.

From where might they receive light? Either from external sources or from other cells. Does this offer us the possibility for coordination and communication between cells – at the speed of light?

What is a biophoton?

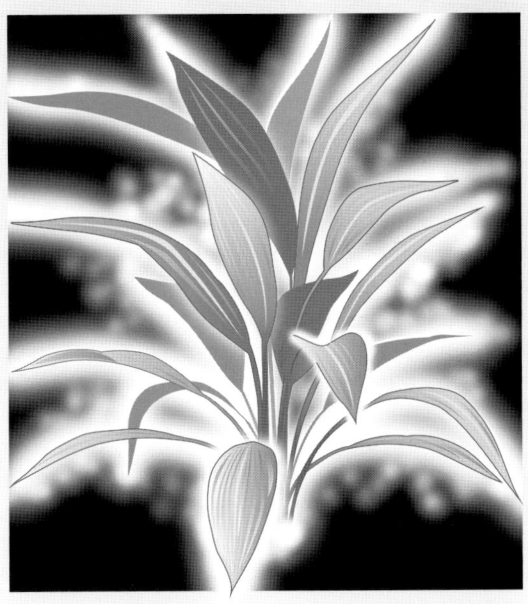

Figure 9.2

All living organisms emit light in the UV range of the spectrum

A photon is a quantum or 'bit' of light from the visible spectrum. It is the smallest bundle of light possible. Photons have no mass and no charge and they behave both as particles and waves, some saying they move as particles and act as waves (Fleming and Colorio, 2003). Because they are a form of energy, they can be transformed into another type of energy, such as in a solar panel where, by bumping into particular atoms they will cause them to lose an electron and the energy released is converted into electricity.

There are other wavelengths from the electromagnetic spectrum as well (Fig. 9.3). Our eyes 'see' light waves from a narrow range of the spectrum we call visible light, we can feel the heat from infrared (whose wavelength is longer), or witness the change in skin colour after exposure to UV light.

Biophoton is the term that has been coined for the ultraviolet low-frequency radiation that can be measured coming from organisms and not seen by the naked eye.

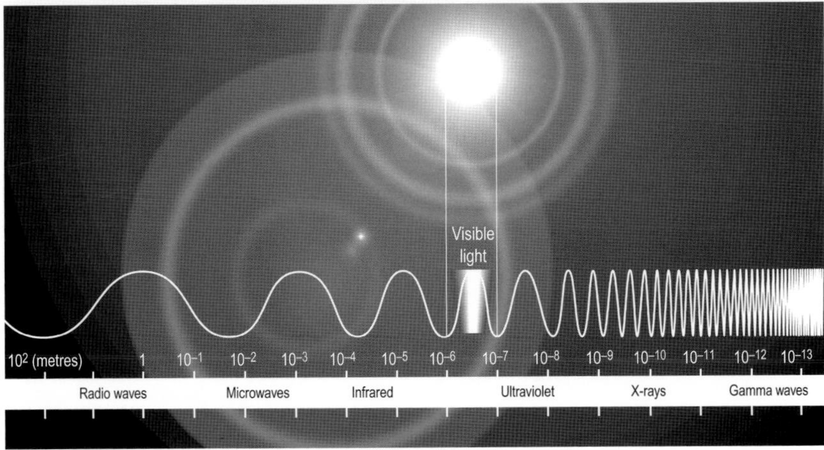

Figure 9.3

The different wavelengths of the electromagnetic spectrum

What we now know is that every atom, every molecule and every larger structure that subsequently builds will emit a biophoton of a particular wavelength and respond to a particular wavelength. This is called its 'resonance'. We also know that waves from the electromagnetic spectrum, when they intersect or combine together, either reinforce each other or cancel each other out (Fig. 9.4). If our cells are emitting (on average) 8–10 photons per second that can combine to create resultant waves, these could lead to cellular signals being transmitted, which could trigger different chemical reactions (Kim, 2015). We don't yet know which frequencies instigate which reactions, but Popp's son says that his father's work shows it is quite possible that with newer technology that lets us filter for different electromagnetic wavelengths we may be able to map them (A. Popp, 2012).

Coming back to Oschman's assertion (2015) that travelling by blood is too slow, we can now ponder instead that if molecules have their own electromagnetic frequency, the radiation they emit could be received by target receptors that are 'tuned', through their own molecular structure, to receive or 'hear' this frequency. As instantly as the molecule is activated to emit the biophoton, the wave is 'sent', like the ripples of a pebble in a pond, but at the speed of light, to activate anything that resonates to its frequency. Importantly, this also allows for feedback – a co-resonance would occur and feedback would be instantaneous. Does a molecular message in fact not need to 'arrive' but just biophotonically announce its presence? Is this a more likely possible scenario? If so, then the other beautiful part to it is that it can be received everywhere at once, so that there can be a whole-system response. It is enabling our cells to create communicating networks.

Here is another way of coming to understand this phenomenon as a whole and put it, and perhaps the importance of it, into perspective. Whilst all the things we understand from molecular biology are happening, just envisage that there is a whole other system of activity going on at a level just below this (I say 'below' only because it seems it occurs on the smaller level size-wise). Imagine the hive of activity going on beneath the earth to make a plant sprout or a flower bloom, or perhaps imagine all the activity going on in a busy kitchen of a busy restaurant – you will just see the constant delivery of meals to the right tables, and (hopefully) not hear the communicative shouts that get issued for all to hear but the appropriate person to respond to! Our cells are constantly emitting radiation, a sort of instant messaging that informs the other cells in the body what is happening, but only those that need to respond specifically will do so.

As we know, plant cells also emit light: this translates into the fact that food also contains biophotons that we can absorb – not surprisingly, much more so from raw, organic and naturally grown foods than food that has been modified in any way.

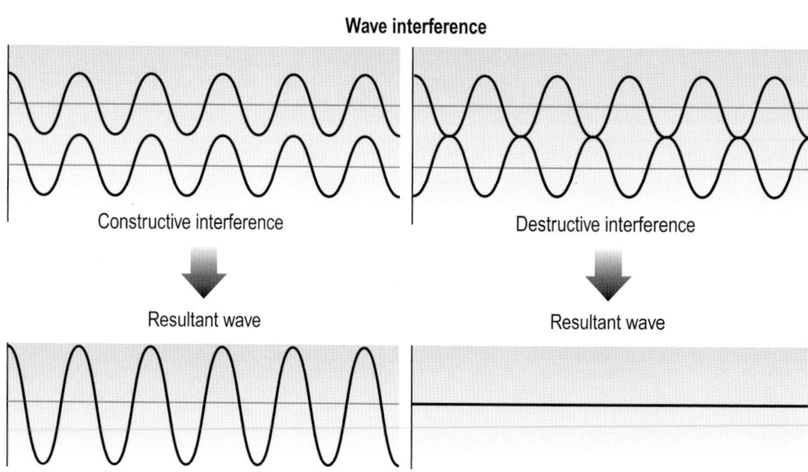

Figure 9.4

Wave interference: interference in the same phase leads to a larger amplitude (constructive interference), and in the opposite phase to lower amplitude or destruction of the wave (destructive interference)

The possibility of light pipes? A madcap idea!

Oschman (2015) also reflects on another possible mechanism for the action of photons working with a cell by taking a good few steps back in evolution to red and blue–green algae. Studying their physiology has shown that they have light-absorbing structures within their cell membranes that consist of many alpha-helical proteins, affectionately known as 'light pipes'.

An alpha-helix is a region in a protein that forms a tunnel by twisting into a right-handed spiral or coil, sort of like the old-fashioned telephone cords. In the algae it has been shown that photons go directly through to help them to absorb as much light as possible from the darker regions they commonly inhabit. Oschman comments on the distinct likelihood that nature would conserve this process.

How light travels is an ongoing question in physics. It is mentioned above (in the box 'What is a biophoton') that photons move as particles and act like waves. Physicist Richard Feynman stated that it travels in particles and that those particles travel in a helical fashion. If this is indeed the case then is it plausible that the many transmembrane proteins that we find in our cell membranes made up of alpha-helical spirals might act as our light pipes?

I find this a poetic idea, yet I heed Guimberteau's (2015) warning, mentioned in Chapter 5, that we must avoid being seduced by theories that are conceptually attractive but may be wrong. I have been a little seduced by the lovely idea of light pipes. I am sure science will eventually shed more light on the matter. (Indeed.)

From coherence to consciousness?

Another really interesting thing that Popp (2003) asserts, after decades of work in this field, is that whilst many of the biophotonic messages are sent and received unconsciously, our consciousness, should it so choose, is able to influence the potential information available and turn it into actual information. He explains this by saying that a photon is like a coin flipped up in the air – it could land on heads or tails. Our consciousness can influence which side it lands on. Marcel Vogel suggested that the patterns of our mind (thoughts, intentions) as well as other forces around us create biophotonic messages that enter

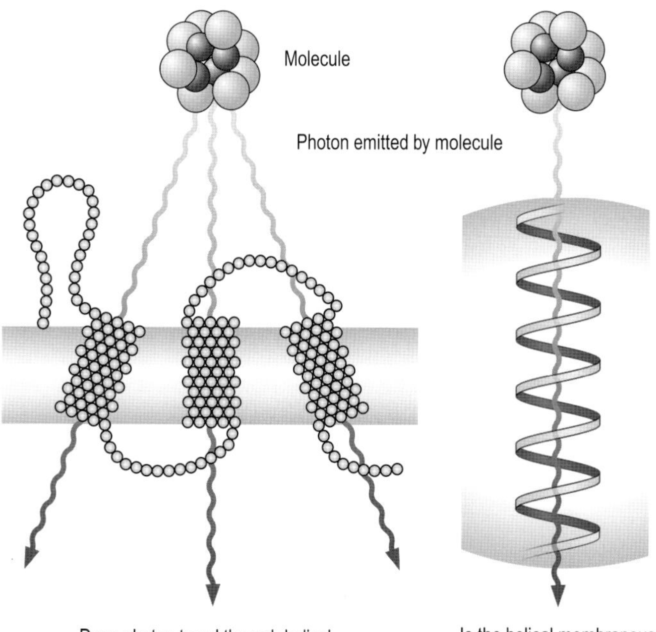

Figure 9.5

Is it a helical segment of a transmembrane protein – or is it a light pipe?

into our cells. They will then influence the receiving cells and affect the oscillations that occur there.

A recent review by Salari and team (2015) also suggested that neurons contain many 'light-sensitive molecules' and thus it would be hard to imagine how they would not be affected by biophoton emissions. How we do these things we still do not understand, but maybe it gives us an avenue to wander down if we want to think about what might have happened at times like my fire walk experience, the extraordinary changes that people can make in their health and wellbeing after what we might call big 'aha' moments, and a myriad other experiences that we have not really had a scientific explanation for before.

So how does this relate to stillness?

Alexander says from all his years of meditation and stillness practice, teaching many students, that the place they report *feeling* stillness most in their body is the abdomen – some say solar plexus, others say below the belly button, or what I know of as the hara.

An experiment by Van Wijk and colleagues (2006) measured the ultra-weak electromagnetic emissions from people who meditated regularly and compared them with those who did not. They found that emissions from experienced meditators were lower. They postulated that this may be because they are generally less stressed; previous researchers have suggested higher levels of this energy may be due to oxidants and increased chemical reactions that cause damage to cells and tissues – which may of course amount to a pretty similar thing. Others have also asserted that less healthy cells have higher emissions. So this suggests our cells are engaging in less activity when we are stiller.

If there really is communication between all systems at this energetic level then it explains some of whole-body reactions we achieve in regular stilling practice. Plus, I wonder, if through our stilling we are able to create a greater level of coherence of biophoton emission, and if that does indeed last up to days, it shows how we can hold a stiller state and, with more practice, hold it more effectively and for longer, re-finding the resonance of it faster next time. Perhaps we are also conserving the energy for the really vital processes, thus the feeling of greater vitality and health that can arise from regular practice.

Maybe, even, my experience of stillness as being dynamic and potent is simply an in-touchness with the vibration and oscillation at this level, before getting in touch with other parts of this phenomenon, which may feel even stiller as we move within the scale of stillness. If we follow the physics in the quantum paradigm we get to nothing! That's probably pretty still. This is all indulgent conjecture on my part, but there are some lovely parallels to the philosophy, as Alexander has covered when he talked in Chapter 2 of the different aspects of cognition falling away and that the 'facets of the mind become utterly still and coalesce'.

Just one more thing I found interesting from the above study: looking at the body overall, the lowest readings were in the abdomen and the solar plexus (second lowest). Is this why we feel our stillness here?

Is there a relationship to disease?

Dr Vlail Kaznacheyev has experimented (repeatedly) with cells exhibiting disease processes or which are dying (see Bearden, 1988). When healthy cells are placed near the unhealthy ones with quartz glass (which lets UV light through) in between them, the healthy cells start exhibiting the disease pattern – usually 70–80 per cent of them within about 12 hours. When there is normal glass (does not let UV through) between them they do not. Furthermore, when the second infected sample was left in contact (through the quartz window) with a second healthy set of cells, the second ones became infected – fewer, only 20–30 per cent and only after 18–20 hours (Fig. 9.6).

At first Kaznacheyev did not know what the agent of infection was, then he realised the key was the UV light being emitted. The message of disease was being passed, and was 'received' and acted upon, by previously healthy cells. We do not, of course, see this as obviously in everyday life, despite the fact that our cells are constantly being subjected to photons from all aspects of our environment, perhaps because we are more complex and have other recovery processes available. In this instance the healthy cells were becoming subject only to the photons produced by the dying cells and were overwhelmed by them.

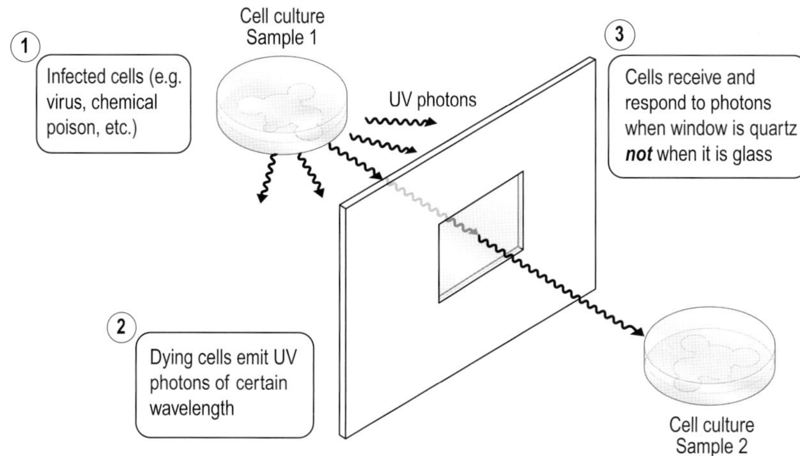

Figure 9.6

The Kaznacheyev experiments

'It is well documented that at high cell densities, large differences in ... photon emission exist between normal cells and tumor cells originating from the same parental tissue' (Alvermann et al., 2015). What is also interesting is the observation that as more cancerous cells accumulate, the emission rate of each cell continues to increase. Vogel (2012) adds that malignant cells have lost their connection to the 'network', their sensitivity to the other cells around them and their knowledge of what the correct organisation of things should be.

Popp's early observations of why the 3,4-benzopyrene was carcinogenic turned out to be because this structure absorbs (and scrambles) the frequency of light our DNA needs to function. The same is true of other carcinogens. There have been a range of studies that show that the 'dis-ease' that can be inflicted by removing a specific frequency can be 'eased' by reintroducing that frequency.

Georges Lakhovsky (1869–1942) was a very forward-thinking Russian scientist and inventor. He believed that cells produce and radiate oscillations of high frequencies, and that they respond to outside energies. In health they are in harmony and 'dynamic equilibrium', but disease, he said, 'is the oscillatory disequilibrium of cells, originating from external causes. It is, more especially, the struggle between microbic radiation and cellular radiation' (Lakhovsky, 1939).

Now, this was written in 1939, so the terms are used in a different way from current definitions. However, he invented a device called a multiple wave oscillator to essentially emit a broad spectrum of frequencies into a system (the body), which, in a similar fashion to the ideas of resonance above, gave each cell the chance to resonate with its own 'proper frequency', enabling it to restore its vibration. If this sounds way out there, bear in mind that this device was present in hospitals in Europe and the US until the middle of the 20th century and, it has been suggested, achieved a 98 per cent survival rate for many types of cancers (see reports listed by Farrell, 1982). Versions of these technologies are gradually becoming available today – can we imagine a world where this paradigm and technology could seep into every local surgery?

What is so exciting about this field is that we are on the edge of a shift in understanding, and once we have toppled over that edge as a collective we will have a set of diagnostic and treatment tools that I suspect will leave future generations looking back on today's medicine the way we look back at bloodletting (for example). We have covered only the tip of the iceberg here but I hope it gives some sense that in some quarters change is afoot. Techniques are still in their infancy, says Popp (1998), but 'can be considerably improved in order to develop biophotonics into one of the most powerful non-invasive tools of investigating life with light'.

Let me remind you of the essence of this chapter. That our cells emit light and that other cells receive it. We really do have an inner light! Our ability to have conscious influence over this becomes more important as we come to understand ourselves better, perhaps using the experiments in these pages as one way to bring our light into stillness and coherence. The universal teachings of philosophy support this.

Many people who work with their hands in whatever type of healing capacity are likely to already be aware that something is going on that should fit in this chapter – the science has not quite reached it yet, but it is getting ever closer. Popp says that if it were not for light we would literally fall apart physically. Ponder the quote attributed to physicist Nikola Tesla: 'If you want to find the secrets of the universe, think in terms of energy, frequency and vibration.' And I would add feel from your place of stillness.

Summary

- We are able to make very fast changes within our biology that the molecular biological models of cellular activity alone do not support.
- All living cells emit, take in and respond to light in the UV spectrum, which we call biophotons.
- This creates coherent connectivity between all cells and communication at the speed of light.
- Maybe we have light pipes!
- Our consciousness and intention can direct our biophotonic activity.
- Biophoton emission is lower in meditators and the lowest of all is seen in the hara.
- Disease gives dis-equilibrium in our biophotonic emissions; technologies still developing may lead us to use light non-invasively as medicine in the future.
- We are truly beings with inner light!

Experiment

Take a moment to tune into the idea of the biophotonic activity of your every cell. Play with envisaging the instant, coherent communication pathways between cells near and far and the never-ending resonances of this energy level.

Become your resonant beingness …

Imagine yourself as messages of light.

How does it feel?

If you are messages of light – what are you saying?

Final thought

The waiting oocyte

When I was first thinking about the concept of stillness-memory and where it might 'exist', it struck me that there is one very obvious place for it: in the waiting oocyte! (Actually the waiting primordial follicle – but this doesn't have quite the same ring to it!)

I remember my surprise when I first learned that all the primordial follicles, only some of which will eventually become eggs (or oocytes), undergo their cell division and thus production from 15 weeks to about 6 to 7 months in embryo. They reach a peak in number (roughly 7 million), then many die before birth, so that a baby girl will be born with about 1 million, by puberty there will be about 500,000 and by menopause only a few hundred or perhaps a thousand left.

Whichever egg eventually made us was dormant for, well, anywhere between 16 and 40-something (occasionally more) years! Is that not stillness? How can that not hold memory of potential, of patience? We do not yet know what the trigger is for awakening the cells as they begin further development after puberty, nor what mechanism 'chooses' which of the 30 or so that start out developing during each cycle (which in total lasts about 60 days – not just the 28 days we think of as the cycle) becomes 'the one'. But whatever causes the one to fully develop into a mature oocyte to be blasted out of the ovary at ovulation has spent many years lying in stillness.

The waiting oocyte, if a holder of our essence of stillness, brings us cellular memory of quiescence, laced with potential. Perhaps this is coded into those very DNA molecules that sat waiting to complete their meiotic division and were then replicated into every one of our cells.

References

Alvermann, M., Srivastava, Y., Swain, J. and Widom, A. (2015). Biological electric fields and rate equations for biophotons. *European Biophysics Journal*, 44(3): 165–170, www.arxiv.org/pdf/1407.4689.pdf [accessed Mar. 2016].

Bearden, T. (1988). *AIDS: biological warfare*. Greenville, Tex: Tesla. Chapter 5: Extraordinary biology, www.cheniere.org/books/aids/ch5.htm [accessed Dec. 2015].

Farrell, K. (1982). Hyperthermia for malignant disease – a history of medicine note – the work of Georges Lakhovsky. In: H.I. Bicher and D.F. Bruley (eds). *Hyperthermia*. New York: Plenum Press.

Fleming, A.H.J. and Colorio, E.B. (2003). *The photon and its energy*, www.biontology.com/wp-content/uploads/2012/10/The-photon-and-its-energy.pdf [accessed Jan. 2016].

Guimberteau, J.C. and Armstrong, C. (2015). *Architecture of Human Living Fascia*. Edinburgh: Handspring Publishing.

Kim, W.H. (2015). 3D wave explains 'water memory'. *Journal of Vortex Science and Technology*, 2(117), www.omicsonline.com/open-access/3d-wave-explains-water-memory-2090-8369-1000117.php?aid=60307 [accessed Mar. 2016]. doi:10.4172/2090-8369.1000117.

Lakhovsky, G. (1939). *The Secret of Life*. London: Heinemann.

Lipton, B.H. (2005). *The Biology of Belief*. Santa Rosa, CA: Mountain of Love/Elite Books.

Oschman, J.L. (2015). Vortical structure of light and space: biological implications. *Journal of Vortex Science and Technology*, 02(01).

Popp, A. (2012). Biophotons and consciousness [video], 16 August, https://www.youtube.com/watch?v=ST6cVA-VUak [accessed Apr. 2016].

Popp, F.A. (1998). About the coherence of biophotons. In: *Proceedings of the international conference on macroscopic quantum coherence: Northeastern University, Boston, 11–13 July 1997*. Singapore: World Scientific, http://meridianenergies.net/wp-content/uploads/2012/04/CoherenceOfBiophotons.pdf [accessed Mar. 2016].

Popp, F.A. (2003). Properties of biophotons and their theoretical implications. *Indian Journal of Experimental Biology*, 41: 391–402.

Salari, V., Valian, H., Bassereh, H., Bókkon, I. and Barkhordari, A. (2015). Ultraweak photon emission in the brain. *Journal of Integrative Neuroscience*, 14(03): 419–429.

Vogel, M. (2012). *Bio-Photons*. YouTube tutorial, 29 August, https://www.youtube.com/watch?v=dMvfwqgr94o [accessed Mar. 2016].

Wijk, E., Koch, H., Bosman, S. and Wijk, R. (2006). Anatomic characterization of human ultra-weak photon emission in practitioners of Transcendental Meditation™ and control subjects. *The Journal of Alternative and Complementary Medicine*, 12(1): 31–38.

3

The insightful self

Stumbling blocks and obstacles

What we need to know

Perception

Getting to neutral

Stumbling blocks and obstacles 10

The theory trap

Knowledge has become the topmost priority for many people, and in today's world is seen as the key to personal and professional success. However, knowledge is like a double-edged sword, especially when it is simply acquired and retained as theory. To know does not mean to understand, and without true understanding knowledge never has a chance to inform us and our work or become part of our being. Unlike our being, which is our subjective nature, or what we simply are at any given moment in time, our knowledge is separate from us, because we can visualise what we know and put it on paper or into other modalities, such as images, recordings and words. The Fourth Way philosophy points out that we comprise both what we know and what we are, yet we do not necessarily understand all of what we know, because we haven't made the right connections that can shift knowledge into our being. However, like most of the observable, there is scale to knowledge.

That is, knowledge exists on many different levels, and we usually only have access to knowledge that exists in and belongs to our own level, which fluctuates according to the state of our being (subjective nature). Depending on our inner state, mood or feeling, being can limit knowledge to a great extent (specifically when we are biased), which means we won't be able to utilise it, consciously connect with it or properly understand it.

For example, during my studies of movement, yoga and bodywork, most of the knowledge of anatomy I acquired was derived from anatomy lessons, attending lectures and studying anatomy books. Hence, I was in possession of a lot of book knowledge, which at that time I took for granted. Initially, this knowledge gave me the confidence to work with people in a safe way. However, only when I participated in actual dissection, palpating the anatomical structures with my own hands, did I truly realise and understand the interconnectedness of everything within the human body. I could see that muscles do not necessarily attach at the exact locations displayed in the anatomy books, and that some people might not even possess a certain type of muscle. I simply could not make the right connections through book knowledge only; it required this life-changing experience of human dissection, which put my understanding of anatomy into a totally different perspective. What then furthered the deepening of this newly acquired understanding was decades of experience in movement, which led to the knowledge of applied anatomy and a much more realistic understanding of anatomy in the moving body. I therefore progressed and evolved from the initial book knowledge, which is two-dimensional, to a three-dimensional knowledge derived through dissection of a passive body, to a four-dimensional understanding of anatomy through movement in space, which is active and created a connection between all three types and levels of knowledge.

The example above shows us that if we are not exploring and utilising the whole scale of knowledge on our own level, our understanding will not be mature enough to access higher levels and dimensions of knowledge in the future. This means that our understanding will remain forever limited. My personal enquiry into the philosophy of knowledge, which I studied from an ancient teaching point of view, has changed my belief that 'I' know, which I try to apply to all other kinds of knowledge acquired in the past, as well as knowledge that is still waiting to be explored.

Now, due to the fact that our position in life and our professional expertise as practitioners is based on what we know and what we have learned and studied, we are inclined to acquire a tremendous amount of theoretical knowledge, which has very little to do with the real world. That is, without higher knowledge that enables us to study things in relation to the whole, and helps us to fully understand the real world, all our theoretical knowledge is of very little

ONLY KNOWLEDGE THAT CAN BE
APPLIED
IS OF GREAT VALUE

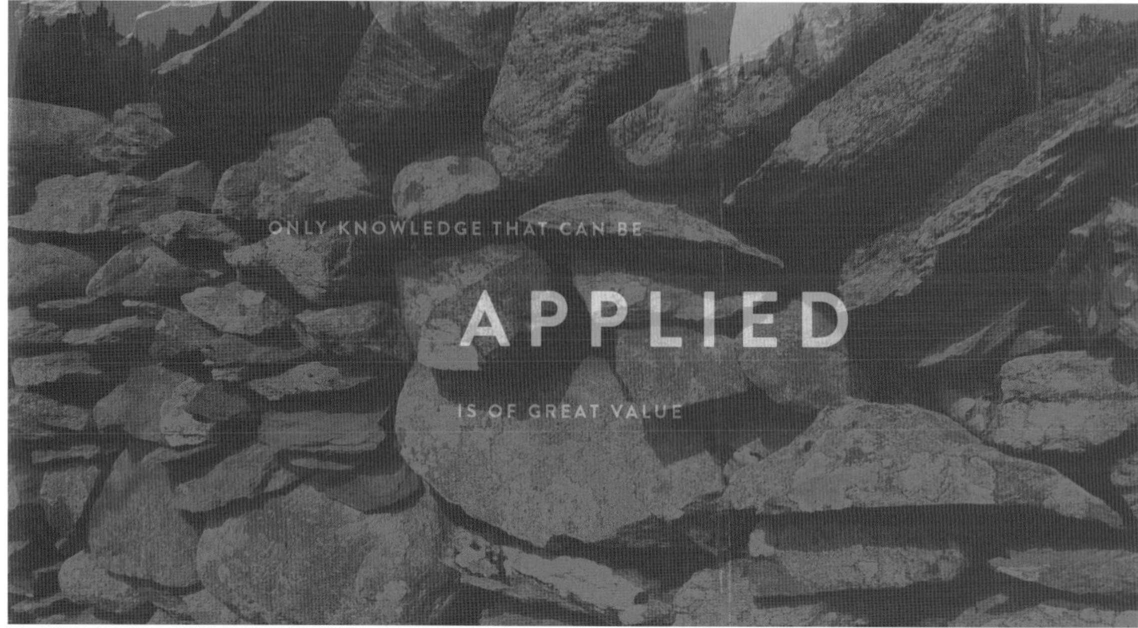

Figure 10.1

Artwork Victoria Dokas; photography Alexander Filmer-Lorch

value and can easily turn into a theory trap that is preventing us from truly understanding and reaching our full potential in our work as therapists, teachers and practitioners, as well as people. To be able to genuinely evolve the knowledge we possess, it needs to shift from different parts to a general whole, as well as from the imaginary to the actual. The reason for this is that most of the knowledge we accumulate consists of different parts that never connect and interact with the greater whole. For example, we gain knowledge of muscles, bones, organs and cells without appreciating that they are parts of a whole body that is alive and moves in space. However, the moment we come into contact with higher knowledge, it does not only show us the different parts and their location, but the actual meaning and function of all parts in relation to the whole, which will ultimately lead us to true understanding. This principle is not only true when it comes to knowledge of things we use in our work and our profession, but also applies to the knowledge we have acquired about ourselves (self-knowledge). If we start working on both (knowledge and self-knowledge) and gradually shift from the particular to the greater whole, the great divide between knowledge and truly knowing how to 'be' will finally fall back into balance. This is work that is well worth pursuing.

Habits

One of the main objectives of reflective practitioners is to prevent our work from becoming mechanical. From an ancient philosophical point of view, becoming mechanical means that we have 'fallen asleep'. To avoid falling asleep, we want to start working towards a definite direction and objective, through which manifestations that have become mechanical in us and our work render themselves passive. In other words, we first have to fully wake up to our habits to be able to gradually change or neutralise them.

According to the *Oxford Advanced Learner's Dictionary*, a 'habit' is defined as 'a thing that you do often and almost without thinking, especially something that is hard to stop doing'. Habits are acquired by means of repetition, and we usually repeat the kinds of actions and behaviours that work for us and enable us to get what we want to achieve our goals and objectives. 'Habits develop when people give a response repeatedly in a particular context and thereby form associations in memory between the response and recurring context cues' (Neal et al., 2011). An average of 40 per cent of our daily activities are habits, which usually take place automatically; that means we do have time to contemplate or think about other things. We can easily observe the habits of other people, but are rarely aware of our own habitual behaviours and responses to the different context cues in our environment. The older we become, the higher the chances of us becoming more habit driven. Just as our body tissue can calcify under repetitive stress and ultimately ossify, so our response mechanisms and common behaviours can crystallise. According to the study by Neal and his team (2011), 'In neuroscience research on the brain systems activated during behavioral tasks, performance of stimulus–response habits is localized in the basal ganglia, especially the putamen, whereas control of goal-directed actions is localized in other brain regions, often involving the prefrontal cortex.' (See also Ballaine and O'Doherty, 2009; Yin and Knowlton, 2006.) This means that the creation of habits requires a neural shift from evaluation-driven circuits to circuits that are engaged in performance (Neal et al., 2011). In addition, there seems to be a competition between brain systems that control habits and systems engaging in performance. The former may actively suppress goal-directed control actions whilst we execute habitual behaviours. Neal and colleagues went on to compare evidence from various research studies and concluded that, whilst 'habits are cognitively represented as context–response associations, habit strength had these effects only when habits were assessed from frequent performance in stable contexts'. This means that we need 'specific conditions that enable the formation of habit associations in memory' (Neal et al., 2012).

Yet, it is encouraging to know that 'participants continue to perform habits with minimal influence from goals, but only so long as they continue to live in the

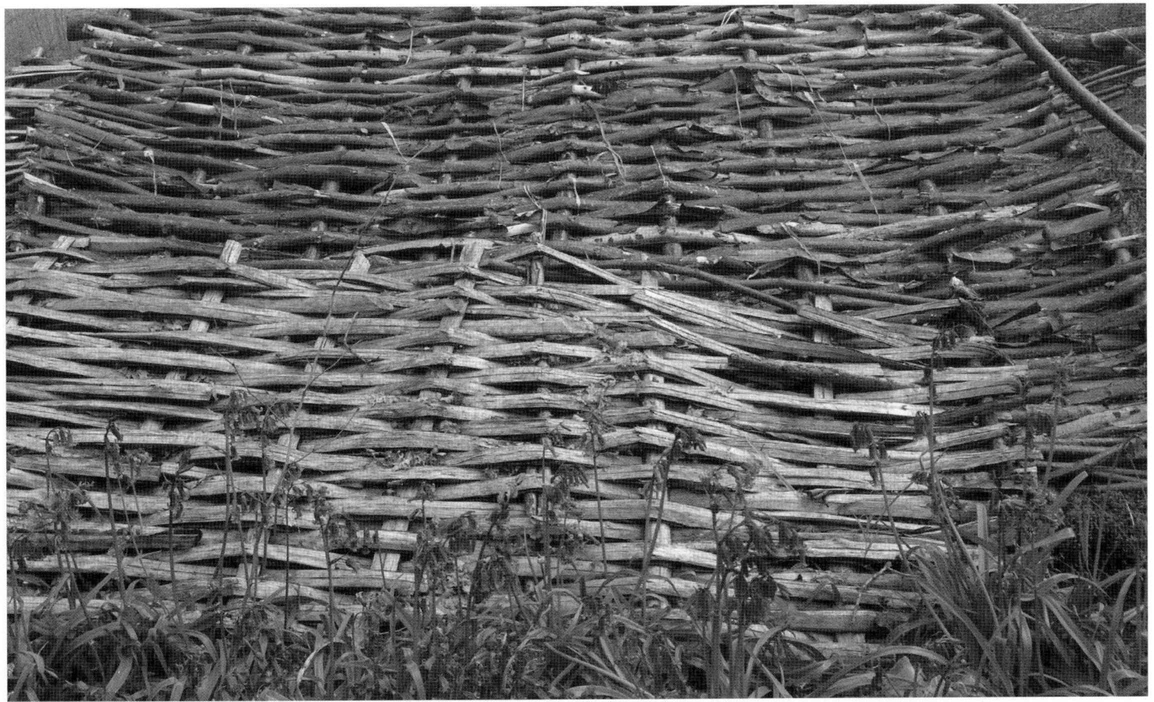

Figure 10.2

Deeply engrained habits interweave with the patterns of life, creating the mechanical structures of our everyday life

same context' (Neal et al., 2012). The paper further explains that participants are apparently freed from their habits the moment they move to a new location, due to the absence of cues to habit performance. Neal explains: 'Even if habits are not responsive to changes in motives, they should be disrupted by challenges to habit cuing' (Neal et al., 2011). (For further information see Part 5: Chapter 24.)

From an Eastern psychology point of view, the unconscious and mechanical nature of habits creates a tremendous force that continuously acts on our state of consciousness, limiting our possibilities of acting and responding more consciously. The universal teachings say that we can only neutralise or change our habits if we are connected or attached to a stronger force, which in philosophical terms is called 'the force of meaning' (see Part 3: Chapter 11). However, in today's world, positive news and encouragement can be found in recent studies. Laurie Aznavoorian (2013) comments that, in his 2012 book *The Power of Habit*, Charles Duhigg refers to several different studies that clearly demonstrate that 'the only way to break a habit is to replace it with another activity that will respond to the same environmental cues that instigate the "habit loop".' However, according to Duhigg's research, they need to 'provide the same reward at the end', and that 'once we understand our habits, we can change them'. Aznavoorian continues by referring to good news he found in a new study from MIT, where neuroscientists have found 'that a small region of the brain's prefrontal cortex, the infra-limbic (IL) cortex, is responsible for moment by moment control'. Aznavoorian then explains that 'the IL cortex therefore has the ability to determine which habits are switched on at a given time'. Jane Taylor, a professor of psychiatry and psychology at Yale University, says of the study: 'We've always thought of habits as being inflexible, but this suggests you can have flexible habits, in some sense' (Trafton, 2012). In addition, the IL cortex seems to favour new habits over old ones. This is consistent with other studies which show that, once we have broken a habit, it is not forgotten but is replaced by something new instead. Now, if we have broken an old work habit with something more conscious and less mechanical, like quietly sitting with the unknown for a few moments instead of habitually accessing what we already know intellectually, we might be able to respond to the actual 'is-ness' of the situation much more objectively than through the lens of our subjective knowledge. At this point, you can probably well imagine the important role that inner stillness plays when it comes to the transformation of habits. How to ignite this process will be discussed in Part 5: Chapter 21.

Challenge: mindfulness, meditation and being present

Experiment

Are you conscious, present and aware right now?

... Of course you are, because this simple experiment question shocked you into the present moment for a millisecond. Now think of being fully present and you will realise that the momentary experience of 'being fully present' has more or less turned into a concept or idea, which still leaves you under the illusion of being fully present. It becomes very obvious that the concept or idea of being fully present is worlds apart from the actual experience, which does not last long enough for us to fully grasp what has happened in a moment of complete presence.

Whenever we look at topics such as research on stilling, mindfulness and meditation, we have no problem at all in analysing and understanding the always astonishing and promising effects these ancient techniques can have on a physiological and psychological level. We are also able to envisage how these findings can profoundly change and benefit our work as practitioners and enhance currently taught training modules and professional standards in different fields of expertise, including our interactions with others and the whole work environment in clinics, hospitals and education centres. To make these findings and their great potential less theoretical and more accessible, as well as give them more credibility in health, therapy and treatment sectors, a whole new vocabulary has been created, such as therapeutic presence, mindful interaction, the reflective practitioner, self-reflective practice, therapeutic dialoguing, observing presence, self-evolution practice, Socratic discussions, secular mindfulness, compassion-centred intervention, contemplative listening, and so on. Each term is used in a specific line of work that includes evidence-based knowledge and a conceptual framework that we can study, utilise and apply to our own practice and work environment.

However, what we don't usually grasp or understand are the actual means that led to the research results. That is, the ancient practices and teachings themselves. This is partly because of the innumerable books that theorise and philosophise about the ultimate state of mindfulness and meditation in great detail, leaving us with a massive amount of theoretical knowledge, too much to consider, and the impression that these states of being are very elaborate, elusive and unachievable.

Experiment

Now, before you keep on reading, take a minute to shift yourself into a complete state of therapeutic presence ...

You have probably realised that therapeutic presence is merely a theoretical concept for a state that is not based on an actual experience that would enable you to verify the truth of your theoretical concept.

The second experiment shows that we are dealing with something we haven't ever experienced before, something that can't be put into words due to its formless nature, and which can only be expressed through allegories and parables. Hence, most of what we know about a thoughtless state, therapeutic presence, mindfulness and meditation is based on theory, preconceived ideas and quite a significant amount of imagination as well. And, the moment we start putting things into action, the very idea and theoretical understanding we have formulated in our mind about being mindful and manifesting therapeutic presence prevents us from experiencing the actual state. This is one of the main reasons why being mindful, as well as being fully 'present' to things, or staying put in a deep thoughtless state of meditation for a prolonged period of time, has become such a great challenge. However, it does not matter that we initially might not grasp or understand these refined philosophical ideas, because what is much easier for most of us to understand is the concept of stillness and acquiring stillness-memory.

It took me decades of teaching Eastern philosophy, presence, mindfulness and meditation, and of seeing students and trainees struggle with the concepts, techniques and ideas, to realise that there is a missing link – something so utterly simple that no one can possibly see it. Something that gives rise to all these different states of presence, mindfulness and meditation.

So why start with the second or even third step, if it is the first step that carries, nourishes and ultimately gives rise to the others?

References

Aznavoorian, L. (2013). Breaking habits. Futuresrambling [blog], 4 October (74), http://futuresrambling.com/2013/10/04/breaking-habits/.

Balleine, B.W. and O'Doherty, J.P. (2009). Human and rodent homologies in action control: corticostriatal determinants of goal-directed and habitual action. *Neuropsychopharmacology*, 35(1): 48–69. doi:10.1038/npp.2009.131.

Duhigg, C. (2012). *The Power of Habit*. New York: Random House.

Neal, D.T., Wood, W., Wu, M. and Kurlander, D. (2011). The pull of the past: when do habits persist despite conflict with motives? *Personality and Social Psychology Bulletin*, 37(11): 1428–1437. doi: 10.1177/0146167211419863.

Neal, D., Wood, W., Labrecque, J. and Lally, P. (2012). How do habits guide behavior? Perceived and actual triggers of habits in daily life. *Journal of Experimental Social Psychology*, 48(2): 492–498. doi:10.1016/j.jesp.2011.10.011.

Trafton, A. (2012). How the brain controls our habits: MIT neuroscientists identify a brain region that can switch between new and old habits. *MIT News*, http://news.mit.edu/2012/understanding-how-brains-control-our-habits-1029 [accessed Mar. 2016].

Yin, H. and Knowlton, B. (2006). The role of the basal ganglia in habit formation. *Nature Reviews Neuroscience*, 7(6): 464–476.

What we need to know 11

> *We can't find the 'now' in the domain of time, due to the superiority of our past and notions of our future. That's why we have to look elsewhere – possibly somewhere above time.*
>
> Alexander Filmer-Lorch

The triad of time, state and space

A triad is a symbolic image that can help us understand the dynamics within the cosmos (including our internal cosmos). Once each of the three elements that comprise the triad meet in equal quantities, size or strength simultaneously, this leads to a new proposition, manifestation or result. In the academic field, thesis, antithesis and synthesis are used to represent the three different elements of a triad. Yet, the idea of the triad, and its dynamic and practical application, can be found in almost every philosophical and psychological system in medicine, physics and cosmology. In Christianity we find the idea of the triad represented by the Father, the Son and the Holy Spirit. The Yoga Sutras of Patanjali illustrate the idea of the triad through the dynamics between purusha, prakriti and citta. The great trinity or trimurti in Hinduism comprises the three gods Brahma, Vishnu and Shiva. In Mahayana Buddhism the triad is represented by trikaya (the Buddha's three bodies), Dharmakaya, Sambhogakaya and Nirmanakya. The Fourth Way philosophy offers an accessible, as well as very applicable, explanation of the different dynamics within a triad that we can use in our work and observe in our life and psychological makeup.

The dynamics of forces within a triad

Inspired by the Fourth Way philosophy, and based on my own extensive studies, observations and workings of the triad in life and within ourselves, three powers or three forces of creation must come together simultaneously to bring things into being. This is explained well by Peter Ouspensky in his 1949 book *In Search of the Miraculous*, who says, according to my understanding, that these three creative forces are not only at work in nature, but are at work within us, as well as throughout the whole universe. One of the three forces could be seen as the initiating force, which is active; the second could be defined as the force that resists, which is passive; and the third could be described as the connecting force or the relating balancing principle at the point of application, which of course is neutral. However, they are only truly creative at the point of their conjunction. If only two of them meet, they will cancel each other out, hence nothing will be created or become manifest.

In other words, taking the example of the triad of water, dam and turbine, the initiating force is represented by the power of the water, the resisting or passive force is represented by the dam containing the water, and the turbine at the point of conjunction of water and dam represents the relating or balancing principle that leads to the creation of electricity, which is the manifestation of a totally new proposition.

A thorough understanding of the triad of time, state and space can completely transform the way we work. Looking at the overall makeup of our body–mind unit from a physiological/psychological point of view, one can say that we consist of a physical body and a body that exists within us made up of our psychology. The physical body exists, lives and moves about in a world that is based on a time continuum, which gives rise to a past that can be remembered, a present moment we rarely visit or acknowledge, and a future that can only be imagined because it lies somewhere in the unknown. Even our sense of self is usually found somewhere in 'time', where it moves or jumps back and forth between the past and the future. Hence we live in the triad of time that is past, present and future.

The psychological body, however, exists in a world of countless different psychological states. That is, different states of mind, perception, consciousness and being that can fluctuate from higher to lower. Manifestations of these higher and lower states are mainly determined by what we are dealing with in the triad of time. Additionally, our whole way of thinking is based around the concept of time. We usually think of the past and the future in chronological terms, which is the reason why we possess hardly any memory of higher or lower states of perception that take place at any given moment in time. That is, we remember what happened at a certain point in the past, including things, scenes and people around us, but we usually don't remember the particular state of our perception, being or consciousness. However, this does not change the fact that we have these two different lives simultaneously – the psychological internal and the physical external. We rarely use the incredible potential that lies in our higher states because we are pretty much asleep to them, can't remember or access them and so know very little about them.

Why is this important for us as therapists and practitioners? Because the wellbeing of our clients and the people we work with is affected by their psychology and fluctuating states, just as our work is affected by our own state or level of perception at any given moment during a treatment or session. For example, stress profoundly affects the way we experience time, which easily turns into a vicious circle of trying to catch up. As a result, we actually do much less within this greatly diminishing timeframe. Time has become a currency of incredible value in our modern world. Even for facilitation and treatment, the value of our work is often judged on the results we can achieve in the shortest amount of time. Sadly, people rarely now see any value in simply achieving more refined states of perception and consciousness. This means that precious things such as balance, inner peace and contentment, as well as our treasured inner values, are eroded or destroyed by the ever-increasing demand on time. What makes things worse is that we usually don't believe or even consider that we can establish a substantial amount of living memory outside of the predominant domain of the time continuum.

So how do we bridge the great divide between the world of states and our lives in time, and start developing imprints of memory that might exist beyond the idea of time? The answer is simply *by means of space.*

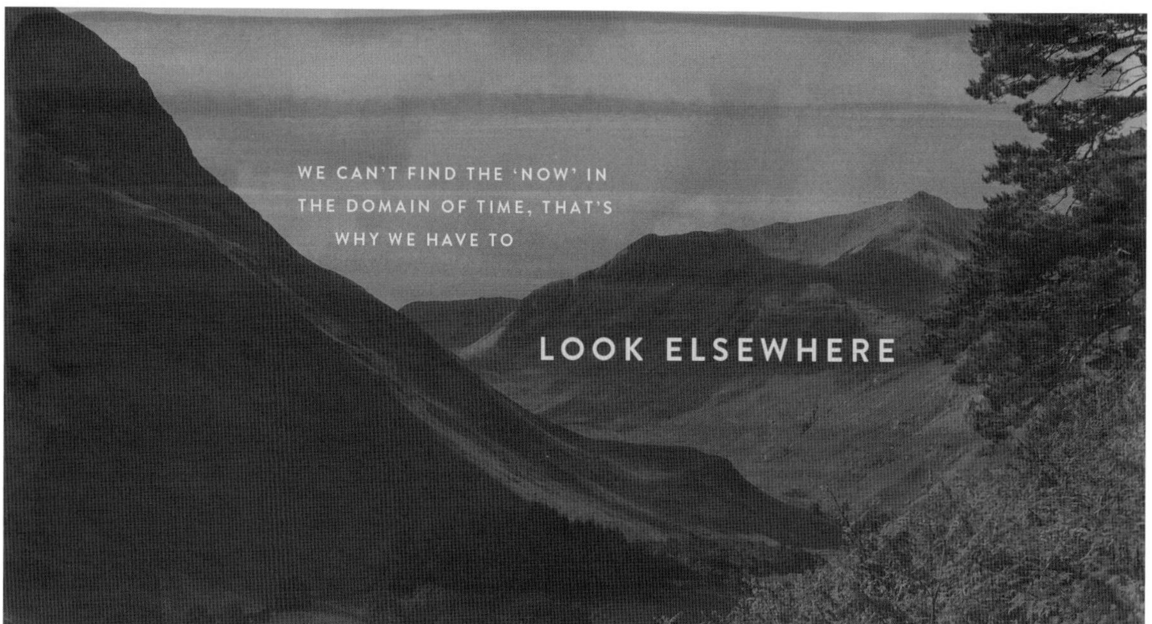

Figure 11.1

Artwork Victoria Dokas; Photography Alexander Filmer-Lorch

It is 'space' that needs to enter into our here-and-now lives, and this is accomplished by accessing inner stillness. That is, this respective space is synonymous with stillness. In due course, this gives rise to a natural state of presence. In the presence of inner stillness our sense of time becomes very spacious and transforms into a state of lucid cognition. In this lucid state of heightened perception, precious memories of short moments of our 'inner awakening' (a higher state of objectivity) or a flickering of the non-dual nature of the 'inner self' are experienced. These valuable moments accumulate, gradually elevate us and take us towards the experience of a different modality of existence that takes place outside of the continuum of time.

Objective

The moment we consciously apply and work from the time–state–space triad through inner stillness, we experience an all-encompassing equilibrium that gives rise to three movements. A spontaneous internal movement creates the connection to higher states of perception (passive force). A subtle external movement keeps up the connection between our client and our work in time (active force). An expanding vertical movement creates sufficient separation, from which all movements can be perceived within the field of lucid and spacious awareness (connecting force), effortlessly sustained and nourished by the inner power of stillness (transcending force). Hence, we are genuinely working from a place that lies above the dynamics of time and non-conducive states, a place of greater objectivity, through which we can meet and start working with information that relates not only to the effect, but also to the cause, and can then be put into the context of the whole as well.

Experiment

First, explore the workings of the three forces in nature and life. Second, once you have gained a better understanding of the three creative powers, choose a good time when you are working with a client and explore the dynamics between you (the practitioner representing the initiating active force), the client you facilitate or treat (representing the passive force) and what might represent the balancing third force that neutralises both active and passive forces, possibly leading to a new proposition or outcome.

The universal idea of scale

In our everyday life, scale is something we mainly use on a practical level, like using the scale of a map to find our way around, or the musical scale we use to learn to play an instrument, or the scales we use to weigh ourselves. However, we rarely consider the idea of scale as something that can be consciously applied to ourselves and our work with our clients.

We can find symbolic expressions of the universal idea of scale in ancient traditions such as the tree of life (Kabbalah), Jacob's ladder, the chakra system, the bodhi tree, the eight limbs, the eightfold-path, the ray of creation, as well as in modern psychological systems such as the egg of being in psychosynthesis and Jung's work on archetypes. Furthermore, the universal idea of scale is expressed in different yantras, mandalas and stupas, as well as in the architecture of temples, mosques and churches. Even art, science and music contain pointers towards the universal idea of scale. However, most of the above-mentioned require in-depth study and a personal interest, so I prefer to use parables and storytelling that we can all easily relate to, which gives us insight into the idea of scale.

A parable

Dean is a very busy freelancer, but has reached an absolute dead end in his work and knows that things have to change. Like most of his colleagues around him, he genuinely wants to develop and improve his understanding, his skill sets and his work with his clients, to be able to offer something special that differentiates his work from others. To keep up with a very competitive market, he knows that he also needs to further his career and expand the business he is running. So, with best intentions, he takes action by putting effort into increasing the scale of lots of things in his work. Once all his plans are finalised, Dean attends several complementary training courses to expand his range of skills and his knowledge in the prime areas of his work. He also invests a significant amount of time and money to learn how to promote his business, improve and extend collaboration with other businesses and make best use of social networking facilities. Furthermore, he moves his business into larger premises, which in his belief meets the high standards required to attract more clients, as well as giving him more space into which his business can grow. Dean works incredibly hard and, of course, the business becomes more and more successful. However, after a couple of years he realises that the quality of his work has started to deteriorate, that his wellbeing and health have been affected, his whole social life is profoundly suffering and he is constantly struggling to maintain his personal relationships. Dean is experiencing the result that everything he has put into action has caused acceleration and is gaining its own, almost unstoppable, momentum. Even the scale of his financial responsibilities has become sky high. At this point, his whole work–life balance has fallen apart, and everything he thought could be improved is now constantly asking for more input, time, money and so much more attention. Facing up to his situation, he acknowledges that, without intending it, he has become the victim of his own success. But what has become even more aggravating is the realisation that he has turned into someone he never wanted to be. Dean realises in his heart of hearts that the only way out is change. He also knows that he does not know how to bring about change or what has to change.

In his helplessness he decides to take a break, and arranges a trip into the mountains. On his train journey he happens to sit opposite an elderly woman. His first impression of her is that she carries an air of understated sophistication and a presence he finds difficult to place. Just at the next stop, lots of people get off the train and they find themselves the only remaining passengers in the carriage. He can't help looking at the woman time and again, which makes him feel ever more self-conscious. The stillness and peace she radiates starts filling the whole space around him, slowly penetrating into his burdened mind and heart. It feels to him as if his whole being is being lifted in the company of her peaceful presence. When her softly spoken words reach him in the form of a question about his present life, the floodgates open and he starts telling her all that has happened to him throughout the past couple of years, finishing his story with the words, 'I know in my heart of hearts that things have to change, but at the same time I don't know what to change or how to change it.'

After a long silent pause she replies, 'The answer to your question is very simple, and I am very sorry to say that, even with your best intentions at heart, you only focused on increasing the scale of all aspects of your work on a horizontal level, which of course only increases the scale of your responsibilities and commitments in your life and at work. What would really need to happen is for you to evolve vertically, not only horizontally.' She pauses and then continues, 'You see, by only expanding horizontally, people spend all their lives on the horizontal scale of time, which is very linear and under the order of countless different laws.'

Here she stops, and her peaceful presence seems to increase even more, soothing Dean's busy mind until it becomes astonishingly still and spacious. Within this unfamiliar inner stillness he hears himself asking, 'But what will happen in this vertical evolution?'

She looks at him and he realises that her dark brown eyes have become full of an almost celestial radiant light. 'Well,' she calmly replies, 'you simply need to start looking inwards to connect with the vertical scale within. This scale consists of higher and lower levels, of unknown things above and of buried things below, with many layers that are arranged vertically in the perfect order of meaning and higher value. Sincerely connecting with your vertical scale means that you connect with the whole scale of your possible potential and development as a person and a professional.' She points towards the sky and says, 'The vertical scale is infinite, and what you will experience along its higher levels are higher states of perception, higher states of being and, of course, higher states of consciousness. On its lower levels you will experience all kinds of mechanical manifestations, increasingly limiting states of perception and ways of thinking and, of course, all that lies buried in your non-conscious state. So the more you work towards what lies above your current way of being, the more you will attract a different kind of life that lies high above your current existence.' She smiles, whilst a luminous spark in her eyes is piercing into the core of Dean's very existence, obliterating the last remaining traces of thought patterns, and she continues, 'This means all your decision-making and the way you work and interact will be informed by what can be found along the higher levels of vertical scale.' She rests back into her seat and brings this dialogue to a close by saying, 'You have to always remember that the possibility of change lies in your own conscious effort that is fuelled by the transformative force of meaning.' She gets up and, in passing, Dean hears her whispering to herself, 'No more needs to be said than that "help" is always there, wherever we are.'

With this she disembarks onto the platform, leaving Dean behind in an all-encompassing state of pure being. A little taster of what might lie ahead. This is when Dean is woken up by the conductor saying, 'Sir, you have arrived at your final destination', whilst smiling at him with a very familiar spark in his eyes. From here onwards, it is up to Dean to *remember*.

Experiment

Frequently try to take a little break from the horizontal scale of life by retreating into your inner sanctuary of stillness, and contemplate your present state of perception, your being and your current state of consciousness. In time this will make you think differently, leading to less horizontal and more vertical thinking. Observe where that takes you.

Evolving observation

Observe always that everything is the result of a change, and get used to thinking that there is nothing Nature loves so well as to change existing forms and to make new ones like them.

Marcus Aurelius, Meditations iv 36

Observation is one of the most fundamental principles in both our work with other people and our work on ourselves. Once fully established, observation will become one of our most important tools.

A study guide for experimental psychology defines observation as 'the conscious acquisition of information from a primary source. In living beings, observation employs the senses. In science, observation can also involve the recording of data via the use of instruments' (Cram101 Textbook Reviews, 2014). Guimaraes (undated, p. 92) says that 'observation in philosophical terms is the process of filtering sensory information through the thought process'. On a physical level, he continues, 'Input is received via hearing, sight, smell, taste, or touch and then analyzed through either rational or irrational thought'. However, Hanson (1958) states that observation is theory loaded, and that the physiological process of observation is claimed to be irrelevant. Based on his enquiry, seeing (observing) is an experience, and not a physical state, and it is people and not only their eyes that see (observe).

In today's world, only the observable is usually recognised as real and true. However, one aim of this book is to unite conventional science with the great knowledge and insights of Eastern philosophies.

The greatest discoveries and developments in science, medicine, physics and cosmology are based on observation. Through dedicated observation, conscious effort and focused attention, the world and our lives can be transformed.

From the point of view of a therapist and practitioner, we can look at observation from two different angles.

First, observation to study the theoretical, technical and academic aspects of our work through which we can acquire vital knowledge and information, including the latest insights into anatomy and physiology and the science behind them. During the process of observation, our attention is directed outwards through our five senses gathering all possible information about the subject that is the centre of our enquiry. This newly acquired knowledge can be creatively utilised, leading to new developments and changes in the environment in which we work. That is, observation of the environment around us is a real means to change, and can profoundly improve the overall conditions of our life and external world. Furthermore, prolonged observation in our own field of expertise over an extended period can lead to the development of entirely new methods, which improves and enhances our own professional skills, and of course will benefit the people we facilitate or treat.

Second, when it comes to our human nature, the greatest insights and developments in philosophy, psychology and the arts are based on self-observation. Through dedicated self-observation it becomes possible to transform and change ourselves.

Self-observation looks at our inner world, which includes our psychological makeup, our personality and everything that takes place within us. Throughout

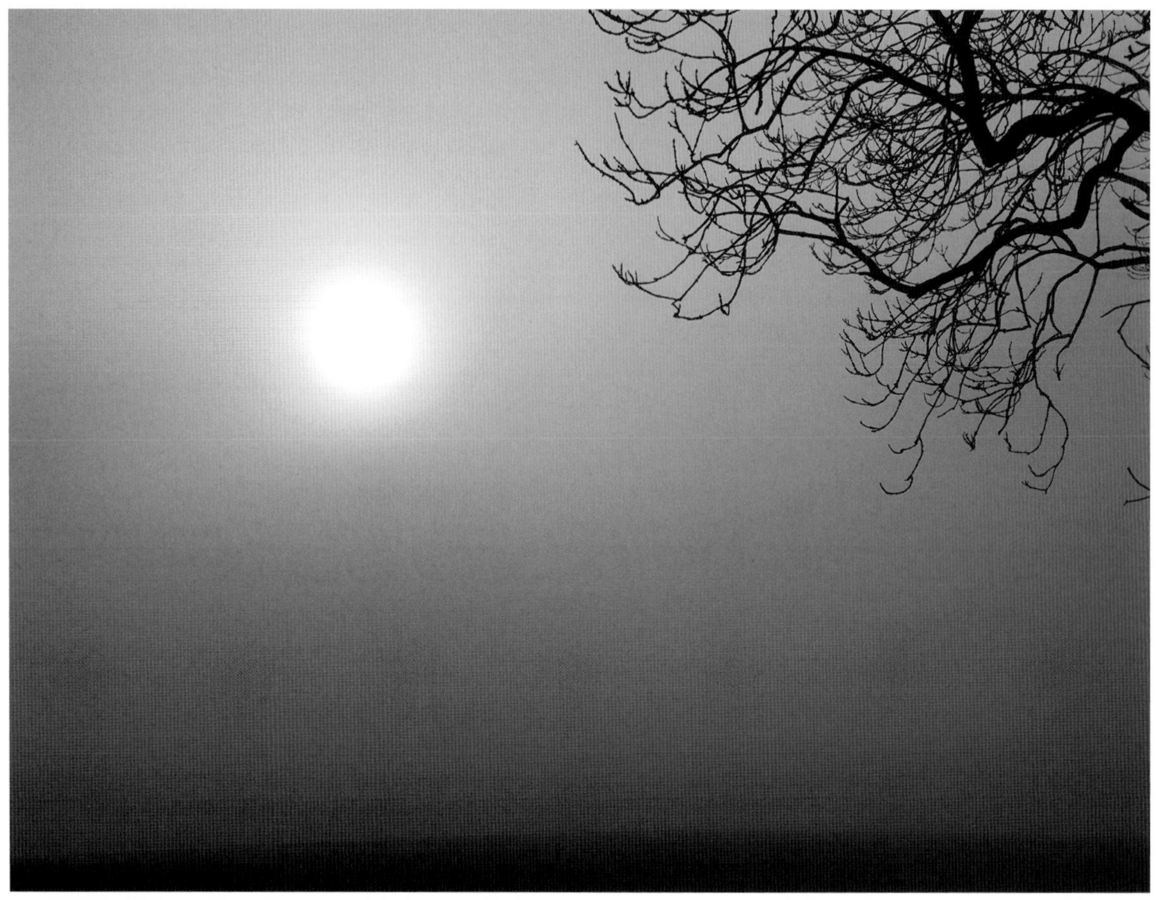

Figure 11.2

Even if we consider the observable as the truth, there might be a deeper truth beneath the visible, concealed by the so-called 'veil of ignorance'; photography Alexander Filmer-Lorch

the process of self-observation our attention is directed inwards by means of conscious effort and through introspection, which does not require our five physical senses. We can gain great knowledge and gather vital information about ourselves, which gradually leads to greater self-knowledge, and once utilised will enable us to change what is not required or not conducive for our own inner evolution, as well as our work with our clients.

However, what is important for us to know is the great difference between the internal and the external. According to the Fourth Way philosophy, our outer and inner worlds represent two totally different realities; the former can be seen and shared by anyone, whilst the latter is completely invisible to everyone else around us. In other words, everybody can observe each other within the outer environment, but only we can truly see what is happening within ourselves. If we apply this to our work with our clients, it becomes very obvious that we can observe and assess all physical and external manifestations in our clients, and through conversation and palpation we might even be able to gather some valuable knowledge of the inner physical and physiological conditions of our clients' bodies, but we are not able to observe what takes place inside the inner world of our clients, which includes their psychology and state of perception, their being and their state of consciousness. However, the more we know about and understand our own inner world and the functioning of our own mind and psychological makeup, the more we will understand the frictions, conflicts and struggles that take place in the mind and in the inner world of other people. In addition, we need to remember that both our inner and outer realities exist and unfold simultaneously, and each of them has its own momentum, yet we mainly see and interpret the outer reality through our inner world of experiences. This is the reason why the fundamentally objective external world is perceived by us as something entirely subjective and personal. In other words, this truth is what we bring to our work, to the treatment table or to the classroom. However, to be able to get out of this dilemma of fluctuating subjectivity, we need to study the different types of observation we can apply to our work.

Both observation and self-observation can be divided into seven different types if we apply the idea of scale. The first three types of observation take place on the same level of perception, they all include biases and all three of them are subjective. Furthermore, they usually arise out of default mechanisms, depending on whether we are more intellectually, emotionally or movement orientated. The remaining types of observation, however, evolve in four progressive stages of refinement.

1 Movement-biased observation

The first type of observation is informed by movement and function, including body mechanics, compensation patterns, postural alignments, body language, facial expressions and demeanour, as well as physiology.

2 Emotionally biased observation

The second type of observation is informed by the observer's interest in emotions, feelings and psychological manifestations, as well as the emotional response that is being evoked by the object currently observed. The observer is mainly interested in the emotional states, their psychological impact and the feelings of the individual being observed, as well as emotions and feelings that take place between different individuals and groups.

3 Intellectually biased observation

The third type of observation is informed by what the observer knows in the form of theoretical and academic knowledge, including hypotheses, concepts, systems, mathematical equations, strategies, statistics and pathologies. The subjects observed are continuously analysed and verified by the ever-increasing knowledge of the observer.

4 Balanced observation

The fourth type of observation is informed by the first three types, leading to a more integrated and holistic view of the observable. The actual process of observation is sustained by an evolving centre of gravity (gravitates towards neutral) that generates an element of separation from biases. The fourth type of observation is the gateway to 'know thyself' through self-study and introspection.

5 Neutral observation

The fifth type of observation is informed by 'a place of no position'. It is sustained by a permanent centre of gravity that is inner stillness. The observer's attention does not need to identify with the subject observed, hence labelling and editing has ceased to interfere. If this type of observation is applied in self-observation, it leads to the state of self-consciousness, in which the truth of shadow and light within us, as well as what we are at the core of our being, are illuminated, fully realised and understood.

6 Objective observation

The sixth type of observation comes after years of sincere work on ourselves through introspection, some help from others and through utilising universal knowledge that facilitates change. It is informed by the unchanging nature of the self. Here, most of our psychological layers that previously acted as filters on our perception have been removed, and we observe what exists in its totality and 'is-ness'. This type of observation will gradually lead to objective consciousness in which we fully realise the transcendental nature of all things, manifest and hidden, including the transcendental nature of ourselves.

7 Transcendental observation

Figuratively speaking, the seventh type of observation is informed by the non-reflective nature of our 'non-self' (the complete absence of any remaining traces of a sense of 'I' or 'me'), in which all subject and object dynamics have ceased to exist, giving rise to a complete state of direct perception in which the observer, the observed and the process of observing have merged and become one.

The three Os

To be able to observe and self-observe we need to apply the principles of the three Os:

- Open body
- Open heart
- Open mind.

Open body means a body free of tension and stress, which we can accomplish through regular physical exercise in the form of sports, dance, yoga, Pilates or regular strengthening walks.

Open heart means a heart free of upset, self-pity and negativity, which can be accomplished by our own inner work, as well as regular supervision, or by using suitable approaches that work with our psychology and tissue memory.

Open mind means a mind that is spacious and without limiting biases, a mind that is free from affirmation and negation, as well as being free from trying to explain everything through what we already know theoretically and intellectually. This can be accomplished by achieving stillness-memory through the second stream of influences (see Part 1: Chapter 3), breathing exercises and different stilling techniques (see Part 5), as well as practical work on consciousness that might require some initial facilitation.

Experiment

1. Observe which type of observation is your default, and how this affects work with your clients. Keep observing the different trigger points for a couple of weeks without any attempt to judge. Remember observation is simply gathering valuable information that can be used for change.

2. After two weeks, whenever you happen to catch yourself falling into default mode, simply connect with the stillness generated by the space around you. Observe how this affects you, your work with your clients and the outcome of each session, treatment or class.

Working with the unknown

Nothing holds a greater mystery than the unknown, and whilst life itself simply happens, the unknown accompanies us wherever we are and wherever we go. Most of the time, we live in fear of it or resist it. To avoid having to face the unknown, we are busy following a multitude of routines, habits and patterns in our everyday life, as well as subconsciously creating new ones, which gives us the feeling and confidence that our life has become a lot more predictable. If we meet the unknown during our work with our clients, the usual default response is to fill and cover it up with what we already know. All of this creates the illusion of a safe life lived in the known, a life in which nothing out of the ordinary can happen or change. To put this into greater perspective, we usually don't do this on purpose, but because of what we have learned, mimicked and acquired during our upbringing, as well as the deeply engrained patterns that were set by our parents and social environment at a very early stage in our life. Later in life we keep creating patterns because it has become a strong habit to do so. That is, from a philosophical point of view, we simply don't know better. However, on a far deeper level, the fear of the unknown is rooted in a subconscious fear of death. This fear relates not only to the death of our physical body, but also to the death of our 'I-believes', our personal philosophies, and the fear of the death of what we believe or imagine ourselves to be as a person and as a professional.

This is one of the reasons why philosophical ideas, including the teachings of psychology, are based on one fundamental idea, which is the possibility of evolving and changing. Change requires work, and to be able to change we have to go through a process of transformation that consists of three different stages. According to ancient teachings and philosophy, we first have to wake up, then we have to die, and then we have to be newly born again. Through observation and self-observation we become more conscious and see things in a different light.

That is, through an increase in consciousness we wake up to a new truth or possibility within us or around us. In this new light of awakening, we first come to realise that the only possibility is to truly change, then we have to die to the old, and only then can we transform to be reborn.

> *The unknown is the sum total of possibilities that lie outside the field of our awareness.*
>
> Alexander Filmer-Lorch

Working with the unknown means bringing more light of consciousness into the field of our awareness. Nothing moves us faster into the present moment than the unknown. However, if we keep working only from what we know, we exclude ourselves from the possibilities that lie outside our limited means of perception, simply because there is not enough space for anything else to enter.

So, how do we utilise the unknown in our work as therapists and practitioners? In fact, the unknown will present itself in plenty of situations during a treatment, session, or class when we find ourselves in a position in which we feel completely lost or inadequate. Situations where we have no idea of what is happening right now, what to do next or what to fall back on. We are held in a place of suspension, and it is here that the appearance of the unknown, in the form of a totally unexpected situation or development, acts as a powerful conscious shock, which in psychology is also known as a shock of change. This unexpected shock, which leads to our inner awakening by suddenly expanding the field of our awareness, separates us from any intrinsic default response, and for a brief moment renders any conscious and subconscious need to know passive. Throughout this moment (approximately three seconds!) we feel very lucid, incredibly awake and open. It is this very moment, which takes place within the heart of the unknown, that we need to use to listen to what the present moment is saying. It is here that the unknown is offering us new possibilities we haven't come across or considered before, possibilities that might relate much more to the actual physical and psychological needs of our clients, yet they did not form part of our repertoire of skills and protocols that we normally work with or know. These are the possibilities that have not been limited and excluded by what we know already or what we think is 'best'.

However, to avoid any misunderstanding, it is important for us to appreciate that, as always in philosophy, we are dealing with another paradox. That is, to be able to truly collaborate with the unknown, we first have to study and accumulate a tremendous amount of knowledge, skills and best practice, and apply all these protocols, theories and tools that we have studied and come to know until they become second nature. This is when we become a true professional and expert in our field of work. Then, once we have mastered what we have studied and practised, we have to start undoing what we have learned to become free of all default knowledge after all.

The unknown teaches us to undo what we know by waking us up to a higher level of consciousness and perception. This inner awakening allows more of the light of consciousness to enter. This new and increased light of consciousness radiates far beyond our usual scope of perception, illuminating knowledge that lies above our ordinary knowledge, which in ancient philosophy is called higher knowledge and meets us in the form of possibilities that

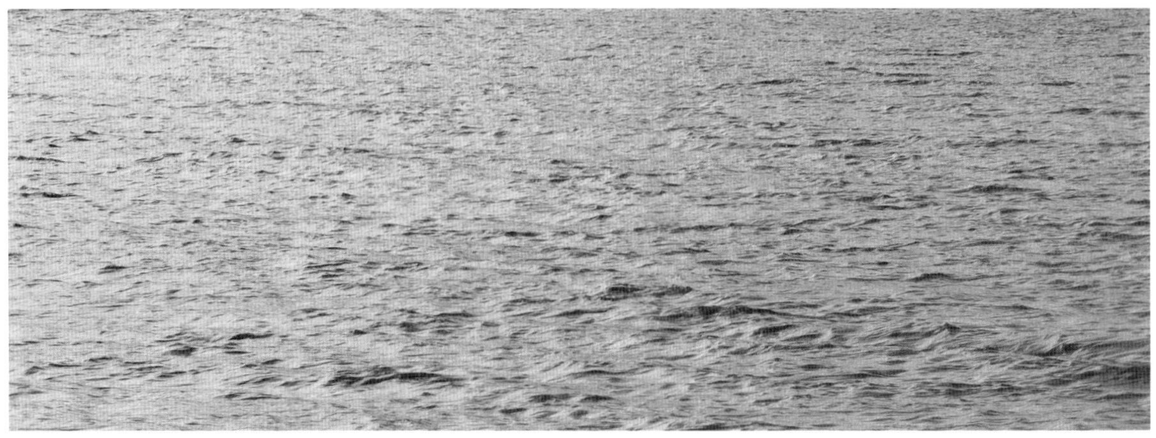

Figure 11.3
The sea is a great example of how the unknown represents itself to us through nature; photography Alexander Filmer-Lorch

carry a depth of insight and wisdom that has the power to transform and deliver change. Additionally, there is another aspect that is worth mentioning. Higher knowledge can only reach us in a moment of self-remembering (the very moment of inner awakening) that takes us into the depth of our self or inner stillness. Here, transformational knowledge is perceived by two higher faculties that are known to us as *inspiration* and *intuition*, which belong to the 'insightful self'. Once we abide *in spirit* we can receive *inner tuition* (one of the philosophical meanings of intuition) generated by the omnipresence of the unknown. This is the true meaning that all ancient teachings talk about in stating that 'the truth can only be found within ourselves'.

Conclusion

In the presence of the unknown, both our clients and ourselves can transform and change. We do this by stepping out of our own ways, facilitating and treating from a place of no position (see Part 3: Chapter 13) in which new possibilities can enter, and which activate the self-healing response in our clients. The clients change through activating their inner self-healing ability, which can now respond to possibilities on a different scale, and have become available through the shift that took place vertically within us as their facilitator.

Experiment

1. On holiday abroad (provided you don't speak the native language of the country that you are visiting), go to a bar or restaurant that is mainly used by native speakers who might speak very little of your own language. Initiate a conversation, which will put you into a situation in which you are faced with the unknown. Let yourself be surprised by the scale of new possibilities you will find at your disposal to hold a meaningful conversation with the people around you. Acknowledge the change in you.
2. The moment you are faced with the unknown during a session or treatment, use your heightened state of perception and your increase in consciousness. Simply pause and listen in inner stillness to the totality of what the present moment is saying. Then watch, be guided by and collaborate with whatever unfolds. This is how you transform a work pattern that is based mainly on knowing and doing into a new proposition that gives rise to allowing and being.

A short note on the force of meaning

> *To know is to know that you know nothing. That is the meaning of true knowledge.*
>
> Socrates

Without the force of meaning behind everything we do in life, things will turn pretty shallow and mechanical. However, meaning does not equal likes and preferences, which are short-lived and far too subject to change. Just as a simple like or preference does not get us anywhere in life, so an aim without meaning is an aim not worth pursuing. From a philosophical point of view, everything in this universe is striving towards completion, and it is usually those things we meet in life that carry the force of meaning that take us closer to completing what we are *supposed* to become in life and in our work, rather than what we *think* we have to become, which can turn out to be completely meaningless once we have arrived at our objective. The latter only makes us go round in circles, which become more and more difficult to break. In other words, it is not us but the depth of meaning in our work with others that enables us to evolve as practitioners and therapists, just as it is the depth of meaning we find in life that makes us evolve and grow as a person.

The scale of meaning is infinite and its force reaches us from a very high level, carrying the power of transformation that brings about real change. In addition, change requires work, and if our real aim is to do some sincere work on ourselves at a very deep level to inform and transform our work as therapists, teachers and practitioners, initially a lot of time and dedication, as well as a great amount of force and effort, will be required to make that happen.

The force of meaning, therefore, is the fuel that drives our conscious effort and builds the foundation on which we grow 'real aim', which takes us from disciplined effort to inspirational effort, and ultimately from inspirational effort to selfless effort.

This means that real aim can only be achieved if it carries the transformational force of meaning, because without meaning we would stumble and give up at the first hurdle. What has made the aim of writing this book so meaningful to us is the belief that some universal idea or technique transmitted through this book might bring a spark of meaning to our readers and consequently to their dedicated work with others.

Experiment

The next time the force of meaning ignites a spark in your life at work, use it by exploring the scale of possibilities it offers. This new meaning, possibly in the form of higher knowledge that can be applied to you and your work, will take you into a deeper meaning, which will take you further into a deeper meaning, which will take you ... and so on infinitely.

References

Cram101 Textbook Reviews (2014). *E-study guide for: experimental psychology: a case approach by M. Kimberly MacLin*. 8th ed. Cram101 Textbook Reviews.

Guimaraes, F. (n.d.). *Research: anyone can do it.* Pedia Press.

Hanson, N. (1958). *Patterns of Discovery: an inquiry into the conceptual foundations of science.* Cambridge University Press.

Perception 12

> *The only true voyage of discovery ... would be not to visit strange lands but to possess other eyes.*
>
> Marcel Proust in *Remembrance of Things Past*

The most important tool in our work is our faculty of perception – everything we perceive through our five physical senses and our inner sense. In philosophy, perception consists of two different subfaculties that have to work together in perfect harmony and balance to shed enough light of consciousness onto the object perceived for it to be seen, acknowledged and recognised in full and for what it truly is. Those two subfaculties of perception are known to us as *awareness* and *attention*. Modern psychology knows a lot about attention, but only very little about awareness. Every month it seems we hear about new research looking into different attention disorders, and the fact that more people are being affected by them. However, the same is not true of awareness disorders that don't stem from brain injury or malfunction. To be able to fully develop our sense of perception, and utilise its full potential in our work, a thorough understanding (not mere knowledge) of both awareness and attention on a physiological and psychological level is paramount.

Attention

Through attention we are able to concentrate on one specific aspect or task within our environment whilst filtering out all other incoming stimuli. As already mentioned in the first part of this book, our attention span is rapidly decreasing every year due to the increase in stimulus caused by mobiles, tablets and computers. According to ancient philosophy, during any kind of work project or task that requires our full attention and input, our brain can keep focusing on a particular task for only 45 minutes before it needs a break to assimilate and recover. Our productivity and clarity of thinking will lapse shortly after that and, allegorically speaking, our brain will be longing to switch from beta brainwave activity to any other brainwave pattern, which we usually override due to lack of time. So, what actually happens in the brain during attention?

Our most common understanding about the physiology of attention is that our brain uses two different kinds of attention that are allocated to two different areas in the brain. If we are in focused concentration, the prefrontal cortex will be active, and if we are faced with an unexpected or unsettling experience, the parietal lobe (which has lots of other functions as well) will spring into action. According to an article from Inside the Brain (2013), neurons need to emit electrical pulses of a lower frequency to sustain concentration in the prefrontal cortex that relates to work based on intention, and electrical pulses of a higher frequency when it comes to sustaining concentration in the parietal cortex based on automatic processing. In addition, there are three networks in the brain that relate to different aspects of attention, namely *alerting*, *orienting* and *executive attention* (Posner and Fan, 2008). According to Posner and Rothbart (2007), alerting achieves and maintains a state of high sensitivity to incoming stimuli. Research has found that the alerting system is associated with the thalamic, frontal and parietal regions of the cortex. Orienting is the selection of information from sensory input. It aligns attention with the source of sensory input. Executive attention involves mechanisms for monitoring and resolving conflict amongst thoughts, feelings and responses (Fan et al., 2005).

According to Posner and Rothbart (2007), lots of questions have been raised about the degree to which attention is inherited. There are strong suggestions that specific genes may be involved in the development and efficiency of the attention networks, which recent studies have confirmed. This leads to the assumption that 'because parenting and other cultural factors interact with genes to influence behaviour, it should be possible to develop specific training methods that can be used to influence underlying brain networks ... Several such attention-training studies have shown improved executive attention function and produced changes in attention-related brain areas ... The practice of a form of meditation has been used to change the brain state in a way that improves attention, reduces stress, and also improves functional connectivity between the anterior cingulate and the striatum …' (Petersen and Posner, 2012). Just recently, two further independent networks have been discovered that help us control behaviour, thought and feelings. In developmental psychology this is known as self-regulation, and in adulthood it is known as self-control. During conflict tasks, areas of the anterior cingulate gyrus are active, for cognitive tasks the dorsal portion is active, and for tasks that relate to emotions the ventral area is active (Botvinick et al., 2001). 'We now have the opportunity to go from genes to cells, networks, and behaviour and to examine how these relationships change from infancy to old age' (Petersen and Posner, 2012). Furthermore, it is worth mentioning that 'In development [from infancy to adulthood], the number of active [attention] control systems increases and their influence changes' (Petersen and Posner, 2012). I would not be surprised at all if stillness practice leads to greater synchrony of and within the different attention control systems. But this is for the scientists to prove.

The way our attention works and how we use it in our life has a major impact on our psychology, as well as on our interactions with others. Let's remember that it is our attention that helps us to focus on different things and their details, by allowing us to zoom in. However, if we become completely absorbed and swallowed by attention, we will completely lose our connection to a greater perspective and get lost in the details. As a consequence, our sense of self is switched off. An article in *New Scientist* magazine commented on research by Goldberg and team in 2006: 'The team conducted a series of experiments to pinpoint the brain activity associated with introspection and that linked to sensory function.' This led to the result 'that the brain assumes a robotic functionality when it has to concentrate all its efforts on a difficult, timed task – only becoming "human" again when it has the luxury of time' (Vince, 2006). Goldberg's paper describes a complete segregation of regions in the brain that are involved in introspection and sensory perception, yet they are also well connected. However, according to Goldberg, the moment the brain needs to execute a challenging task, it needs to divert all of its resources to it, whilst the self-related cortex is inhibited.

If a person's sense of self is impaired by constant attention, it can lead to dogmatism and an extremely narrow way of thinking, as well as to all different kinds of compulsive behaviour. Because we habitually spend most of our time in attention, it's easy to see how the slightest impairment or disconnection to our sense of self impacts upon our treatments and our work with others, gradually culminating in mental and physical depletion, over-identifying and ultimately even burn-out. Hence, the main reason that most of us are struggling to keep a natural connection with our inner sense of self, a neutral state of mind and inner stillness is the great divide between awareness and attention.

Eastern philosophy on attention

In philosophical terms, attention symbolises the masculine energy, or the active force, which is always ready to act. From an energetic point of view, attention is represented by the light of the sun that manifests as pingala, a nadi (energy channel) that runs along the right side of the spine. The ancient teachings say that, in our everyday life, attention has become the slave of our five senses. However, through specific stilling techniques (see Part 5), attention can be brought back into balance, re-establishing the homeostasis in our body–mind complex, which is exactly what Tang and team proved in their recent research (2007, 2009).

Experiment

For the next couple of hours, observe how much time you spend in attention, how much you zoom in to the details of things, and how often you lose your connection to your sense of self. Keep coming back to this on a daily basis for a while.

Awareness

In his book *Psychiatry and the Human Condition* Bruce Charlton (2000) writes that the definition of awareness is 'the ability selectively to direct attention to specific aspects of the environment, and to be able cognitively to manipulate these aspects over a more prolonged timescale than usual cognitive processing will allow'. That is, 'to hold in mind selected aspects of the perceptual landscape. Technically, awareness is attention plus working memory … a mechanism of integration

... Hence working memory is the anatomical site of awareness.'

Neuroscience shows that awareness and self-awareness are associated with the medial prefrontal cortex, the insula and the anterior cingulate of the brain. Yet, research by Philippi revealed that a patient who suffered from extensive bilateral brain damage to these areas could preserve a high sense of self-awareness: 'He has a stable self-concept and intact higher-order metacognitive abilities', which suggests 'that self-awareness is likely to emerge from more distributed interactions among brain networks including those in the brainstem, thalamus, and posteromedial cortices' (Philippi et al., 2012). Philippi's research seems to explain that people suffering from complete locked-in syndrome are retaining a clear sense of self, including the experience that they exist as a fully aware being within a body that has completely shut down.

However, Casey Blood, Professor Emeritus of Physics at Rutgers University, estimates that there is a 90 per cent chance that awareness does not originate in the brain at all, which he bases on the fact that it conflicts with the law of probability (Blood, 2008). This implies that unamended quantum mechanics cannot properly account for awareness. In his view, the most likely picture is that awareness cannot be based in the physical brain, and that its origin must be outside of physical reality. Blood says: 'The most straightforward way to picture this result is to suppose that we each have a non-physical "Mind" that "looks in" from outside physical reality and focuses on just one version of the quantum state of our brain.' He concludes that 'the highly successful theory of quantum mechanics gives *many simultaneously existing versions* of the physical world, including many versions of our brain'. Hence, awareness only *perceives* the wave function and does not alter it in any way, which takes us right into the psychology of this state, and how it affects us and our work with others. If we follow this reasoning on quantum mechanics, our faculty of awareness simply perceives things, without having to edit or label whatever it perceives. Its intrinsic nature is to view the whole that includes the parts. It sees things purely as they appear, and has no inclination or need to change whatever enters its extensive field of perception.

Therapists and practitioners are very conscious of what is happening when it comes to their work with others, and in my experience as a table assistant during CranioSacral Therapy (CST) training, as well as when teaching, I have been struck by how prone most therapists are to falling far too much into awareness. I have witnessed sessions when all sense of time got blown out of the window, the lines of communication broke down even whilst communicating through palpation, no real dialogue between therapist and client took place any more, and the client stopped processing altogether. As a result, the treatment or session came to a complete halt. That is, falling too much into awareness during a treatment session leads to 'dis-identifying' and detachment from the client and the therapeutic process, a state in which nothing can happen. A wrong understanding of detachment, the state of therapeutic presence and the practice of mindfulness is one of the most common reasons that practitioners fall too much into awareness. We have to be very careful, because regularly falling into either one of these faculties of awareness or attention can, in the long term, easily turn into a deeply engrained habit that might be difficult to break.

In everyday life, however, it simply disconnects us from our common sense, diminishes our ability to respond, and makes it very difficult to stick to our commitments and responsibilities. Clients who are in a constant state of indecisiveness, or who seem to float aimlessly around in life, showing no sense of being grounded and displaying a diffused, blurry sense of self, might have fallen too much into awareness.

Eastern philosophy on awareness

In philosophical terms, awareness symbolises the feminine energy, or the passive force, which does not need to act. From an energetic point of view, awareness is represented by the light of the moon that manifests as ida, a nadi (energy channel) that runs along the left side of the spine. According to ancient philosophy, awareness has no ability to become aware of itself. In addition, it is so utterly still and motionless that it usually gets buried below powerful waves of attention. However, through specific work on attention (see Part 5: The practitioner's toolkit), the waves it creates start phasing out, culminating in a genuine balance between awareness and attention.

Experiment

1. Every day, ideally on a walk in nature, spend some time working on spatial perception. That is, instead of looking at the details of things, be aware of the whole picture that enters your field of perception. In this more spacious state of perception, find out as much as you can about the power and the workings of your attention without formulating a conclusion.
2. Once you have settled into this practice, apply the same technique during your treatments or sessions whenever it fits the process or situation.

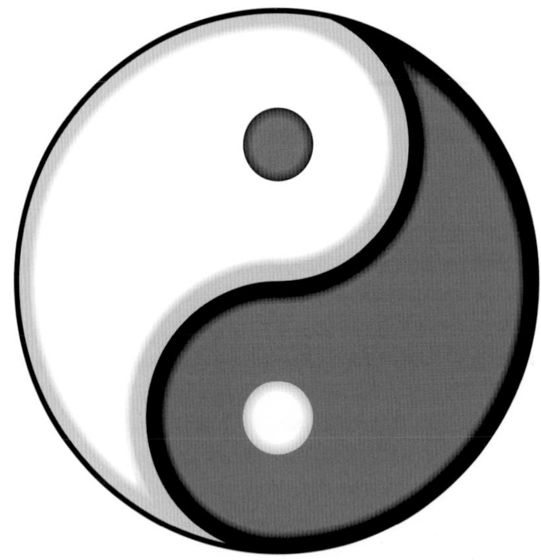

Figure 12.1

Yin Yang, a symbol of balance, referring to the middle or the centre

The fulcrum in the middle

It is very obvious by now that, whichever direction we take on this linear plane between awareness and attention, the moment we have moved too much into either one of them, they will cancel each other out. That is, the deeper we move into attention, the more restrictions and laws we will meet, whilst the deeper we move into awareness, the less we will be able to act and respond due to ever-increasing passivity. Hence, neither is conducive to our own work as therapists and practitioners.

Now, if there is homeostasis in all our physiological functions, our body will be healthy and well. So we have to create a genuine homeostasis between awareness and attention that can only be established once we start working from a different place altogether, possibly a place somewhere in the middle. This train of thought takes us back to philosophy, where the main emphasis lies on balance. Throughout history we find pointers symbolising a perfect state of balance in the form of archetypal expressions, such as the yin and yang symbol in Chinese philosophy, the bindi or dot in Hinduism, and the hara or tanden in Japanese traditions. The main focus in Eastern and Western psychology today lies in becoming a 'balanced person', which according to the former is accomplished by working on the dynamics between awareness and attention. In other words, it is neither one nor the other but both simultaneously held and sustained through the still-point, giving rise to the fulcrum in the middle, an imaginary gravitational pivot point around which awareness and attention can gyrate and coexist in perfect balance.

The best term that describes the state that emerges from this balance between awareness and attention is *lucid cognition*, and what is interesting for us to understand is that, presented as a philosophical idea, this is a state comprising the quintessence of both active/male and passive/female that springs into being when awareness and attention fully comprehend and perceive each other simultaneously for a prolonged moment in time, consequently ceasing to oppose each other, and finally coalescing and merging. To be able to utilise lucid cognition in our work as therapists, we have to start working with the philosophical idea of action through non-reaction that will be discussed in Part 5.

Experiment

Direct your attention inwards (you might like to close your eyes) with the help of your proprioceptive sense (sensing the relative positions of internal sensations and neighbouring parts) and be aware of different tensions, tightness, pulses or rhythms in your body, then shift your perception to what you experience or perceive as space within your physical body. Rest within this inner sense of spaciousness and get a sense of both your awareness and your attention. Do not edit, grasp or analyse what you perceive or experience.

Consciousness

What is consciousness, and how does it work? It is undoubtedly an unresolved mystery that has been occupying many thinkers, philosophers and scientists throughout the entire history of humankind. Based on archaeological findings in burial sites, built by our Cro-Magnon ancestors, historians assume that the origins of modern human consciousness date back 40,000 to 50,000 years. Even today's notion of consciousness is vague and speculative. However, we might gain a better understanding of consciousness by looking at it from three different perspectives. That is, from the point of view of neuroscience, quantum physics, and philosophy and psychology.

Neuroscience on consciousness

Where do we exist within our physiology? Is perception of the world we live in a result of changes in neural activity, or is consciousness based on the workings of a much broader neurological network? Is the seat of consciousness in our brain, and if so, is it focal or global?

Recent research on network theory has shed new light on the origins of consciousness. Moran (2015) writes: 'Modern theories of the neural basis of consciousness fall generally into two camps: focal and global. Focal theories contend there are specific areas of the brain that are critical for generating consciousness ...'. She then points out that 'global theories argue consciousness arises from large-scale brain changes in activity'. The study in question applied graph theory analysis to adjudicate between these theories, defined by WhatIs.com (2016) as 'the study of points and lines. In particular, it involves the ways in which sets of points, called vertices, can be connected by lines or arcs, called edges.

The lead author of the research told Moran: 'With graph theory, one can ask questions about how efficiently the transportation networks in the United States and Europe are connected via transportation hubs like LaGuardia Airport in New York. We can ask those same questions about brain networks and hubs of neural communication.' Moran continues: 'The research suggests that consciousness is likely a product of this widespread communication, and that we can only report things that we have seen once they are being represented in the brain in this manner.' Moran concludes 'Thus, no one part of the brain is truly the "seat of the soul" ...' (Moran, 2015).

However, other researchers, such as Christof Koch, have different views. In his interview with Brandon Keim, Koch explains that 'consciousness arises within any sufficiently complex, information-processing system. All animals, from humans on down to earthworms, are conscious; even the internet could be. That's just the way the universe works' (Keim, 2015). Koch ties his radical theory with the ancient philosophy of panpsychism, which is based on the view that 'all things have a mind or a mind-like quality' (IEP, 2015). Koch talks about a theory, called integrated information theory, which was developed by Giulio Tononi at the University of Wisconsin, 'that assigns to any one brain, or any complex system, a number ... Any system with integrated information different from zero has consciousness ... In the case of the brain, it's the whole system that's conscious, not the individual nerve cells'. Koch continues: 'For any one ecosystem, it's a question of how richly the individual components, such as the trees in a forest, are integrated within themselves as compared to causal interactions between trees' (Keim, 2015).

Other research suggests that the seat of our consciousness can be found in the claustrum, which is 'a thin, irregular sheet of grey matter on the underside of the neocortex in the center of the brain (located sagitally between external and extreme capsule and mediolaterally between the putamen and insula)'. The research also found that this thin sheet has 'widespread connections throughout the cortex and the rest of the brain' (Bromer, 2014).

Around the same time, the findings of a similar study by Koubeissi and colleagues in 2014 were reported: 'Researchers at George Washington University are reporting that they've discovered the human consciousness on-off switch, deep within the brain. When this region of the brain, called the claustrum, is electrically stimulated, consciousness – self-awareness, sentience, whatever you want to call it – appears to turn off completely.' The study also found that 'when the stimulation is removed, consciousness returns. The claustrum seems to bind together all of our senses, perceptions, and computations into single, cohesive experience' (Anthony, 2014). It is interesting to note that, whilst consciousness was switched off, the person undergoing the procedure in the research remained fully awake but did not retain any memory of what had happened afterwards.

Bromer (2014) suggests that the research by Koch and previous work by Francis Crick 'promote the idea that the claustrum could perform what they term "sensory binding", namely a process of aggregating relevant information to develop a single, uniform experience'. The same research also suggests 'that this makes the claustrum an attractive candidate structure for the "seat of consciousness"'.

In spite of all the above theses and new propositions, neuroscience has not yet found a conclusive explanation that verifies the functions of consciousness in our physiology.

Quantum physics on consciousness - the brain in quantum space

Dave Mason FSRP kindly contributed the following section.

Quantum science was formulated in the early 1900s and continues to create radical changes to the way in which we think about our world, particularly the behaviour of molecules and subatomic particles. It has enabled us to harness new technologies and advance those that existed before. We are beginning to see quantum science being applied to computers and in the world of biochemistry. It is also the stuff that we can dream about to create pseudoscientific explanations of our world that may suit our particular paradigm. Yet it is important to speculate. This challenges our thinking and enables new ideas and models to develop. It is only when we structure our speculation into a rational hypothesis that we can begin to formulate a means of interrogating the predictions that we make and offer some scientific analysis, modelling and measurement to lend support to our ideas. Quantum explanations are being applied to biochemistry to explain the role of enzymes in speeding up biochemical reactions and the efficiency of chlorophyll reactions. In relation to the functioning of the brain, ideas are in gestation, with a few scientific hypotheses being explored relating to the transfer of electrons in the microtubules of the neuron.

First of all let us explore what quantum science is, propose how this may be related to the functioning of our brain and then discuss meditative processes.

Science begins with the observation of the physical world and asks questions about why we see things the way we do. So, for example, why do an apple and lead weight fall from the same height at the same rate? When steam is used to create mechanical work, what is it that limits how much energy we can extract from the steam? Each question demands an hypothesis that will explain what we can observe and predict what else will happen. Through repeated observation and painstaking measurement we have built many models to explain the world around us. When we reach the limits of one hypothesis we develop another until we find one that again explains our world, as we currently understand it. So whilst science is always painstaking and precise, it isn't always accurate, simply because we discover more about our world that demands more explanation.

Over the years we have developed quite sophisticated models of the world that explain a lot. Humankind advanced technologically very quickly using these so-called classical models of science. Classical physics worked fine until we started to explore the world of the atom and it failed to explain what was being observed. New thinking and new models were required.

Work by Einstein on the photoelectric effect, where light impacting on a metal released electrons, showed that this was a quantised effect involving discrete packets of energy, quanta. Einstein also proposed a wave-particle duality for light suggesting that it behaved both as a particle and an electromagnetic wave. Models of the atom suggested that electrons surrounding a nucleus held discrete quantities of energy. Electrons were also shown to have the properties of waves by creating interference patterns when a beam of them was aimed at a diffraction screen. This duality was subsequently proposed for all matter.

Mathematical models were developed to describe these quantum phenomena and wave-like properties, with quite surprising implications. The wave functions were of a probabilistic nature, describing probability amplitude of position, momentum and other properties, leading to outcomes with multiple states, such that a system can be in all states simultaneously up until such time as it is measured. The wave function also allows two particles from a coincident event to entangle their wave functions and exist in multiple states until the property of one is measured, when instantaneously this determines the property of the other event, even if separated by vast distances. Einstein didn't like this concept of 'spooky action at a distance' since it ran counter to his theory of relativity that limits communication of events to the speed of light, but entanglement has since been shown to be so, with instantaneous transformation. Spookier things happen too. When a beam of electrons is fired at a double slit target it will produce interference patterns on a detector directly behind the double slit, thus showing electrons have wave-like properties. If a detector is installed so as to examine the waves before they hit the interference detector then the waves instantaneously disappear, the interference pattern disappears and the electrons behave as if they were particles. This mystery is as yet unexplained.

In classical physics if a particle has insufficient energy to overcome a barrier then it can't. Yet in practice it can and it occasionally does and this can be explained by wave mechanics and is known as quantum tunnelling. Fusion requires two atoms that would naturally repel each other to be joined by overcoming the repelling energy. The fusion of the nuclei leads to a mass difference that is equivalent to the energy released – $E=mc^2$ and all that. Within the sun it is calculated that there is insufficient energy to bring the atoms together, but quantum tunnelling allows subenergetic fusion reactions to take place that provide the energy of the sun.

In summary, in quantum physics there are some new concepts and phenomena that apply to the world as we observe it:

- Particles and matter have a dual nature as either a wave or a particle.
- Quantum particles can be in multiple states and places until measured.
- Quantum tunnelling is a probabilistic phenomenon where matter can exist on either side of a barrier without traversing between the space.
- Quantum entanglement is an interconnection between quantum events that allows the measurement of one to define the others' complementary properties, irrespective of the distance between them.

So does our brain function on a quantum basis?

Neurons are an important component of our central nervous system. They are complex single cells that are the information highway of the brain. They can be electrically stimulated and respond by sending onward an electrochemical signal. They receive electrical signals that they transmit along microtubules within the axon of the cell to terminal buttons. The terminal buttons on receiving a signal respond by emitting further electrical signals or by releasing chemicals in the form of neurotransmitters. The nature of their operation depends at a molecular level on the concentration of calcium, potassium, sodium and chloride ions. The functioning of the neurons determines our brainwave pattern.

So, right at the heart of our brain's functionality we have at a molecular level the transmission of small particles that will behave as either a wave or a particle and may well function on a quantum basis in quantum space (quantum physics is being used to develop an hypothesis for consciousness).

Recent research has shown that biochemical reaction rates involving enzymes are faster than expected from a classical perspective. It is only when quantum tunnelling is invoked that the observed reaction rates can be explained. In the chlorophyll process the efficiency of energy conversion is far higher than expected. It is only when consideration is given to quantum wave properties that an explanation can be given for how a photon selects the most effective and efficient route for energy exchange. Within the brain it has been suggested that the electron within the microtubule of the axon can exist in two states, one that contracts the tubule and the other extending it. In quantum space the electron has a probability of being in both places. Thus the microtubule can be both collapsed and elongated at the same time. The electron transmission can then find the favoured route as more electrons summate to form the most effective route.

The fact that we are dealing with a biochemical electromagnetic system at a molecular level that forms thoughts and images in a fraction of a second suggests that quantum phenomena take place within the brain and probably help explain the speed at which our brains do work, and maybe even more!

Quantum tunnelling could allow new neural pathways to form: entanglement of coherent quantum events would allow instantaneous information transfer within the brain and, since distance is no object to entanglement, outwith the brain. This may not be so crazy since there are developing schools of thought that our brain functions outside of our skull anyway (just as when we form the image of our world inside of our brain, we perceive it to be outside of our bodies).

Could this quantum space of tunnelling, entanglement and multistate existence explain flashes of inspiration?

Why should there not be a correlation between brainwave activity and the functioning of the neuron in quantum space? Does one come before the other, or is it a symbiosis that we can influence through meditation?

Now, let us speculate further that our brainwave activity, an electromagnetic field, influences the quantum field and so determines the probability amplitude of the electron transmission and biochemical exchanges and so influences our conscious state and our process of thinking. We know that meditation can change our brainwave activity, so could it be that meditation not only controls our thinking but also changes how we think in quantum space? A change in our process of thinking will influence our values, our values will change our beliefs, our beliefs will change our behaviours and our behaviours become our destiny.

Philosophy and psychology on consciousness

Consciousness refers to many different phenomena, and each one of them is asking for a more detailed explanation.

According to Chalmers (2010), 'The easy problems of consciousness are those that seem directly susceptible to the standard methods of cognitive science, whereby a phenomenon is explained in terms of computational or neural mechanisms'. Chalmers continues: 'The hard problems are those that seem to resist those methods.' The 'easy' problems explained in Chalmers' book, however, do not resist those methods but include and explain phenomena such as:

- being able to categorise, discriminate and respond to external stimuli
- that a cognitive system can integrate information
- being able to report mental states
- that a system is able to access its own internal states
- that attention can hold a focus
- being able to deliberately control behaviour
- differentiation between sleep and wakefulness.

Chalmers concludes that 'all of these phenomena are associated with the notion of consciousness'.

All other phenomena of consciousness, such as experience, the intrinsic nature of consciousness and what might be conscious within us, fall into the category of so-called hard problems, because we can't determine a specific mechanism that would solve them. Instead, we have to explain a mechanism that gives rise to consciousness that might consist of something unknown or nothing at all. In philosophy this is known as phenomenology, and some people argue that a hard problem can't be solved at all, because we do not possess access to the whole scale of information required that would piece everything together and resolve the problem. Albert Einstein said that no problem can be solved from the same level of consciousness that created it. That is, we have to gain access to a much higher level of consciousness that gives us a bird's-eye view to be able to look at this phenomenon from a much higher perspective. High enough to shed light on the whole.

To explain certain inner experiences, a new approach is needed. The common explanatory methods of cognitive science, as well as neuroscience do not suffice. However, mystics, philosophers and ancient psychology might give rise to new possibilities for scientists to work with. Buddhanet's study guide (undated) on the Abhidhamma philosophy explains: 'The Buddha succeeded in reducing this "immediate occasion" of an act of cognition to a single moment of consciousness, which, however, in its subtlety and evanescence, cannot be observed, directly and separately, by a mind untrained in introspective meditation.' The article goes on: 'Just as the minute living beings in the microcosm of a drop of water become visible only through a microscope, so, too, the exceedingly short-lived processes in the world of mind become cognizable only with the help of a very subtle instrument of mental scrutiny, and that only obtains as a result of meditative training.'

A Christian perspective on consciousness by Struthers (2001) states: 'Consciousness is a topic that combines the simple essence of our self-awareness with the complexity of the neural system that underlies it. As Christians, I believe that our task is to approach consciousness with a respect for the recent discoveries made in cognitive science and neuroscience.' Struthers continues: 'We must be careful, however, of adopting definitions that might lead to a consciousness that leaves God out of the picture …' He concludes by saying: 'Consciousness is not just survival and reproduction, but is the vehicle through which we enter into relationships with our environment, each other, and, most importantly, our Creator.'

Raman (2011) outlines the theories of mind and consciousness from a Hindu point of view in a beautiful article: 'In the framework of modern science, there is no distinction between mind and consciousness: both are emergent properties of the brain. In classical Hindu theories, mind is different from consciousness', which from a universal teaching point of view is a distinction of great significance. The article continues: 'The mind has a material aspect which is super-subtle in its substantiality. The mind is seen as the instrument through which consciousness perceives physical reality ... The quest for transcendence is not just thirst for a fantasy.' This does not take us very far. 'Even as a heliotrope is drawn to light, the evolved brain may be reaching out for the transcendence that made it conscious. The thirst for transcendence is the yearning of the human spirit to remember its own pre-physical origins.' Raman concludes by saying: 'Such is the Hindu view of consciousness.'

We can all agree that someone who gets knocked out in an accident can lose consciousness and then regain it after a while. Hence, we are able to remain alive with or without consciousness, which means it is made of a different substance or energy than our life energy that keeps us alive. That is, no amount of the latter will produce the former.

In ancient teachings and philosophy, consciousness ranks high on the scale of energies. Each is on its own level, yet none of them merges with the others. Maurice Nicoll illustrates this perfectly in his *Psychological Commentaries*: 'A baby has vital energy before it has psychic life, and has a psychic life before it has consciousness' (Nicoll et al., 1956).

Consciousness could be defined as a matrix-like substance of utter autonomy, which perceives, processes and assimilates information with relative freedom from external impressions. Each of us is a unique conscious system, and our level of consciousness can increase or decrease at any given moment in time. Nicoll compares consciousness with yeast, which under the right circumstances can multiply itself indefinitely. We all possess a certain amount of this substance of consciousness, which is known in quantum physics as 'perceptronium', which has been called 'the most general substance that feels subjectively self-aware' by Tegmark (2015). He further states: 'If Tononi is right [about integrated information theory], then it should not merely be able to store and process information like computronium [the most general substance that can process information as a computer] does ... but it should also satisfy the principle that its information is integrated, forming a unified and indivisible whole.'

SELF-EVOLUTION IS TO GO ROUND AND ROUND THE EVER-EXPANDING
HELIX
OF CONSCIOUSNESS

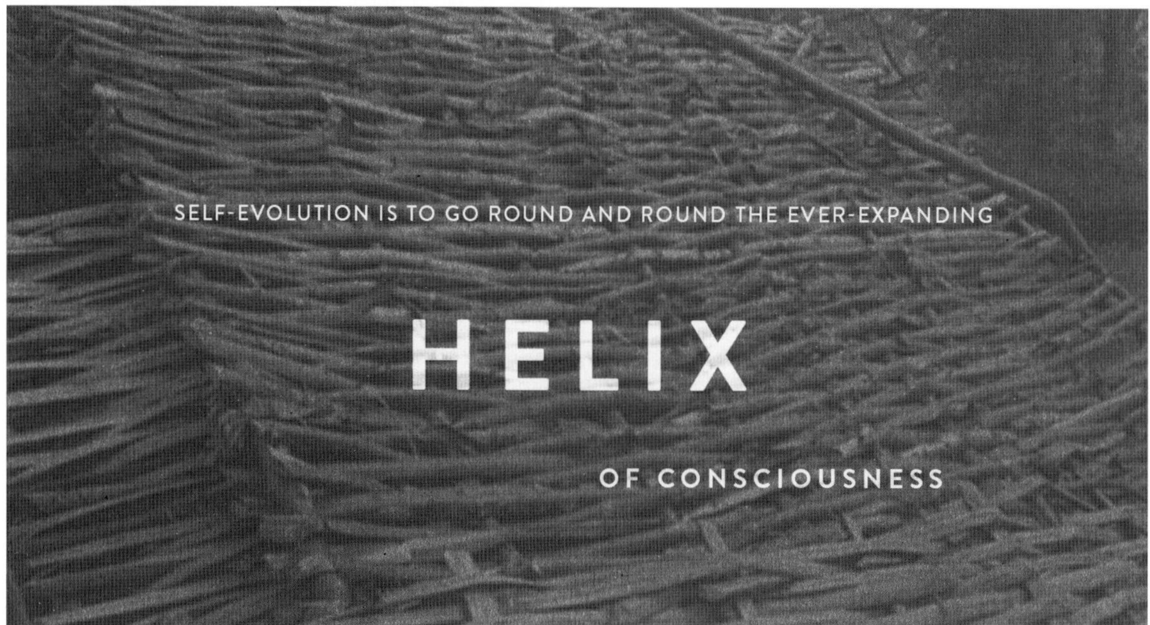

Figure 12.2

Artwork Victoria Dokas; photography Alexander Filmer-Lorch

The definition of consciousness according to Max Tegmark (2015)

Tegmark's definition of a conscious system is based on six principles, of which the first four are conjectured necessary conditions, with two additional principles.

- The first principle necessary for a conscious system to work is called the 'information principle', meaning it must hold sufficient storage capacity for information.
- The second necessary principle, called the 'dynamic principle', requires an ability to process a great amount of information.
- The third necessary principle, called the 'independence principle', means the system must be mainly independent from the rest of the world.
- The fourth necessary principle, called the 'integration principle', means the system cannot comprise almost completely independent parts.

The two additional principles are called the 'autonomy principle' and the 'utility principle':

- The autonomy principle has, according to Tegmark, substantial dynamics and independence.
- The utility principle means that an evolved conscious system records mainly information that is useful for it.

When it comes to our own evolution, we have to make a clear distinction between consciousness and mind. We need consciousness whilst we are treating, teaching and facilitating, as well as when studying the world, our own mind and our psychology. Whichever form consciousness might ultimately take, it is clear that it exists as something definite and distinctive, and that it does not comprise just our mind and those things that we are conscious of. The great psychologist Maurice Nicoll (1956) says: 'Consciousness is not your memory, thoughts, feelings or sensations. Through consciousness you become aware of them as contents. In fact consciousness can exist without any content ...' He continues explaining in more philosophical terms that consciousness 'is something unique. It is something we come in contact with'. Furthermore, he defines consciousness as 'a group of vibrations of high frequency and like light it exists apart from our contact with it ... it is not the light that is to be increased but our contact with it'. Nicole concludes his take on consciousness with a pointer saying: 'The receptive point of consciousness has to be changed. Then more consciousness is received.'

Now, why is all of the above so relevant to our work as therapists and practitioners? Because, without increasing our consciousness, we will forever remain within the linear dynamics of awareness and attention. To become more conscious to what is actually required at any given moment throughout a treatment, session or class, we first have to become still. Through inner stillness we find the fulcrum in the middle, the still-point in which both awareness and attention are naturally held in frictionless balance within the sudden influx of increasing consciousness. Within this heightened state of consciousness that lies above the horizontal and two-dimensional world of experiences (subject–object dynamic), we truly wake up to our three-dimensional world of experiences, which is perceived and observed through the eyes of the fourth dimension, the home of the 'I am' or the self. It is here, high above all knowing and doing, that the required action or insight is given in perfect accordance with each situation or event that unfolds. This 'inner awakening' or emergence of the fourth dimension is promoted by the gradual increase in consciousness by means of our own *conscious* effort, sustained by the idea of 'a place of no position' (see Part 3: Chapter 13), as well as 'action through non-reaction'. Hence, with the help of the amount of consciousness we already possess, and some dedicated conscious effort on our behalf, we can gradually bring much more of the light of consciousness into our self, our life and our work.

Experiment

When you meet a new situation, refrain from being immediately drawn into a subject–object dynamic with the people and things around you. Let one part of you keep an overview of the whole situation whilst you interact.

References

Anthony, S. (2014). Scientists discover the on-off switch for human consciousness deep within the brain. ExtremTech, www.extremetech.com/extreme/185865-scientists-discover-the-on-off-switch-for-human-consciousness-deep-within-the-brain [accessed 13 Oct. 2015].

Blood, C. (2008). Unamended quantum mechanics rigorously implies awareness is not based in the physical brain. Poster for the 12th annual meeting of the Association for the Scientific Study of Consciousness (ASSC 12), www.theassc.org/files/assc/ASSC12_Poster.pdf [accessed 28 Oct. 2015].

Botvinick, M., Braver, T., Barch, D., Carter, C. and Cohen, J. (2001). Conflict monitoring and cognitive control. *Psychological Review*, 108(3): 624–652.

Bromer, C. (2014). The conscious claustrum. NeuWrite San Diego, http://neuwritesd.org/2014/08/08/the-conscious-claustrum/ [accessed 13 Oct. 2015].

Buddhanet.net (n.d.). Buddhist analysis of consciousness in the Abhidhamma, www.buddhanet.net/abhidh05.htm [accessed 14 Oct. 2015].

Chalmers, D. (2010). *The Character of Consciousness*. Oxford: Oxford University Press.

Charlton, B. (2000). *Psychiatry and the Human Condition*. Abingdon: Radcliffe Medical.

Fan, J., McCandliss, B., Fossella, J., Flombaum, J. and Posner, M. (2005). The activation of attentional networks. *NeuroImage*, 26(2): 471–479.

Goldberg, I., Harel, M. and Malach, R. (2006). When the brain loses its self: prefrontal inactivation during sensorimotor processing. *Neuron*, 50(2): 329–339.

IEP (2015). *Internet encyclopedia of philosophy* [definition], www.iep.utm.edu/panpsych/ [accessed 13 Oct. 2015].

Inside the Brain (2013). *Understanding attention deficit/hyperactivity disorder (ADHD) part 2*, http://inside-the-brain.com/2013/03/06/understanding-attention-deficithyperactivity-disorder-adhd-part-2/ [accessed 3 Feb. 2016].

Keim, B. (2015). A neuroscientist's radical theory of how networks become conscious. *Wired*, Science, www.wired.com/2013/11/christof-koch-panpsychism-consciousness/ [accessed 13 Oct. 2015].

Koubeissi, M., Bartolomei, F., Beltagy, A. and Picard, F. (2014). Electrical stimulation of a small brain area reversibly disrupts consciousness. *Epilepsy & Behavior*, 37: 32–35.

Moran, M. (2015). Network theory sheds new light on origins of consciousness. Vanderbilt University, http://news.vanderbilt.edu/2015/03/213466/ [accessed 13 Oct. 2015].

Nicoll, M., Gurdjieff, G. and Ouspensky, P. (1956). *Psychological Commentaries*. London: Stuart & Watkins.

Petersen, S. and Posner, M. (2012). The attention system of the human brain: 20 years after. *Annual Review of Neuroscience*, 35(1): 73–89.

Philippi, C., Feinstein, J., Khalsa, S., Damasio, A., Tranel, D., Landini, G., Williford, K. and Rudrauf, D. (2012). Preserved self-awareness following extensive bilateral brain damage to the insula, anterior cingulate, and medial prefrontal cortices. *PLoS ONE*, 7(8): e38413.

Posner, M.I. and Fan, J. (2008). Attention as an organ system. In: Pomerantz, J. (2008). *Topics in Integrative Neuroscience*. Cambridge University Press.

Posner, M. and Rothbart, M. (2007). *Educating the Human Brain*. Washington, DC: American Psychological Association.

Raman, V. (2011). Theories of mind and consciousness. Metanexus.net, www.metanexus.net/essay/theories-mind-and-consciousness [accessed 14 Oct. 2015].

Struthers, W. (2001). Defining consciousness: Christian and psychological perspectives. American Scientific Affiliation, www.asa3.org/ASA/PSCF/2001/PSCF6-01Struthers.html [accessed 14 Oct. 2015].

Tang, Y., Ma, Y., Fan, Y., Feng, H., Wang, J., Feng, S., Lu, Q., Hu, B., Lin, Y., Li, J., Zhang, Y., Wang, Y., Zhou, L. and Fan, M. (2009). Central and autonomic nervous system interaction is altered by short-term meditation. *Proceedings of the National Academy of Sciences*, 106(22): 8865–8870.

Tang, Y., Ma, Y., Wang, J., Fan, Y., Feng, S., Lu, Q., Yu, Q., Sui, D., Rothbart, M., Fan, M. and Posner, M. (2007). Short-term meditation training improves attention and self-regulation. *Proceedings of the National Academy of Sciences*, 104(43): 17152–17156.

Tegmark, M. (2015). Consciousness as a state of matter. *Chaos, Solitons & Fractals*, 76: 238–270.

WhatIs.com, (2016). What is graph theory? [definition], http://whatis.techtarget.com/definition/graph-theory [accessed 3 Feb. 2016].

Vince, G. (2006). Watching the brain 'switch off' self-awareness. *New Scientist*, Daily news, https://www.newscientist.com/article/dn9019-watching-the-brain-switch-off-self-awareness/ [accessed 30 Sep. 2015].

Getting to neutral 13

'I'd rather meet on neutral ground,' is a common phrase when people try to resolve a conflict. Seemingly unresolvable situations may even require a mediator, who represents the neutralising element aiming to negotiate a resolution that finally might solve the problem. Throughout a creative process people find somewhere that feels neutral to regroup. Hence, 'neutral' is required in all aspects of our life. Here are some examples of how we commonly use the concept of neutral. Peace conferences are usually held in a neutral country. The final of a sports competition is held at a neutral ground. I have to remain neutral when my friends fall out with each other to prevent myself from being dragged in. In chemistry, pure water is considered a neutral substance, and because it has a pH of 7, it is neither an acid nor an alkali. There is no electrical charge in a neutral object in physics, and an atom consists of a negatively charged electron, a positively charged proton and a neutral particle known as a neutron.

These are all examples of 'neutral' as physical places, a substance, energy or person that represents the neutral element. But our interest here lies in how neutral functions psychologically as a genuine faculty within ourselves.

In this chapter we will discuss the obstacles and laws that prevent us from becoming neutral, as well as practical solutions, techniques and the 'work' required that will ultimately get us to neutral.

The universal idea of neutral

The idea of a genuinely neutral state of mind gives rise to the same problems and misunderstandings as for the ideas of therapeutic presence, mindfulness and meditation due to the divided nature of our 'self'. We all understand neutral as a concept, but when it comes to *being* neutral in the literal sense, we do not possess a reference point, and have nothing to access that is based on the actual experience of neutral, not just as a fleeting state of mind but as a genuine state of *being*. We all know that by keeping an objective view of things throughout a treatment, class or session, we have a much higher chance of staying connected with the greater truth and reality of whatever unfolds beneath our hands or during the process. However, from the viewpoint of Eastern philosophy, without equal proportions of neutrality and objectivity, a truly objective view on things can't be sustained. That is, the former informs the latter, or both are a different side of the same coin.

Now, all those philosophical ideas sound great and might excite our intellect, yet without another vital element they are not worth a penny, because they don't tell us how they can be practically applied, hence they could remain forever passive. This is the reason why most ancient philosophy schools incorporated an incredibly refined body of psychological teachings. The philosophy gives meaning to the psychology, and the psychology teaches how to apply the philosophy and put it into action. Sadly, most psychological teachings that formed part of the ancient philosophical systems have been lost in history, and are waiting to be discovered again at some point. But, from an ancient philosophy point of view, 'neutral' is seen as the middle. The Vedas talk about 'neti neti', which means 'not this, not that', which brings about a state that is experienced as the middle. There is a similar concept in Buddhism: 'the search for the Middle Way can be considered a universal pursuit of all Buddhist traditions ...' (Soka Gakkai International, 2015). This is the reason why Buddhism itself is sometimes referred to as the 'Middle Way'. The Fourth Way philosophy speaks about the importance of becoming 'the middle man', describing the balanced person that interacts in the midst of the ever-changing nature of life, whilst Aristotle uses the 'golden mean' as the desirable middle between two extremes. It is well worth exploring the different takes on the 'middle' of as many different traditions and schools of thought as possible, yet to gain a much clearer understanding of

neutral in our field of work, we want to dive into the cosmological side of Eastern psychology, and explore the forces and dynamics between opposites.

Opposites

The world we live in is ruled by opposites, starting with ourselves as the subject and everything else as the object, which gives rise to the concept of duality. Dual, of course, means two, a binary involving two components that oppose each other. We usually bounce back and forth between them, feeling good and healthy at one minute, and bad or ill at the other. In philosophy this is known as 'living in the swing of the pendulum of life' (Nicoll et al., 1956). As long as we are moving back and forth, we will achieve great things and fame in life, but we are pretty much guaranteed to lose them again at a later stage, certainly at the time of our death. Continuously bouncing back and forth between opposites will forever keep us on the same plane of our current existence. Our planet earth would not be what it is without the law of opposition. Our summer would not be followed by winter, and there would not be a day that would turn into a night. This law causes us to inhale and exhale and makes our heart contract and expand, it gives rise to our different moods and contradictions, as well as frictions such as 'shall I?' or 'shouldn't I?' and the many dilemmas of choosing between 'yes' or 'no'. When the swing is taking us towards the positive end we feel recharged and exhilarated, but in times when we are taken towards the negative end we feel deflated and even paralysed.

However, if we look at the swing from a greater perspective, we realise that we might not be able to change the course of life and the way it moves us back and forth, but we can change our response to it. This means, according to Ouspensky's teachings, that *both negative and positive movements are occupied and illuminated by the light of consciousness*. This allows us to contemplate and stay centred, rather than feeling that we have reached the ultimate dead end of life, void of possibilities. This deep sense of centredness enables us to see things from a totally different place within us, which means that we are able to see ourselves, as well as other people, with different eyes and from a far more all-inclusive perspective. In Jungian therapy, we are encouraged to acknowledge both sides – the shadow and the light – within us, within the world and within other

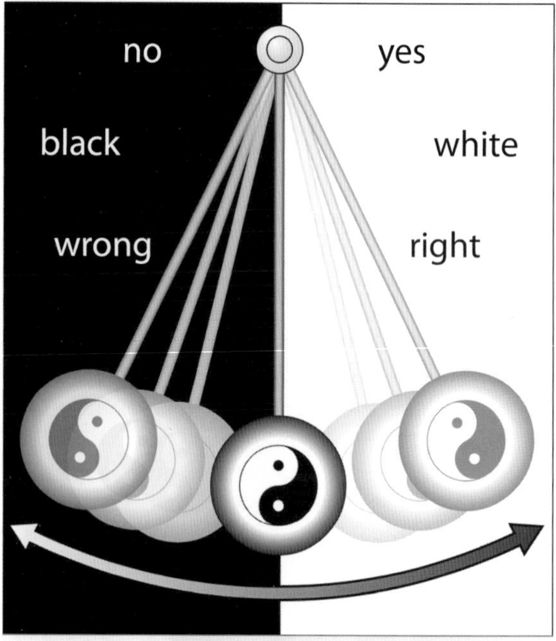

Figure 13.1

We are constantly bouncing back and forth between opposites

people. Hence, the opposites in our psychology are transcended, and our life no longer feels or appears to be randomly disconnected by the shadow and light within us, because we have finally reached the fulcrum in the middle where higher possibilities can be met. Here, we have stepped out of the momentum of the pendulum swing and entered the cyclical motion of life, in which our different 'seasons' are organically unfolding one after the other, and within the cycle of the seasons we go round and round the ever-expanding helix of consciousness. (A practical example of the helix of consciousness can be found in the 'cycles of life' in psychosynthesis.)

In physics, says Matthews (2005 p. 377), 'a "simple" pendulum may be considered as a point mass fastened to the end of a massless cord ... It is then allowed to swing in a plane, its motion being constrained to one dimension.' However, the moment we increase the force of velocity on the mass, the pendulum moves around in a full circle transcending the law of opposites.

The ancient Chinese philosopher Zhuang Zhou (Zhuangzi) is quoted as saying: 'When there is no more separation between "this" and "that", it is called the pivot of the Tao. At the pivot in the center of the circle one can see the infinite in all things' (Li, 1999).

This pivot point of the Tao can be found right in the fulcrum, in the middle between our faculties of awareness and attention. This still-point is the place of application, where awareness, attention and the balancing principle of *space/stillness meet, a place of no position* that gives rise to *lucid cognition*, which is neither active nor passive. So, let's make use of this idea and explore how this changes our perception and how we can utilise it in our work.

As we have mentioned before, at work, as well as in life, the bit of time we don't spend completely absorbed in attention is usually spent in the dynamic between subject and object. That is, we simply alternate between our own sense of self and everything else. We reference what is happening in the external with the knowledge, history and memory that lies in the internal. However, sometimes whilst we are in this linear dynamic, our attention unexpectedly divides, especially in situations where we need to briefly focus on both subject and object simultaneously. For example, during a treatment, if we palpate an unexpected or sudden change in the tissue and don't want to mentally and energetically disconnect from the process in the body tissue, but have to access some anatomical knowledge simultaneously, we instinctively divide our attention between the information we receive through our palpating hands and the knowledge we receive internally. But because our mind is not capable of maintaining a genuine state of divided attention for very long, we simply fall back into the linear subject–object dynamic in which attention will keep the upper hand, which is clearly not neutral. In addition, many mindfulness practices and meditation techniques unintentionally and involuntarily give rise to a brief but genuine state of divided attention, which the practitioner tries to sustain by sheer will power. This force-absorbing attempt is based on the desired objective of mindfulness and meditation to manifest an internal 'witness'. Unfortunately, we soon find ourselves swinging back and forth between trying to sustain the witness and the objects that are witnessed or observed, simply because the neutralising factor or balancing principle is absent, rendering our sheer-will action effectless by depleting its force.

But what would happen if our attention were tripartite – or 'trivided' (invented verb) instead of divided?

It's very simple: we would soon start working from 'a place of no position', which will be discussed in the following section.

Experiment

1. Mindfulness practice: whilst washing up, stay fully present to what your hands are doing. Avoid becoming distracted by anything else around you. Be aware of what happens between you, the observer, and the observed.
2. Choose a book, an apple or any other object and place it 1.5 metres in front of you. Be aware of your own existence, whilst keeping your focus on the object for two minutes without allowing any other distraction to interfere.

You might find that you can't keep this up for very long before you start moving back and forth again between your own sense of self, the respective object and possibly everything else around you that is asking for *attention*.

Working from 'a place of no position'

In 'The triad of time, state and space' (Part 3: Chapter 11) we said that three powers of creation must come together to make something manifest, and the same is true of revealing the quality of 'neutral' that has a genuine balancing effect on our psychology, including our whole mental makeup and different representations of our personality in the form of little 'me's', 'I-believes' and 'personal philosophies'. Our psychology is nourished and informed by what it receives from our awareness and attention in the form of countless impressions that, in succession, are perceived as different events in our lives. But as we already know, awareness (passive power) and attention (active power) on their own can't manifest as neutral, because together they form a binary or opposite, which can only take us into a state of divided attention that, after a brief moment, throws us back into the momentum of the pendulum. However, the moment we utilise the initial appearance of divided attention to 'trivide', by creating *separation* from awareness and attention through the neutralising force of space induced by stillness, lucid cognition comes into play, through which we are able to see what truly lies in front of us. In lucid cognition we naturally shift into a place of no position – a higher psychological state that is quintessentially neutral. Unfortunately, we usually experience ourselves at a much lower psychological state – that of 'I'.

'I' gives rise to duality, because the condition, state or manifestation of 'I' is always separate from everything else. 'I' is not neutral, because the moment it comes into existence it occupies a position of 'me', 'my', 'I' and countless substates. This position can fill a lot of space. However, in a place of no position, the 'I' has profoundly diminished, and has moved into the background, because it has rendered itself passive. Hence, the diminishment of 'I' gives rise to something that is intrinsically neutral. Within this something that is void of any form or shape, only that which sees and perceives without any connotations attached to it exists, possibly as a modality that could be called 'non-I'.

But what do we practically need to do to settle into lucid cognition and work from a place of no position? We have to apply the practice of …

Action through non-reaction

Action through non-reaction involves both active and passive qualities in equal measure. It is a powerful consciousness inducer that enables us to pause, without becoming too passive and falling into awareness, as well as preventing us from mechanically responding to the situation we are in by becoming active and falling into attention.

The following process outlined in the next paragraph happens within less than a couple of seconds.

The moment we meet the unknown during a treatment or session, the higher level of consciousness that the unknown has induced in us allows us to 'non-react', pause and be still. This highly conscious pause (non-mechanical) brings awareness and attention into perfect balance and brings forth a brief moment of genuine divided attention in which the swing of the pendulum *stops*. The stop of the swing gives rise to the fulcrum in the middle, the still-point (neither awareness nor attention but an interconnectedness of both), the place of conjunction through which the neutralising force of 'space' induced by stillness enters, leading to a new proposition of awareness, attention and the infinite space surrounding them. We might experience this influx of space as a liberating sense of expansion, movement or shift in consciousness that separates us from the pendulum swing, because in this expansion our sense of perception suddenly 'trivides'.

We could say our perception transforms, forming a perfect triad sustained by a place of no position somewhere in space that can be felt in the form of inner stillness, and is located between the solar plexus and the lower abdomen (there is no actual physical location), with the faculty of awareness in the background and attention in the foreground, giving rise to a new proposition of lucid cognition and all-encompassing coherence. In the light of lucid cognition we can understand both parts that form the opposite simultaneously, including the opposites that exist in the internal, as well as the opposites that act on us in the external world of experience. Hence, we are leaving the world of bouncing between right or wrong, yes or no, and should I or shouldn't I, and entering the world in which both opposites are perceived, acknowledged and allowed to simply interrelate, whilst we keep flowing with the relevant things in life (Fig. 13.2). In philosophy, this process is called inducing separation, which takes us to the exploration of *observing presence*.

Experiment

Whilst you walk to work, or can engage in some people-watching on a bus or tube or in a coffee shop, simply lean back into yourself and watch how the patterns of the scene unfold.

Observing

All ancient philosophies and schools of thought speak about the importance of establishing an inner witness. Why is that? Because without an inner witnessing quality that lives above the world of our different 'I's' or 'me's', self-study or 'know thyself' and inner change would not be possible.

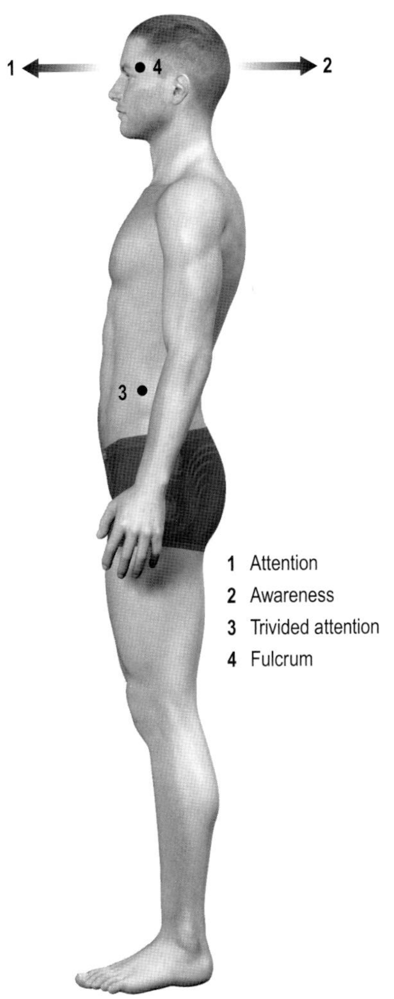

Figure 13.2

The moment our attention 'trivides', we stop bouncing back and forth between awareness and attention

In our field of work, glimpses of this witness are found in complementary teachings on the application of transference and countertransference, as well as in psychological tools that promote healthy boundaries. In life it is usually people who have undergone psychoanalysis or psychotherapy who are familiar with the idea of witnessing. However, here the analysis is synonymous with the ancient idea of the witness, that the witness is neither active nor passive, and is not informed by a past or any kind of psychological state.

As discussed in Part 1: Chapter 3, to be able to change we need a different kind of knowledge that does not belong to the knowledge we usually access by default. We need knowledge that lies above our knowledge, which is, as we already know, higher knowledge that induces change. However, without a witnessing faculty this higher knowledge can't be used or applied, because we haven't established anything within us yet that can remember it for what it is. We can only explain this knowledge by what we know from the level of our relative consciousness, which is biased, and not from the level of consciousness from which this higher knowledge originates. We can find the origin of the idea of the witness and its practice in the Vedas, dating back as early as 5500 BCE.

'The Sanskrit word for the witness is the "sakshi"; and in the teachings of Vedanta the sakshi is used as a pointer to that which is ultimately real' (Dhanya, 2012). The witness is also described as 'a useful device, useful in differentiating That which is ever present in every experience from the changing body and mind' (Dhanya, 2012). In Buddhism, 'the observer or witness is thought of as an aspect of the higher self that is cultivated through meditative practice' (Hill, n.d.). Krishnamurti defines the observer as 'the censor, the experiencer, the evaluator …' (Krishnamurti and Lutyens, 1969).

A more limited definition of the observer can be found in psychoanalytic theory: 'The observing ego is that portion of consciousness that has the ability to observe our actions and behaviors' (Hill, n.d.).

As we mentioned before, observing presence lies above the world of our different psychological states, defined in psychosynthesis as subpersonalities, each one of which possesses its own history, knowledge and memory. The moment one of them becomes activated by a specific internal or external trigger point, we become it (identify), moving it straight into the foreground where it truly believes that it stands for the whole of us. Unfortunately, the currently present subpersonality will witness and observe the world through its own lenses, complete with its biases and 'I-believes'. Furthermore, because our psychological states (subpersonalities) are constantly changing, our state of being will always shift accordingly. Hence, our being will never be experienced nor shine as something independent, clear, distinct and unique within us, forever being controlled by the temporary psychological manifestation of the given moment.

Observing presence, however, can't be developed by simply observing the world through the eyes of our fluctuating personality, which lives in the world of opposites. If we don't neutralise the dynamic between the opposites of awareness and attention to get out of the swing, the observing presence can't reveal itself. Without sufficient *separation* from both our psychological state and all other things that act on us, access to a neutral and objective view of things won't be permitted. This is the reason why the ancient teachings are also defined as the 'work', because inner change is work. When it comes to developing observing presence, our work is to keep applying the consciousness-inducing practice of action through non-reaction, which induces sufficient separation through which we can seamlessly shift into a place of no position. Here, in the all-encompassing light of lucid cognition, observing presence can flourish and grow.

What else can initially help us to establish observing presence, and what makes observing presence so useful in our work as practitioners and therapists?

We can build the foundation for observing presence by studying ideas from different schools of thought, philosophy and psychology. We can also develop it by profoundly deepening our newly acquired knowledge, as presented in the different sections of this book, to transform it into true understanding, as well as by challenging and evaluating our understanding of these ideas by putting them into action at work and in our self-practice. In addition, what makes observing presence so tremendously useful in our work with clients and students is that we can consciously access and utilise it the moment we need to observe from a place of no position, which is its home. That is, observing presence lives outside the dynamics of the ever-changing nature of the divided self, which enables it to keep sufficient separation, so preventing it from identifying with the object it observes, without breaking the dialogue or line of communication through which this so precious neutral information flows.

MY MAIN EMPHASIS IS TO FACILITATE,
TREAT OR TEACH PEOPLE FROM
A PLACE
OF NO
POSITION

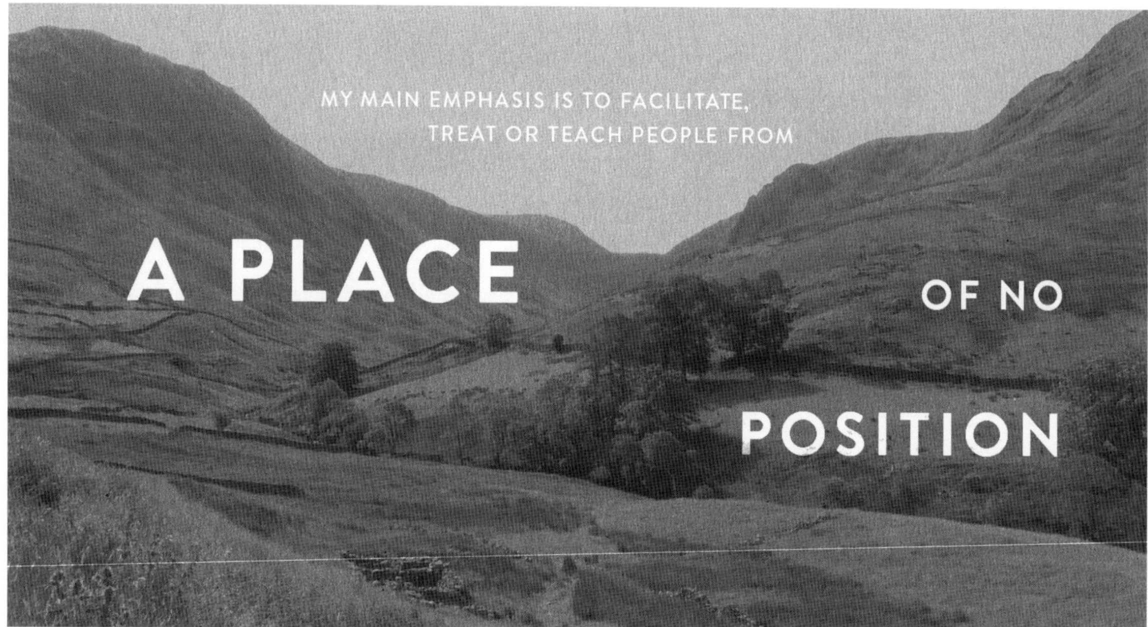

Figure 13.3

Artwork Victoria Dokas; photography Alexander Filmer-Lorch

Another quality of observing presence worth mentioning is that it is able to hold and store the most minute details of what it witnesses, and it remembers things exactly as they were perceived. Hence, observing presence can be compared with a disk that stores all data it receives without compromising the data by taking a position. Additionally, in its non-invasive, unbiased perception, it can't be shocked or compelled by what it observes, even in the most challenging treatments, sessions and classes. In its silent purity and simplicity, once present, observing presence will be highly conscious of all aspects of a treatment or teaching environment. Furthermore, through the extensive higher knowledge it can access, and its utter acceptance of things, it will change and renew the entire basis of our work, as well as our whole concept of our skills, methods and techniques. Because of this our work will grow, flourish and evolve.

Internally, by means of self-study, the objective nature of observing presence frees us from the illusion of what we think we are, and believe ourselves to be, both at work and in life, and gives rise to an entirely new sense and different take on ourselves and the world around us. We no longer need to keep up what prevented us from simply being what we were always meant to be, which lies outside and above our different 'I's' and personality traits. In other words, we can make use of observing presence to promote and further the development of a unique, pure and distinctive inner being.

Experiment

1. Divide your attention between yourself as the seer and the seen (landscape or spacious environment), then gently inhale and, whilst you feel your chest expanding, feel the distance between the seer and the seen increasing. Then give a big sigh of relief. Rest in your solar plexus after the sigh whilst you allow your gaze to soften (soft focus).
2. Let the breath flow naturally for a few minutes before you apply the above again.

Repeat, but leave several minutes before you start with step 1 again.

Thoughts on the relationship between 'observing presence' and 'being'

When it comes to our own personal inner development, observing presence is a powerful means, but not the end. Yet, when it comes to our work as practitioners, choosing to work from a fully established and reliable observing presence during treatments or sessions is more than we could ever wish for, because observing presence is infused, sustained and informed by the inner power of stillness it derives from the inner self. So, the more we work through observing presence, the more it will, just by itself, widen, broaden, inform and enhance our actual being.

The following further thoughts may illuminate our personal understanding of where what we have covered so far in this book can lead to (and might become the subject of a sequel to this book).

In the context of philosophy, observing presence is still considered as an 'I', because it can be perceived by something deep within us. That is, it is a state, possibly even a higher psychological function, that manifests within us in the form of a subjective experience that neutrally observes, monitors, photographs, tapes, stores and registers all it perceives.

However, observing presence is also an 'I' that has the function of a highly conscious and accomplished facilitator, which takes us closer to the formless self and, due to the absence of a history that can project a future, it only exists in the present. That is, in the light of lucid cognition, observing presence highlights and registers what we are not. Neti neti, not this not that, until only what we quintessentially *are* remains as our very existence in the form of a pure and distinctive state of being, through which the formless self finds expression.

To conclude I want to briefly summarise the theory and practice of getting to neutral that we have studied in this chapter.

In ancient philosophy (many different schools of thought) neutral is described as the middle way that leads to the middle or centred person. The centred person has established something within that is not subject to change, which is usually experienced as something utterly peaceful and still, out of which the middle state or neutral can spring into being. This is accomplished through conscious work on our inner faculties of awareness and attention that exist in us as opposites, as well as the many opposites that act on us internally and externally. Through the practice of action through non-reaction, we can neutralise the dynamic forces between our awareness and attention, which gives rise to a natural equilibrium.

Here is how it works in pretty much every situation that keeps us in the dynamic of opposites:

- By applying 'action through non-reaction' the movement of the pendulum swing comes to a stop.
- The neutralising element of 'space' enters, creating sufficient *separation* from all linear dynamics, which enables us to work and act from a centred 'place of no position'.
- The centred place of no position is the abode of 'observing presence', which is informed by the power of inner stillness.

Hence, the repeated manifestation of this entirely new proposition and its imprints evoked by our own conscious effort *will get us to neutral.* A genuine neutral in mind, thought and psychology, allowing us to objectively observe and work in the light of lucid cognition. What more respectful place to work from could there be?

How we utilise what we have covered so far, and how to prepare our body and ourselves to be able to work from the 'insightful self' in a session, treatment or class environment, will be discussed by my co-writer, colleague and friend Maggie Gill (teacher of the Upledger curriculum) in the following chapters of Part 4.

References

Dhanya (2012). *You are the witness – or are you.* Advaita Vision, www.advaita-vision.org/you-are-the-witness-or-are-you/ [accessed 28 Oct. 2015].

Hill, D. (n.d.). *Unity through observation.* Lionserpent.com, http://lionserpent.com/unity.html [accessed 28 Oct. 2015].

Krishnamurti, J. and Lutyens, M. (1969). *Freedom From the Known.* London: Gollancz.

Li, C. (1999). *The Tao Encounters the West.* Albany: State University of New York Press.

Matthews, M., Gauld, C. and Stinner, A. (2005). *The Pendulum.* Dordrecht, the Netherlands: Springer.

Nicoll, M., Gurdjieff, G. and Ouspensky, P. (1956). *Psychological Commentaries.* London: Stuart & Watkins.

Soka Gakkai International (2015). *The Middle Way,* www.sgi.org/about-us/buddhism-in-daily-life/the-middle-way.html [accessed 22 Oct. 2015].

4

Working from the insightful self

From the beginning – introduction and aims 14

In Part 3, Alexander gives us a great deal of information about the characteristics of the insightful self. They enable us to exude a presence of calmness and of grace in our work and our relationships, plus enabling us to live, work and play 'in the moment'. It is important to recognise that this ability to find a point of balance, indeed to be able to embody this insightful self, can make a real contribution to our health and wellbeing.

> *The centred person has established something within that is not subject to change, which is usually experienced as something utterly peaceful and still, out of which the middle state or neutral can spring into being. This is accomplished through conscious work on our inner faculties of awareness and attention that exist in us as opposites, as well as the many opposites that act on us internally and externally. Through the practice of action through non-reaction, we can neutralise the dynamic forces between our awareness and attention, which gives rise to a natural equilibrium.*
>
> Alexander Filmer-Lorch

My aim is to show that through developing a greater awareness of some essentials about our own bodies, we can begin to create the space and freedom to give our minds a chance to think differently. With this sense of space and freedom we can begin to observe from a more neutral place and be more aware of our patterns and habits. We then have a choice open to us – what might we choose to change? What could we replace our existing habits with, and how do we go about putting new ways of working into practice in order for them to become effortless and natural? From this new perception of ourselves, can we begin to take on the characteristics of the insightful self? What do we need to do in order to develop and embody them over time so that we can live them?

Firstly, we need to become aware of who we are right now, to accept that and to gain some insights about what opportunities are open to us on our personal journey. This journey is frequently quite hard work – there is no 'speedy boarding' option or a different and more comfortable 'class' of travel.

> *Your journey is what it is, and it is unique, just as you are!*
>
> Maggie Gill

By sharing his learning and experience, Alexander gives us signposts and insights for our own paths. Make no mistake, achieving lightness and a quiet strength in the very core of our being can take a *paradigm shift*. We might move towards a totally different point of view about what is essential for our own wellness, and what will also support us as we find we can work effectively and effortlessly in our own personal practice, and in our work with our clients and students in our role as facilitator of their self-realisation and their empowerment.

In his introduction Alexander writes about his discovery of the power of accessing stillness-memory during a severe health challenge. Before then he already had his years of study of movement, meditation and bodywork, but he needed to access something else. Something deeper and different. A synthesis of all he already knew. That experience led to the creation of this book.

My aim is to show you, even if you come from a very different background as I did, that it is possible to work towards that place where accessing an inner stillness, referring to it, using it and refreshing and renewing ourselves from it can be a reality.

Early background

My contribution to this book reflects my own journey towards embodying the insightful self. It was not an easy path to move from 'mind over matter' and a successful career path based on 'fixing' and being the 'ideas person', with the certificates on the wall to prove it. It does give me a much greater empathy with my clients and students as they gradually develop trust in their own inner intelligence and develop the presence to be able to access and work with the inner intelligence of their own clients, rather than imposing their own ideas and solutions.

To give some perspective, I believe it's helpful to tell you how things were, how change began and something of the path I have been on.

Quite a few years ago ...

You might have recognised me by my suit, heels and briefcase, but it seemed later that it was my fast walking speed and confident posture that others remembered. My studies whilst training as a teacher of adults from 16 to 90 years old included the philosophy of education and the psychology of the adult learner. I felt a great affinity with the world of communication and learning. My skills in managing teams emerged, and I developed a keen interest in gaining management qualifications.

Studying part-time, alongside working full-time, not to mention family commitments, inspired me to think about managing my time creatively and carefully. At least two mornings a week I studied for exams and wrote essays between 5am and 7am. Promotion came, responsibilities increased, job satisfaction too. Several more initials after my name and I was on a roll to learn more. What next? That's when my body intervened for the first time. Looking back there were other clues it had had enough! But I didn't pick up on the clues; I was too busy of course.

A couple of ribs broken on a very rough channel crossing seemed reluctant to heal. Long story short, I discovered the benefits of holistic massage as practised by a gifted and intuitive practitioner. Intrigued by the modality and even more by the results, I did what came naturally: read all about it and decided to train at weekends for a qualification. The training had a modular structure, and it was extremely well organised with clear timelines for our learning objectives, assessment and examinations. I welcomed those as a clear sign of good-quality, student-centred training. There was a lot to learn, and a really great teacher who inspired us with her knowledge of anatomy and practical massage skills and her wisdom with clients.

I had an affinity with the practical work and quickly gained anatomical knowledge. When my training was complete, I had enjoyed it so much that I took the next step and continued with studying aromatherapy and advanced massage, which brought in techniques from shiatsu, reflexology and acupressure.

Alongside my management career I continued to practise bodywork on a very small group of friends. I found it a great antidote to the stress in my other world.

Promotion again, more responsibility and more job satisfaction.

A couple more years passed and then one of my knees became very painful, walking and driving became really difficult and then, within weeks, the other knee virtually collapsed. Surgery was advised, in the form of a simple arthroscopy to wash out both the joints. I was told that operating on both at once was no problem. A case of getting it over with quickly and then I would be back at work in a week. It seemed to be 'just the ticket', a perfect solution to an uncomplicated problem.

Waking up from the anaesthetic with no idea of which direction my feet were moving in was very strange. As was the pain in both legs, which just went on, and on, and on. Day and night, moving or still, painful spasms appeared in my leg muscles without warning. Around six months later, my career gone, I was unable to walk without at least one stick, and it was painful to sit or stand for long. By now I realised that straightforward answers were not forthcoming. There was no clear advice, other than not to sue the surgeon, but promises started to come from many directions about being able to 'fix' my pain. When various attempts failed, I was told there must be 'something else' causing it. Seeking help from various physical therapists and bodyworkers who made promises was getting me nowhere. Any pain relief was slight and simply temporary.

Reflecting later, I realised that what was in abundance was learning. I had met many principles in practice before I even knew the subject matter! I was immersed in a kind of back-to-front experiential learning about the ethics and the standards of client care in parts of the healthcare business.

The anatomy and physiology I knew? Well, it was pretty useless in the face of what I was experiencing. Most of what I learned was organised according to different body systems. What I now embodied was what happens when one of the major systems is damaged in some way and the wide-ranging effects that can have on the rest of the person.

My mood became pretty bleak as I went from one area of therapy or bodywork to another. Promises from experts and 'gurus', and then there were the folk who seemed like new friends and then showed themselves as 'needing to be needed'. I discovered those who were naturally attracted to others who were in trouble, enjoyed bad news and were not interested in anything positive. I began to realise that communication happens on a much wider field than I had understood before. These experiences were practical applications of psychology that I already knew about. I had the theory in place. The understanding of it began when I was faced with the reality of the disillusionment around all those relationships.

A different educational experience was created as I found others who made no promises but helped me to become interested in the way my body worked. Building on the knowledge I had already, I was now moving towards gaining some real understanding. It was not easy, in fact it was frustrating and sometimes really painful, but it was altogether more useful. Finally, some understanding was gained about why the muscles in my legs were going into painful spasms, and why my posture had changed. I became less alarmed at my lack of ability to balance, and understood why simple tasks like getting up from a chair were such a problem.

To add complexity it seemed that the best ways of managing situations like stairs and walking on sloping ground were counterintuitive, which made them even harder. That was all part of the learning. A huge shift was needed, and it was not going to be a quick fix.

I began to trust word-of-mouth referrals to practitioners I might not have considered, realising that often those who advertise extensively are not necessarily the best. Smart marketing and advertising are no guarantee of quality. I reflect now that it's so easy to say those things, but when we are vulnerable and in pain we look for the fastest route to what we need, based on the world view we have at the time.

Conventional business and marketing practice were part of my old career, so they were a strong part of my default or habit; they were what I trusted first.

Can we pay attention with a soft focus?

I was advised to try a gentle form of yoga in the style of Vanda Scaravelli, and despite my initial resistance – having an entrenched idea of what yoga practice entailed, and knowing that my legs could not do any of it – I found her book made so much sense and offered inspiration. Taught by John Stirk, my understanding of my body and its needs began to develop. John's style of teaching enabled me to gain a much deeper understanding of the mechanics and the fluid movement in the body. His classes are not about superficial movement and pushing into a pose; they go much deeper and enable us to gain an understanding of what potential for movement lies within us and how we can tune into it and gently bring it to the surface. Over many years I have observed students of all ages gaining flexibility and vitality through receiving his inspiring teaching and insights.

> *Experience shows that deeper work has the potential for ever deepening and ever changing. We cannot 'know' it.*
>
> John Stirk, *The Original Body*

After almost two years my GP found another surgeon, apparently one who had a reputation for sorting out surgical 'mistakes', and he operated on both knees separately with about four months in between, and some further healing began.

Can we work without 'trying'?

Now I was able to put into practice some of the work I had already begun in my study of gentle yoga, using gravity and breath to enable movement without strain and stress. The healing after the new surgery was fast and sustained, and the surgeon was intrigued.

Starting with ourselves – preparing to embody a greater awareness 15

When we are in the midst of our full-on world, consider how we view anyone in the family or a work colleague brave enough to mention concerns about us and their perception of a decline in our general wellbeing. The chances are we would dismiss their good advice as competitive rivalry or coming from some negative personal agenda to make us feel inadequate in some way. We might simply smile, shrug our shoulders, possibly thank them, and then work harder to prove them wrong. *Well, I know that's how I might react!*

There is a way to master a bright smile and to reply 'Fine' to any enquiry about one's health. In organisations prone to funding cuts there is always the prospect of staff redundancy and it is often heralded by a restructuring. The 'ministry of rumours' is the only believable word on the street and the pressure to be seen to be well and to be achieving 100 per cent is almost palpable. Uncertainty and change are the only constants in many large organisations.

Any of this seem familiar?

As you can imagine from the previous chapter, when my body got my attention in the past, it simply meant a quest to find an 'expert' to fix it for me, remove any discomfort that might prevent me from working to my capacity, and the sooner the better. My head ruled. The insightful self was a world away.

Becoming interested in the details without losing the whole picture

The chances are that if you are reading this book then something is already drawing you to something different to enhance your lifestyle and your health.

Good intentions are one thing. This kind of change – embodying and working from the insightful self – is not about a *resolution*; it's potentially a *revolution*. Sometimes the prospect of a revolution is something we cannot contemplate. It would cause more stress and more complications than we can handle. So, if we are convinced that change is necessary, we might decide to take an *evolutionary* path and to manage a change in stages, which gives us an intelligent and sustainable process as part of our working towards maximising our health.

Observing how a lack of awareness of our own bodies can inhibit us as we work

Discovering Dr John Upledger's CranioSacral Therapy and beginning to learn in depth about the craniosacral system complemented my gentle movement practice. Inspiration and motivation began to flourish. I began to train as a craniosacral therapist. As my bodywork practice grew I started assisting in Upledger classes and eventually, after some years of training and experience as a craniosacral therapist, I became a teacher of the work. Finding that a lack of body awareness and poor posture were key factors in inhibiting the palpation ability of many therapists in training led me to think hard about ways of helping them by drawing on my own learning experiences.

My belief is that to create stillness-memory we need space in our physical body: space to move, to breathe and to allow fluid flow. We need to be aware of where we are holding tension so that we can release or reduce it. We need to develop the ability and the willingness to 'tune into' our own bodies several times a day and check out what's happening during home and work activities, not simply rely on an hour once a week in a class. Before finding John Stirk as a teacher, I observed yoga classes where students pushed themselves and competed with others, thereby defeating the very name of the work. Creating stillness-memory is unlikely to come from an adrenaline-fuelled activity.

You might be reading this from the point of view of a broad knowledge of anatomy. My challenge would be to ask if, through practical application, you have gained a level of real understanding? The next would be whether through work and effort you are now embodying that understanding and are living it? If you are a bodyworker or physical therapist then please don't ever let your superior knowledge of anatomy, hard-earned though it might be, get in the way of what you are palpating or seeing. That includes your own body as well as your work with clients and students.

So let's start with some reminders around key points in our own bodies and some small but beautifully effective ways of helping them function optimally.

Getting onto our feet – standing up for ourselves and deepening our awareness of how our foundations affect our structure, our vitality and our breath

Our feet are a long way from our heads, and if you think that your head rules and therefore anything to do with your feet is insignificant, or some whacky new-age nonsense, then you might be tempted to skip over the next few pages. If you do then you will miss something really powerful and valuable. The key to our posture, and therefore our mobility, is to be found in our feet. The experiments and exercises that follow will facilitate whole-body change and enable you to feel a greater sense of space in your body. Space enables lightness and stillness.

I didn't believe it either, so please don't waste time on ignoring your feet for as long as I did. Get in on the experience curve, because we really don't all have to start at the beginning, or wait until we are in pain.

Alexander reminds us of three Os: Open body, Open heart, Open mind. I invite you to become acquainted with some basics about your feet, and to be open-*hearted* about them, not to regard them simply as support for the rest of you, but to value them sincerely. Remember the last time you cracked a toe on some piece of furniture? Did that experience open your heart a little towards just how much we don't appreciate the periphery of our body unless something goes wrong and causes us pain?

Now open your *mind* to a few important points about your feet and how, just possibly, you could develop an interest in what they are doing, how they are doing it and whether they could be doing it better with a little more focus from you. I am not going into anatomical detail because there are so many excellent texts available. If you don't have one then I suggest you go to a bookshop where there is a facility to relax, or a café where you can peruse several books whilst enjoying some refreshment. Look out for one that explains how you move, not simply a map of bones, ligaments and the like. Movement is the key, after all, so you might as well get the best book to help you on the quest to find out more about yourself. The very best way to learn anatomy is to discover what something *does* and then find out more.

Our feet are indeed a feat

They are quite simply brilliant. Yes! I can hear the anatomists say, there are 26 bones – most of the time we treat them as though they are made up of very few.

What do you already know about them? You will be aware of toes, arches and heels, but how long is it since you really considered them? They are often tightly controlled in their ability to work – we cover them in shoes that are fashionable rather than functional, thereby we compromise our precious connection to the ground, and our ability to balance. We might well sideline the parts of our feet and legs that are designed to act as load-bearing, and our brilliant body in its quest for homeostasis and equilibrium rapidly starts to adapt. An unskilled observer would see us as 'just fine'. But we are using energy and effort to maintain our equilibrium – and we don't even know it.

Don't believe me? Then, provided you are reading this somewhere safe (don't do it if you are reading on a train or a railway platform), please remove one shoe. It doesn't matter if you are wearing heels, boots or brogues. Now begin to walk slowly around. If you are in a room with a mirror and can catch a glimpse of yourself from time to time that can be useful. If you are not alone and can persuade others to try this, even better still, as you will all be able to observe what happens. Do not try to do anything in particular, just be yourself, just look ahead and simply walk. Perhaps it will help you to take your mind to something else.

After a few minutes what do you notice? The chances are that you will find that you don't notice the absence of the shoe so much; in fact, if you are observing someone else, you will see their posture looks pretty normal. The body is adapting.

Adapting is what we do very well, and we do it naturally. It takes effort and energy to hold adaptive patterns, so the more we can support balance and equilibrium from the ground the better. We have other areas further up our body to become aware of, so if we can focus on starting with this one then we are already getting our foundations in place. After all, a building with a beautiful second storey and roof doesn't stand much of a chance if the foundations are inadequate, does it?

Into practice – working with the potential in our feet

Now some examples of how you can 'take a moment' to make a big difference in your own foundations.

Experiment

Take a moment: before you get out of bed

This exercise really wakes your feet up, and also gets the circulation in your legs and lower body going.

Lie comfortably on your back, with your feet in a relaxed position, which we will call neutral. Next, point your toes away from you and really stretch your feet. Hold this for 10 seconds. Then bring your toes back to the neutral position and wait for 10 seconds. Then pull your toes towards you, pushing your heels away for 10 seconds. Back to neutral for 10 seconds, and repeat the sequence at least three times.

Finally, circle both your ankles slowly in one direction three times, then after a 10-second rest in their starting place, circle in the opposite direction. Come back to the starting place and then it's time to get out of bed. Notice how your feet feel as they connect to the floor for the first time, and how warm your calves are. Great start to the day!

I notice that some students in movement classes are reluctant to touch their feet; at times there is an element of distaste. Are they sweaty, dirty, unkempt? Or simply at a distance and a source of occasional annoyance? This is a sure sign it's time for some renovation and a change of attitude. Make sure your toenails are cared for and you are not harbouring fungal infections

Experiment

Take a moment: after bathing or showering

Dry your toes and the areas in between them thoroughly. Difficult to reach? Stand carefully, then put one foot onto a chair or stool or the side of the bath. Bending carefully to dry your feet is one of the first awareness exercises of the day. Seated or standing, after showering or bathing, please become more aware of your feet and start taking great care of them. Check your nails and skin daily to avoid infection or inflammation.

Experiment

Take a moment: to consider your stability

When you walk, how much attention do you pay to the way you are using your feet? There are three key places to be aware of: your heel, the base of your big toe and the base of your smallest toe. We aim to connect equally with these three points.

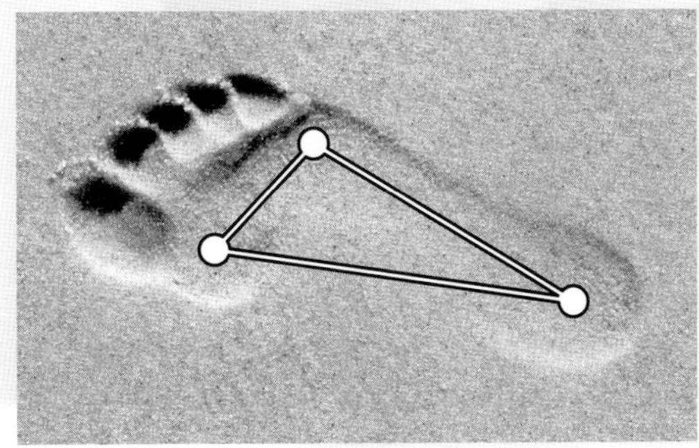

Figure 15.1

Three key places to be aware of

One of these key places is often ignored – the little toe side of the foot and the base of the little toe itself. From where you are now, sitting or standing, just bring your attention to it. Consider how easy it is to move it, to press it into the floor. If you are wearing shoes that prevent any of your toes moving then I hope they are for short-term use only. You need to be able to move them and your whole body posture will benefit.

Experiment

Getting in touch with stability

1. If you have any difficulty with balance, or feel uncertain, stand next to a chair or close to a wall.

   Starting with your feet bare and standing with your feet parallel and hip-width apart, simply wiggle your toes, lift them and spread them out as far as possible. Scrunch them into the surface you are standing on. Notice which toes move most easily. No judgement, just notice – this is all useful information about where we are starting from.

2. Next, lift all your toes straight up as far as you can (Fig. 15.2), keeping the base of your big toes and little toes and both heels firmly on the ground. Count to 10, and then let them relax for 10. Do this at least three times.

3. Bring your feet together so your big toes are as close as possible. Ideally they should be touching at their sides; if they are spreading apart from one another, reach down with your fingers and encourage them to be closer together. Lift all your toes up as you did in step 2 and this time spread them apart at the same time. Do this at least three times.

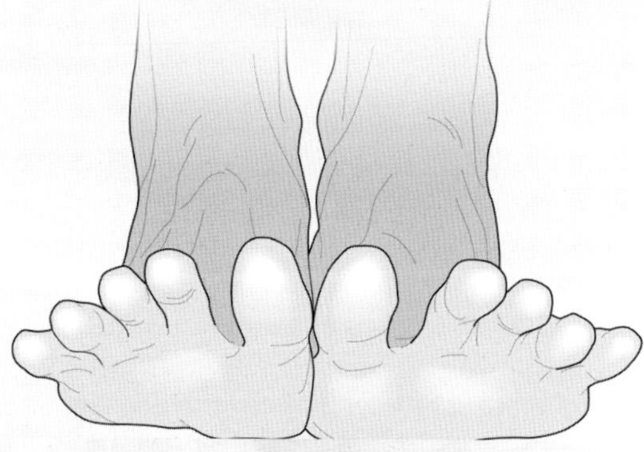

Figure 15.2

Lifting and spreading your toes

Experiment

Take a moment: to consider how you walk

For this exercise keep the gliding movement as slow as you can and really focus on your feet.

In comfortable shoes or sandals that allow your toes to move, or bare feet if you are on a suitable surface, begin by simply standing (feet parallel and hip-width apart). Make sure you have the three key load-bearing points on both feet in your mind. Now, focus on your left heel and its connection to the ground as you take your right foot forward to make your first step. Plant your right heel first and make sure that as you take this slow stride you connect all the way to the top of your right big toe. Leave your left heel in contact with the ground for as long as you can, then as you move to the very end of your left big toe you are ready to lift that foot to take the next slow stride.

Aim to count to four as you take each step. Really work your heels into the ground and make sure you connect with your whole foot as far as the end of the big toe each time.

As you gain confidence in your balance at this slow pace, you can allow the opposite arm to swing, and encourage your hips and shoulders to move freely. Then simply take these principles into your normal walking speed, but challenge yourself to make your strides absolutely even, so if someone were able to listen to your footfalls there would be no difference in pace between them.

When you are comfortable with this, add in the principle of working with a soft focus and feel how quietly you can make your footfalls. Bring in your awareness of your breath, breathing gently through your nose, and feel your shoulder blades move a little towards your pelvis as your sternum lifts. Keep your chin softly towards your chest. Enjoy an effortless walk whilst feeling your calves working and your feet gaining in strength.

Experiment

Take a moment: to take your feet in hand and create some space

No matter how many years you have confined your feet in narrow shoes, or whatever your age, taking your feet in hand on a regular basis will gradually wake up the structures and allow easier movement and fluid flow. If it feels uncomfortable or even quite painful at first then go gently. Do *not* let it put you off. You will not damage your feet, and in fact you are undoing the damage that has already been done! Take any discomfort as a sign that you really do need to do this. Remember the foundations you have are yours and yours alone; no one else's feet can do this for you. Time spent on improving your foundations will be well rewarded, potentially all the way up to your jaw. If you like to use a foot powder or lotion to make these exercises a little smoother, please do!

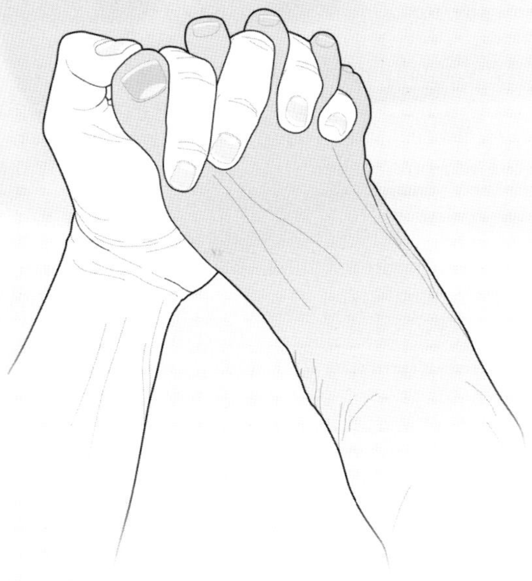

Figure 15.3

Weaving our fingers between our toes

1. Sit on a chair, or on the floor, or on your bed. This is great to do before you go to sleep, or whilst you are watching TV, or generally taking a little quiet time for yourself.
2. Bend your right knee and take your right foot with both hands. Slide the little finger of your left hand into the space between your little toe and its neighbour. (Fig. 15.3) Just support your foot with your right hand. Continue until all your fingers are interlaced with your toes.
3. Wiggle your fingers and toes to make sure you are as close to the very bottom of the space as possible.
4. Spread your fingers to make as much space as possible between them, stretching your toes apart as you do so.
5. Stay there for a few minutes, then change sides. It's really interesting to take a moment to stand after working on one foot and notice the difference in the way you are connecting to the ground.

When this feels smooth and easier, you can stay there longer and take advantage of the position to give your big toes a massage, focusing up and down their sides and all over their back and front.

Experiment

Take a moment: to brighten up and ease compression

This is a great chance to bring in reflex points on the feet; but don't worry if you don't believe in reflexology, you don't have to. Just do the exercise and feel the benefits anyway.

1. Sit on a chair, or the floor, or your bed. This is good to do when you are tired at the end of a working day and want to feel refreshed and vital before going out. It's also great for easing a tired back after a long day of driving, sitting in front of your computer or being on your feet. You can, of course, do this any time you are seated and able to use your hands on your feet.

2. Bend your right knee and take your right foot with both hands.
3. Supporting your foot with your right hand, make a fist with your left hand and work your knuckles all over the instep (think about the supporting arch) and generally all areas of the sole.
4. After working all over that arch and foot, change feet.

To make a change from using your knuckles, or to add a few more minutes to this beneficial foot 'opening', try using both thumbs in a scissoring motion all over the arches and soles.

Experiment

Take a moment: for serious play

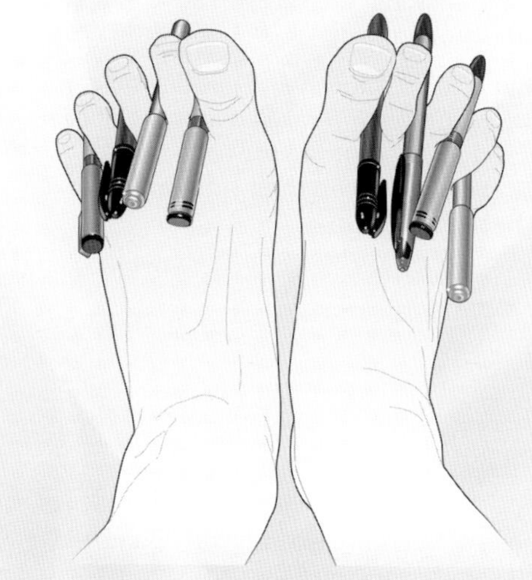

Figure 15.4

Serious play with toes and pens

If you plan to be seated or to have your feet up for a while, then be a little light-hearted and place any pens, pencils or markers you have to hand in between your toes. It's much more fun than using pedicure aids, and you can use smaller ones for any smaller or particularly 'ouchy' spaces. I am not suggesting you are going to walk around with these, so keep the telephone handy, and ignore the doorbell.

or ignoring painful cracks on your heels. A really good time to start a different relationship is after bathing.

The pelvis

After considering our feet we go straight up to our pelvis. Again, if you are interested in looking into the complexity of this beautiful structure then there are lots of anatomical texts. I will refer at the end of this section to some that have informed my understanding over the years. Suffice to say that it's often referred to as the pelvic bowl or basin because that is its shape. It has important links to other structures, including our respiratory diaphragm, the main muscle we use when we breathe. I am going to focus on the bony landmarks that can easily be brought into our everyday actions. My aim is that by being aware of just a few of the structures that link our feet, hips, pelvis, respiratory diaphragm, neck and head, we can work, moment by moment, in our everyday activities to ensure we are in the best position for our body to function optimally. Once again this is about *becoming interested in the details without losing the whole picture.*

If you are sitting down reading this, I wonder if you are using the best bones in your pelvis to support you? Let's see. Slide a hand beneath one of your buttocks and put a little extra weight through that side. Feel a bony support? Try both hands beneath and you will notice you have two of these. Welcome to your ischial tuberosities. If you ensure they are taking your weight rather than your sacrum, the triangular bone at the end of which is the coccyx or tail bone, then your spine has a chance to stack itself up in a balanced way.

Or then again, perhaps you are leaning back, slumping a bit? If that is the case, you will be expecting your sacrum to take your weight. Now, your sacrum is not designed for that, and we need to bear in mind that it has some important relationships with bones around it. If those bony relationships are put under strain then pain and trouble are likely to follow at some stage.

Be aware that the muscles of your abdomen, lower back and pelvic floor all have their role to play in the balance of your pelvis. It is complex. It is very easily put out of balance if your feet are not doing their best work, so rest assured we are already working on your pelvis from the ground up.

Experiment

Take a moment: to connect with your pelvis and balance

One of the most accessible ways of challenging your pelvis is to stand on one leg. This is not always convenient, but you can do some good work when you are standing in a queue at the supermarket or bank, coffee shop or airline desk. If you know you already have problems balancing then do this at home first, standing close to a wall or a chair.

Stand with your feet parallel and hip-width apart. You will be becoming naturally aware of the three points that are vital for load-bearing. Start by checking you have your weight evenly distributed so that both feet feel they are taking the same weight. Now, without lifting your right foot, and keeping your pelvis and shoulders as even as possible, begin to slowly shift your weight towards your left foot. It is interesting to notice whether a part of one of your feet tends to grab the weight. Keep adjusting through this part and you will be developing stronger links between your brain and your feet. Continue until you gradually have all your weight on your left foot. You could, if you wanted to, lift your right foot completely off the ground, and if you did you would be balanced and secure. But you don't, because you don't want anyone in the queue to realise what you are doing!

This is all part of the fun and it makes the exercise more challenging. Now, just as gradually (and this is important), begin to shift your weight from your left foot until it is evenly distributed between both feet again. Rest in this evenly balanced place for a few moments then, just as carefully and slowly, repeat on the other side. This can be a tiring piece, so congratulate yourself afterwards, and don't completely forget where you are in case you need to gently shuffle forward in the queue. Keep a soft, easy breath through your nose as you do this.

Experiment

Take a moment: whilst you are lying down, in bed or on the floor

Be comfortable with a pillow behind your head, your feet flat on the mattress or floor and your knees bent. Have your feet hip-width apart, and close enough to your pelvis so that you can feel just a little tension in your thighs. Now, with one hand feel how much space there is between the back of your waist and the mattress/floor. Aim to flatten the lower part of your back onto the mattress/floor very slowly so that there is no longer a space there. You will need to connect with your tummy muscles to do this, and to curl your sacrum and tail bone towards the front of your body. Push your back slowly, gently but firmly down and hold for at least a count of 10. Then relax for a count of 10 and repeat six times. This very simple exercise is a great way of connecting with your tummy muscles and is helpful for your lower back and your pelvis.

All these connections contribute to your being able to feel freedom and space in your whole body. Within that freedom and space there is the possibility of creating the tissue memory of balance and stillness.

So, back to the pelvis and the ways we can work simply with it – every day.

This is good to do regularly when you wake up or before you go to sleep. Make it a very ordinary part of your commitment to creating freedom and flow in your body. If you are watching TV then get on the floor and do it during the commercials. The more ordinary you make it the better.

If you take a moment to look at Fig. 15.5, please consider the way the psoas muscle creates powerful links between the area of the back of your waist, right down into your hips. You can imagine why this muscle, which is all about core strength and

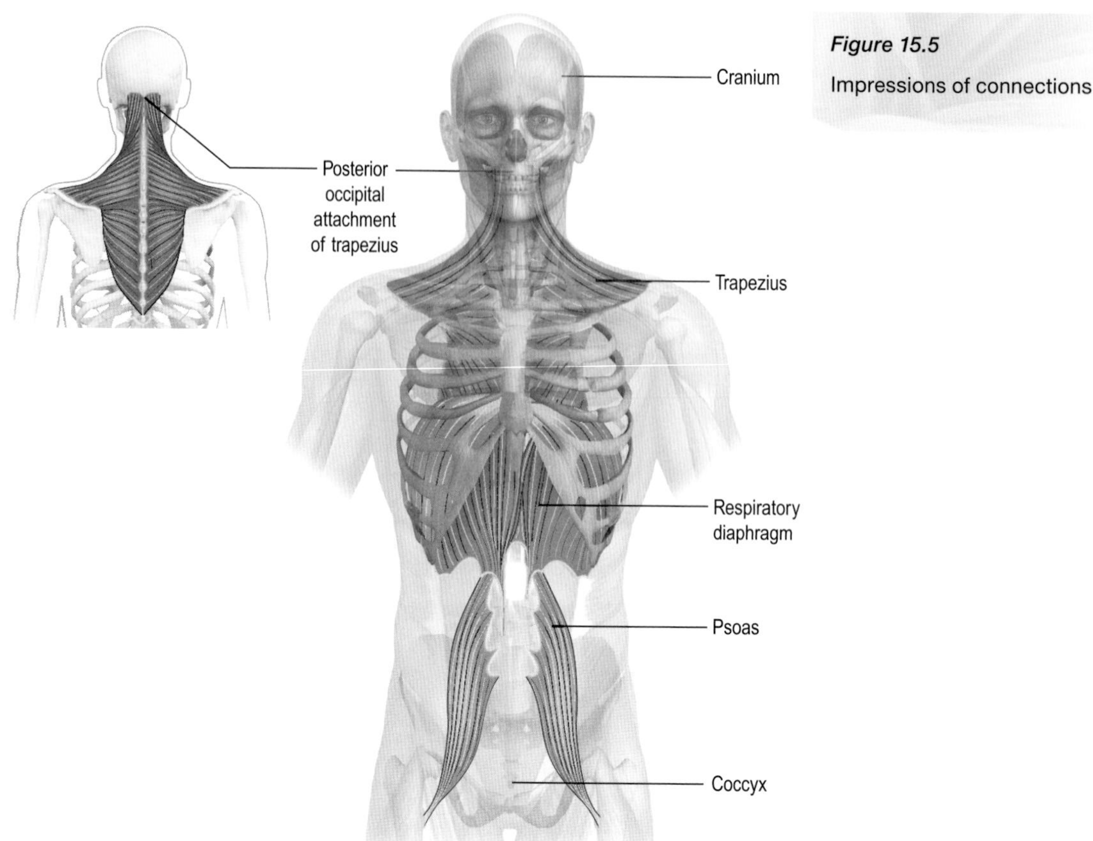

Figure 15.5

Impressions of connections

stability, has a strong focus in the worlds of Pilates and yoga. It is also linked into our stress responses, and it will pull us forward as it spontaneously shortens when we are extremely stressed. Ultimately, it will cause us to roll into a ball to defend ourselves.

When we are not in an extremely stressed state but we are used to functioning at high stress levels, it is easy to imagine that its close relationship to our respiratory diaphragm and our trapezius muscle brings in a very wide area that could be affected, shortened or simply less able to feel spacious and fluid as we move. In fact, when you consider the trapezius and its connection to the occiput, a bone at the back of our head, then I wonder if you could believe that, in some people, persistent shoulder and neck tension might be caused by something as far away as our pelvis or even one of our feet?

Anatomy texts I have found useful:

Atlas of Human Anatomy, Frank H Netter, M.D., published by Elsevier. ISBN -10: 1455758884.

Principles of Anatomy and Physiology, Gerard J Tortora and Bryan H Derrickson, published by Wiley. ISBN - 10: 9780470 565100

As I mention earlier in this chapter - if you are not sure, then go to a good bookshop or library, and take time to relax and browse, then choose the book that suits you. Enjoy!

Looking ahead to Part 5: Chapter 23, Alexander describes the structures, mechanics and stages in our breathing. In Fig. 15.5 we gained an impression of the links between the respiratory diaphragm and the upper and lower parts of our body. As Alexander tells us, breathing happens spontaneously and is controlled by our autonomic nervous system.

We can, of course, bring our attention to our breath and alter its rhythm, and there are many exercises in different modalities where this is practised. Any exercise that involves changing our natural breathing rhythm must be done with great respect and gentleness. He also describes the way we tend to breathe when we are stressed and agitated. If you take a moment to observe the breathing pattern of someone arriving late for a class or an appointment, you will see this clearly. It is always easy to observe this in someone else, and yet it can be really difficult to notice it in ourselves, especially when it is a gradual change over time, rather than a reaction to a short-term situation like trying to catch a train.

What happens to our voice and our expression?

As a teacher, therapist or someone who works with people, it is vital that we are aware of our stress levels. The easiest clue we have is to tune into our breathing rhythm and notice how much of our upper body we are using as we breathe. Without changing anything about your breath right now, just place one hand on your upper chest and one at the level of your umbilicus (that's just below your waist level). Are both hands moved by your breathing or just the top one? If we are using a shallow breath, and our shoulders are being pulled up as our muscles tighten, then we can appear agitated to an observer even if our words appear calm. When we are stressed, our speech pattern generally becomes faster, and our facial expressions tend to be limited. Any effort to smile can make things worse as it does not match the expression in our eyes, which might well appear wide and staring or hostile. The muscles in our throat can become tense and they certainly affect our ability to speak clearly and fluently.

Notice how many people clear their throats in the first few minutes of beginning a conversation with a stranger. You will also see this as some people move up to the reception desk to announce their arrival or ask for an appointment at a doctor's surgery or in a hospital department. If we are not used to speaking in public then, apart from clearing our throats to cope with a sudden tightness or congestion, we often feel as though our tongue has swollen and is taking up far too much room in our mouth. Our words sound strange. We might just begin to panic and forget what we are about to say!

We use the phrases 'choked with emotion' and 'struck dumb' when we are faced with something that limits our ability to speak. This could be a severe shock, such as a fire, earthquake, road traffic accident or sudden death of a loved one. It could also be a tissue memory created by a childhood incident: frightening experiences at home around parents or siblings, or perhaps bullying at school by our peers. It can happen where a child was ridiculed by the teacher (especially if it is one they really liked and admired) in front of the whole class when answering a question incorrectly.

In my practice I have observed several clients who have discovered issues with their voice when faced with making presentations at work or preparing for an interview. They might already have tried singing lessons or some training in presentation skills. When these are unsuccessful they look for another solution. My treatment is based on a whole-body evaluation, which enables me to palpate areas of restriction in their tissues.

Working over that area (not necessarily the throat, as you can imagine after our work with the feet and the connections in the body so far) with gentle techniques can help to facilitate the release of tissue memory, and the client becomes aware of an earlier time when they experienced difficulty speaking. Change begins to happen when the client recognises that their body has held that memory and it has created a tissue restriction, actually preventing their expression in stressful situations. At the time the memory was created, this inhibition was needed to keep them safe from harm or from ridicule. When that can be accepted and acknowledged, their tissue releases and relaxes and from now on they have a chance to work with their voice to restore its power and strength.

Into practice – working with the potential of our breath

Experiment

Working from the back of our bodies

Alexander talks about the power of using the back of our bodies. I would ask you to work with this in combination with your breath. To do this we simply visualise the back of our diaphragm working to bring in our breath. Engaging the muscles on the back of our body to bring in this quieter, calmer breath immediately changes the way we feel. You can do this any time – but especially when feeling uncomfortable, perhaps in a meeting where the chairs are not great, any time you are travelling and whenever you are becoming tired. Taking a nice deep breath through the back of your body enables your sternum (front of your chest) to fill from the inside and to lift naturally.

Experiment

A calming breath to use when we are faced with difficult situations

Sometimes there is an opportunity to use the breath and its effect on our nervous system in order to calm it. Examples would be making a presentation, feeling restless and unable to sleep or visiting the dentist (apologies to dentists, but there are still plenty of people who are nervous about this one).

How do we do this?

We decide to count as we take our in-breath and then make our out-breath last longer. We need to do this for a while, and definitely without stress and struggle, so I would suggest starting with counting four seconds in and six out. You can make it longer, but you should be able to do this easily and not be gasping to take your next in-breath. It really can work. One of my clients who had the worrying combination of being extremely nervous about visiting his dentist for a long procedure and having a serious heart condition, including two previous heart attacks, tried this simple technique and went to sleep during the procedure. His dentist was intrigued, having known my client for a long time, and concluded he must have taken drugs. My client taught this simple technique to the dentist and his nurse, and they now use it with their nervous clients.

Integrating what we have so far and noticing our voice

So – as you bring in your great connection with your feet to the ground, your balanced and relaxed pelvis and soft relaxed breath, notice how your voice is.

My client was feeling undervalued at work. He described his frustration at becoming angry whenever he tried to state his case for a better job and, most importantly, for a salary increase: 'I know what I want to say, but as soon as I am in that office I feel my legs wobble and I can hardly breathe, yet alone speak. I feel an absolute idiot and often don't even start what I really want to say, but simply talk about something else and get out of there as quickly as possible.'

My evaluation showed a restriction in the area of his respiratory diaphragm. As I connected there and allowed my hands to softly blend with his tissue, he described a vivid memory. As is common in my practice, clients who experience this type of memory start by saying something like, 'You'll think I'm crazy but I just saw myself in the headmaster's office.'

My response goes something like this: 'No, I don't think you are crazy in the least. Please tell me more about how it feels to be there.'

'I am so angry. I have been accused of stealing someone's pen. I didn't do it, but in our class, even though I know who did it, we never "tell" on someone else. The head says he is going to talk to my parents.'

I ask him how old he is when he is there, and also to tell me more about the headmaster's office, the headmaster's name and what he thought of the headmaster when he was 12 years old.

A good deal of detail about the place, the character and the client as a 12-year-old emerges gently. I ask him if, with hindsight, there is anything he would like to say to the headmaster, knowing that he was unable to do so at the time. When he has said his piece I ask him to imagine what the headmaster would reply to that.

Later that day I received a message from him to say he had gone straight back to work, and was feeling like a new person. He reported: 'I felt completely connected from top to toe. I went into the office and nothing changed – no wobbly legs or emotional stuff.

My voice was calm and strong and I felt I was able to breathe all the way down to my boots. I have negotiated a new job description, a salary increase and, even better, their full support to do a master's level course which is related to my work.'

Sometimes just one session can make a huge difference to a client, and can really validate our own trust in the style of work we do.

Generally, there is a greater understanding of the situation after this kind of dialogue, and my client's respiratory diaphragm and the area around his occiput freed up considerably.

Our neck, arms and hands 17

Moving upwards from the great foundations of our feet, pelvis and respiratory diaphragm, we now consider the area of the neck, which many of us and our clients describe as 'Where I keep my stress', 'My headaches start from there', or 'That's my weak point'.

If you have already put into practice the exercises with your feet and pelvis then you will be starting to move with increasing fluidity. This will be particularly noticeable as you walk. Your feet will be well and truly on the ground as your focus goes quite naturally to the three load-bearing points and to making sure you are using those points evenly. Our breathing is soft and gentle, not forced, and we are connecting, whenever we need to, to the back of our body and involving the muscles of our back in creating a calming breath.

As we create our soft and even footfalls, our arms start to move naturally, our shoulders become softer and we sense our upper body becoming lighter. Standing for a moment, we can sense our upper body lifting from our mid back, and our lower body with all its strength is grounded and poised to propel us forward when we decide it is time to move.

We are already influencing our neck with our good work so far, and we have considered some of the links between key muscles from our hips all the way to the back of our head. The structures within and around our neck are extremely complex and, apart from the delicate and mobile vertebrae allowing us to move our heads, we have vital fluid pathways connecting our head and our body. Our brain needs this flow to be as free as possible in both directions. We are much more comfortable if the structures in our neck can glide and move well. So, what gets in the way of this perfect situation? Various challenges influence our neck, including the way we sit, especially if we sit to work.

We have developed our individual patterns and habits with posture as we walk and sit. If we are used to spending time working at a computer, or we need to sit when we are working with our clients, then we need to consider once again whether we are using our sitting bones or if we are slumping onto our sacrum. Perhaps the chair we use is meant to be helpful to us and can be adjusted, but we feel a strain in our back after using it for only an hour.

This is something to sort out and manage for the sake of our health. If we find ourselves with our back feeling unsupported then we move into a 'chin forward' posture, thereby encouraging a shortening of our neck muscles. The connective tissues influence the extent to which our vertebrae can move, and then finally there is the possibility that there is reduced space all round, and over time nerve pathways can become reduced. Tension headaches can be a feature too.

We might start feeling some numbness or tingling in our fingers when we wake up, and we are aware of strain and tension, and possibly pain, in our necks, shoulder and hands. There is a real possibility of an unpleasant cycle being created here. You will recall my mentioning that our trapezius muscle links the back of our waist to both our shoulders and to the back of our head. This is just one of the influences on our neck. There are very many muscles involved here, but I wanted to point this one out because it helps to make sense of why clients feel symptoms at a distance from their actual problem.

The occiput I mentioned is at the back of our head and, either side of it, offering a home to our ears, are our temporal bones. The relationship between them and the occiput involves an important gap, which forms a passageway for vital structures, including our jugular vein and three of our cranial nerves. One of those nerves looks after the main muscles of our neck, the trapezius and the sternocleidomastoid. When a nerve doesn't have all the space it needs then it can become irritated, just as you might do if you were in a crowded and restricted space.

So – if our posture as we work encourages our neck to shorten, and this begins to influence the shape of the gap between occiput and temporals, and that brings about an annoyed nerve, which then causes the muscles it looks after to become even tighter … Can you see what I am getting at? It's not an instant thing; it happens over time, but add in some tension around work deadlines, relationship stress and a little anxiety about job security and concerns about difficult clients and the whole thing serves to create a number of possible symptoms, including headaches, migraine and pain in the shoulders, arms and hands. I didn't mention that one of those nerves is the vagus, which looks after many functions in our body. If you take a look at it and check out all the areas it influences then you will soon see that we need our vagus to be as happy as possible.

Another client story to illustrate this

With a diagnosis of irritable bowel syndrome and weekly migraine headaches, my client was pretty miserable and was concerned about whether he was likely to lose his job as a software designer. My evaluation took me to the area of his thoracic diaphragm, in fact to the area of his sternum and clavicles (collar bones). With gentle techniques the tissue in this area began to soften and the next area of tension showed clearly around the base of his cranium. Working there I found the muscles at the back of his head and neck to be very tight and hard. I asked him about his work and, apart from a lot of stress and tension around deadlines and client demands, he mentioned he was concerned about sore eyes. He also worked at home on his sofa or even in his bed as he would occasionally work through the night to get his tasks done.

He really liked the technique at the back of his head and felt his muscles beginning to release and soften: 'I think I am going to be taller after this. I can feel my neck lengthening.'

He came for several sessions, during which we discussed the possibility of eye strain (he needed spectacles) and also the ways in which he could safeguard his posture even when he needed to work incredibly long hours. At one stage, and rather hesitantly, he asked whether the work we were doing could have any effect on his digestion, because it was much calmer. I showed him a picture of his vagus nerve and encouraged him to research it on his computer and see what he made of its influence. We also talked a little about the relationship between this area and migraine headaches, and he mentioned they were reducing in severity and frequency.

This client has sessions around every six weeks now, as he finds that helps him to manage his work challenges. The irritable bowel symptoms are gone, and he has occasional headaches but not migraines. By paying attention to his body as he works and getting regular treatment, he has been able to manage the work he really enjoys so that it doesn't affect his health in a negative way.

Experiment

Take a moment: to keep our necks mobile

We now need to explore some simple, but immensely helpful, ways to keep our necks mobile. Awareness of these could well help us recognise and subsequently avoid, or certainly manage, any patterns we fall into as part of our work.

To make this as effective as possible we are going to combine it with using our breath as we move. When we take our breath in – our inhalation – we do nothing. When we breathe out – our exhalation – we move.

You can do this when you are standing, remembering to connect with your feet, or whilst you are seated, in which case remember to connect with your sitting bones. In both cases we are going to prepare the front of the area by softening your jaw first. This is also a preparation for our next chapter, where there will be more information about why this is so important. Just for now, imagine or intend that the area below your tongue becomes floppy and soft, and allow, with your mouth closed, your lower jaw (mandible) to float gently as though it is suspended very softly from its joint with your temporal bones. This joint is known as the temporomandibular joint or TMJ. You might have heard someone say they have an issue with it.

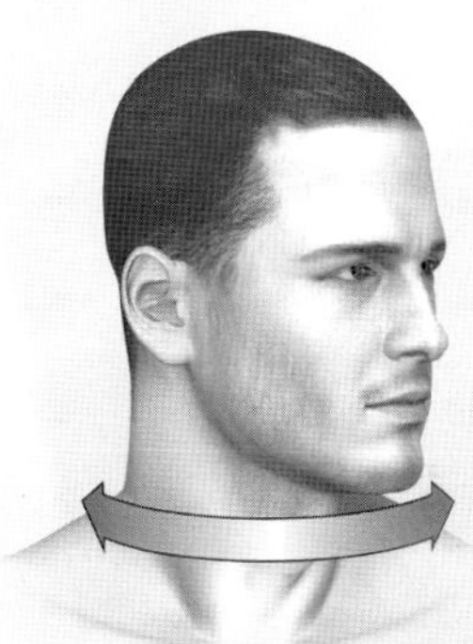

Figure 17.1

Effortless rotation to wake up our neck muscles

Start by looking ahead, take your first soft and effortless inhalation (no need to count) and on your exhalation gently rotate just your head to the left (Fig. 17.1). Do not move your body at the same time; the idea is to keep your shoulders soft and still as you do this. When you are at the furthest point to the left, inhale, and then on your exhalation return slowly and softly to the centre. Once again inhale, and then on your exhalation gently rotate to the right. When at the furthest point to the right, inhale and then on your exhalation return slowly and softly to the centre. Repeat this several times.

It's a pleasant practice to keep the inhalation and exhalation of equal length. This creates a gentle rhythm. Please do not struggle or strain to reach further; if you feel any discomfort, stop at that level. You might well find you can move further and more easily on one side than the other. This is all information, it is your starting point, so no judgement please.

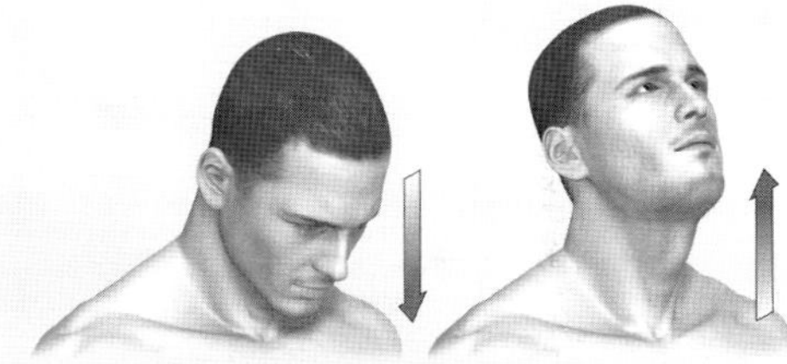

Figure 17.2

Chin to chest without strain

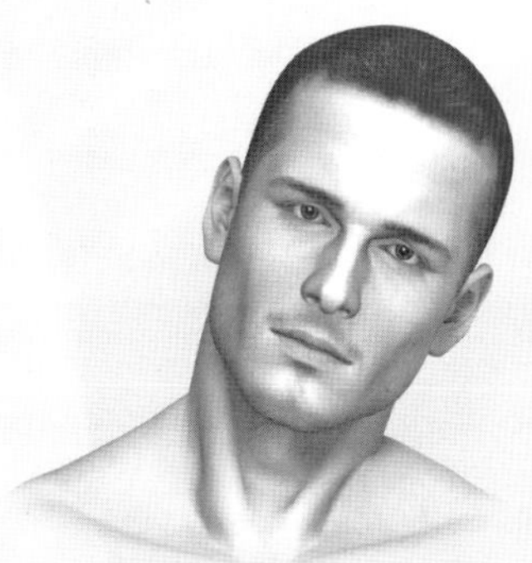

Figure 17.3

The less familiar ear to shoulder move

Using the same arrangement with your breath, and once again with a soft jaw, start by looking straight ahead and move your head slowly so that your chin is down onto your chest (Fig. 17.2). You will feel this stretching the muscles at the back of your neck. Return on the exhale to looking straight ahead, inhale again and then on your next exhale move your head so you are looking up at the ceiling or sky (Fig. 17.2). As you inhale, you will feel this stretching the muscles at the front of your throat and between your chin and your neck. Always return to the starting point.

Finally, and again using the same arrangement with your breath, this time from your straight ahead starting place slowly move the left side of your head towards your left shoulder (Fig. 17.3). Think of taking your ear to your shoulder! This direction offers a gentle stretch to the muscles on the right side of your neck. As in the other movements, return on the exhale to looking straight ahead, inhale softly, then on your next exhale move your right ear to your right shoulder, offering a gentle stretch to the muscles on the left side of your neck. Always return to your starting position and always use your breath. If you are used to doing this exercise by wrenching your head from side to side – simply annoying your already tense muscles – then you will find this gentle, slow and focused way works rather differently.

Bringing our focus to our arms and hands

Many bodyworkers, especially massage therapists, begin to notice strain in their arms and particularly their hands. But you do not have to be a bodyworker for this to occur. Remember the connections all the way from our feet to our pelvis, then respiratory diaphragm and finally the back of our head? We also mentioned the way tight muscles influence the relationship between bones and the possibility of nerve pathways becoming inhibited. It is no coincidence that the spinal nerves in our neck, which emerge from spaces between what are known as our cervical vertebrae, look after many functions related to our arms and hands. Some also look after our respiratory diaphragm, so there's even more reason to make sure there is plenty of glide and flow in the way we move our necks.

Communication in the body goes both ways, so if we are overusing parts of our body and they are irritated or inflamed then we have that information being relayed to our brain. Chronic inflammation is something we need to avoid if possible, so working to release and balance overworked areas is really beneficial on a whole-body basis. If you use your hands on a keyboard, as a bodyworker, or possibly playing the piano then you need to keep them open and flexible. There are some 'everyday' ways of doing this, as follows.

Experiment

Take a moment: to open your hands

1. With your hands together, including the palmar surfaces of your fingers, begin to press and push them closer for a few seconds (I like to do this for about six seconds) and then release the pressure, but keep them together. Gradually increase the pressure, for just a few seconds at a time, using the muscles of your arms and shoulders as you do so. Do this at least 10 times, always taking a moment to completely release the pressure in between each push. Of course, you might also like to combine this with your breath, pushing on the exhalation and resting on the inhalation.

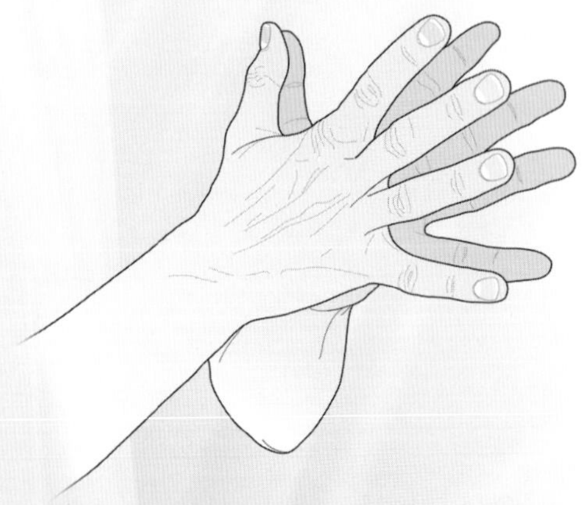

Figure 17.4

Challenging our hands and fingers to stretch

2. From the same position, with your palms and palmar surfaces of your fingers still together, stretch each pair of fingers away from each other as far as you can. Hold each time for a few seconds, and relax the pressure in between. Combine with your breath for extra value!
3. Start from the same position, with your palms and palmar surfaces of your fingers still together, but now as you keep your palms firmly together stretch the fingers away from one another and backwards, opening up a V-shaped space between them. Really work your fingers away from your palms, and remember to keep your jaw soft as you do this. It is possible to work the muscles without gritting your teeth as you do so.

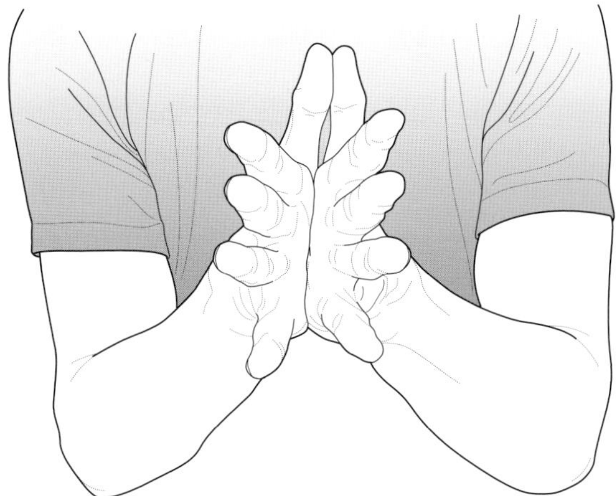

Figure 17.5

Hands stretching and opening

Experiment

Take a moment: to get into the swing of things

At any point – between clients, classes or whilst you are walking (but not somewhere crowded) – allow your arms to move and swing them up in front of you, out to the side, behind you and across the front of your body. Smile when you are doing this and enjoy it. You will begin to feel softer in your arms and hands and in your upper body generally.

Touch

In my practice I use touch, but even if you do not use it in your own work you might be interested just to take this principle into the touch you use in your family or relationships. Palpation enables us to feel what is happening beneath the skin. There are many levels of palpation. I want to be aware of what is going on in the body, as though I was not there at all, so in my work I use a very light touch. It is important that I am able to feel subtle changes in the client's tissue, rather than tuning into the level at which the tissue defends itself. I recognise that at times a light touch can feel irritating or even be misinterpreted, so I always check in with my client regularly and ask how it feels to them. My touch needs to be perfect for my client's body so, as all my clients are unique, I need to be prepared to adapt to the level at which I can feel those subtle changes, and with which they can relax.

How to work with all of them to release tension in our whole body

Focus on our mouth and our face

In the last chapter we released tension in our jaw by softening the area beneath our tongue. We can do this any time we notice tension in our neck or shoulders. There are many strong connections between the muscles in the floor of the mouth and at the front of our throat, right down to our sternum (breast bone), through to the top of our shoulder blades, and to the tissue immediately in front of two of the vertebrae in our neck. That's why we can influence the tensions held in the whole body by bringing a real awareness to this place. It is possible to feel it happening quite easily if we are in a relaxed position, lying down on the floor or our bed. Please don't let that stop you trying it if you are using your computer or as you are walking.

Experiment

Take a moment: to smile

Take a look in the mirror and smile. This is a great way to work the muscles of your face. It also releases tension in the front of your throat and chest. If you are really observant, you might become aware of a releasing of tension in your pelvic floor. There are strong correlations between the tensions we hold in those two places. Whilst you are smiling, take a moment to notice whether the expression contained in and around your eyes is also smiley. If not, that is something to work on. Try to get them to match up, or you might give the impression that you are not sincere.

If you doubt me then observe a salesperson in a department store. Discreetly watch out for any mismatch between the top and bottom of their face as they greet a potential customer.

Please do not be judgemental about any of the staff you notice with this failure to match eyes and mouth. They may be tired, their feet are probably sore and they work in a very competitive environment. It can take work and awareness to make sure your expression offers a client a genuine greeting. If you as a teacher or therapist are at the end of a long day, remember each client needs to get the impression of a safe and neutral therapeutic session. What impression does a mismatch create?

Experiment

Take a moment: to focus on your nose

At the very top of your nose are two little bones, called nases or nasal bones. They meet each other along their inner sides, and meet with your frontal bone (or forehead) at their tops. At their outer sides they both meet with a large area of bone called your maxilla, which goes all the way down and forms a home for your upper teeth. The bones of your face (there are more) are really interesting, so if you don't know much about them then I suggest some research will be rewarding.

You might be aware that when someone has a headache or feels tired, they tend to take the top of the nose and hold it. Well, we can do better than that by paying attention to it with some soft awareness.

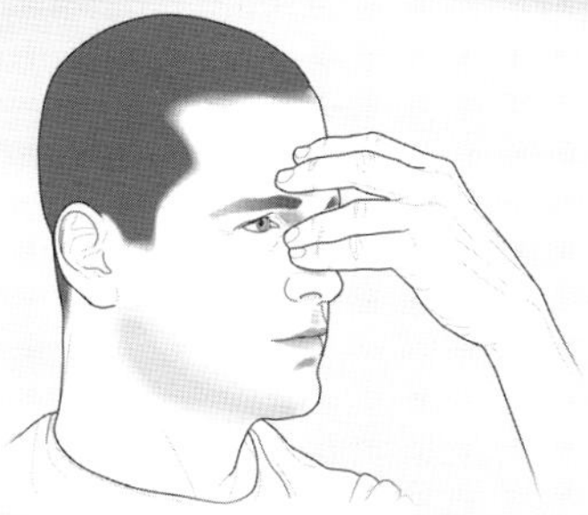

Figure 18.1

Easy release around forehead and nose

Take your thumb and fourth finger and connect either side of the very top of your nose, and let your index and middle finger rest on your forehead, then we are ready to start.

With your gentlest touch, and only a tiny pressure, coax your nasal bones away from the front of your face whilst you stabilise your forehead with the other two fingers. Take a few breaths. Then change your intention so that whilst you stabilise your forehead you gently coax your nasal bones away downwards towards your feet. If you do this really softly then you will feel a pleasant release, generally across your sinuses and the front of your face. If you pull or use a harsh touch it will feel really unpleasant and you will be able to judge just how good your facial bones are at defending themselves. Less really is more here.

Experiment

Take a moment: to focus on our eyes

We need our very precious eyes to glide and move with ease in the environment of their orbits. We need them to use their muscles freely so that, by using them in cooperation with our neck, we can see all around us. Our eyes show a great deal about how we are feeling: the whites appear sore and red when our eyes are strained and there is a dullness and a yellowness when our general health is not great. They need to feel comfortable, not dry, gritty or itchy. It might seem obvious, but when our eyes are strained we tend to get headaches. In my practice, clients come for treatment for those symptoms when they really need to get their eyes tested. They probably need to do both. I send at least six clients a year to an optician to get a test.

What can we do in our everyday activities to ensure we are using our eye muscles and keeping them free and mobile? Are there some easy ways to help them, and to keep a balance when we are challenged with environmental factors? How does air conditioning at work affect us? It might mean dryness in the throat, which is obvious to us, but what about sore and itchy eyes? Perhaps we are lucky and the air conditioning engineers are careful to check any filters and ensure they are clean, and we might be 'just fine' in a well-controlled environment.

Sadly, that is a scenario I very rarely hear from my clients, so we just have to find some ways to manage things as they are.

In many places where summer heat is not extreme, it is possible to work with a window open instead and perhaps use fans, so avoiding the use of air conditioning all together. Some of my clients in the corporate world work in a sealed building and have no choice in the matter.

You might work in a treatment room in a spa, an office, or teach regularly in hotel conference rooms with carpets, and their accompanying cleaning fluids. Perhaps you use public transport or fly regularly? What can we do about dust and traffic fumes? Caroline writes about the power of water in Part 2, and our eyes contain a high percentage of it. So, to protect them from the effects of irritation and dehydration, they might well benefit from regular bathing or from using a protective spray over our closed lids (ask your pharmacist for advice about both of these).

If we use a computer as a main part of our working day it is likely that we already understand the importance of changing our focal length at regular intervals, and of getting up and moving around when we need 'water in or water out'. Keeping hydrated in an air-conditioned building is vital, so we can do both at once.

My observation is that it is best to start our work session looking down slightly at the screen, so that way we can counter any tiredness as we spend a few hours there and our fatigue takes us into our natural tendency to move into a chin forward posture.

Using our awareness about our posture, and putting it into action, means that from now on we will be making sure we are able to use our technology, laptop, tablet and so on whilst we are in contact with our sitting bones and have our feet on the ground or supported on a cushion.

Working with a screen can tire our eyes, though if we are really interested in what's on it or are playing games, we need to recognise that it is stimulating our brain at the same time, so it is best if we avoid using electronic devices for an hour or so before we go to bed.

Experiment

Take a moment: to move your eyes

You will remember the way that we did the 'ear to the shoulder' move for our neck muscles. That is a movement we don't make as regularly in our everyday activities as the rotational ones and the 'ups and downs'. We need to bring any unfamiliar movements into our awareness and remember to practise them as well as the familiar ones. There are some eye movements that are used less frequently, so we will be practising them here.

Please do the following exercises whilst you are seated.

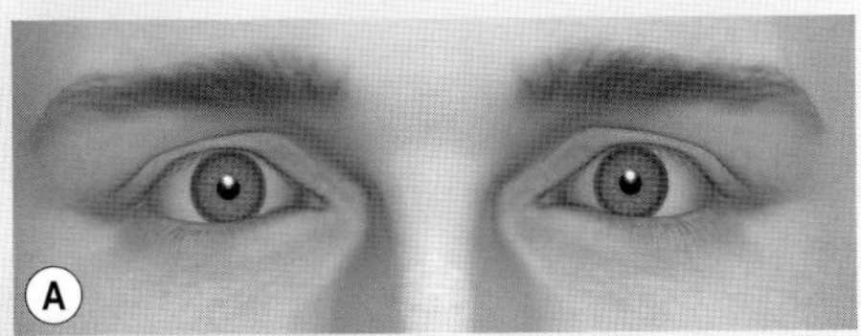

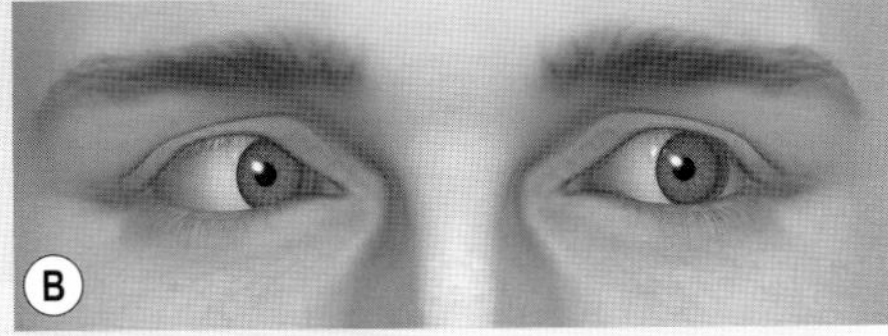

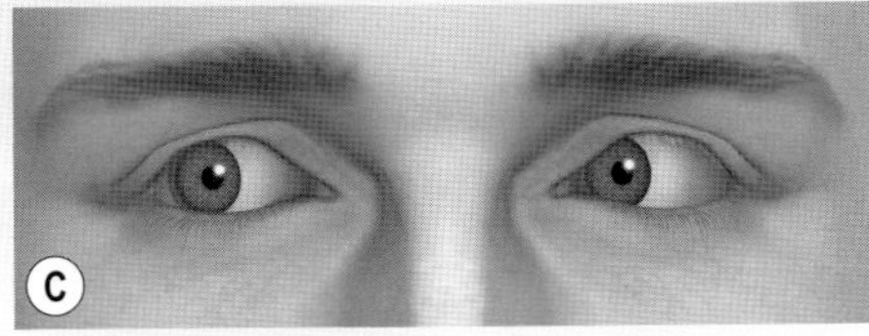

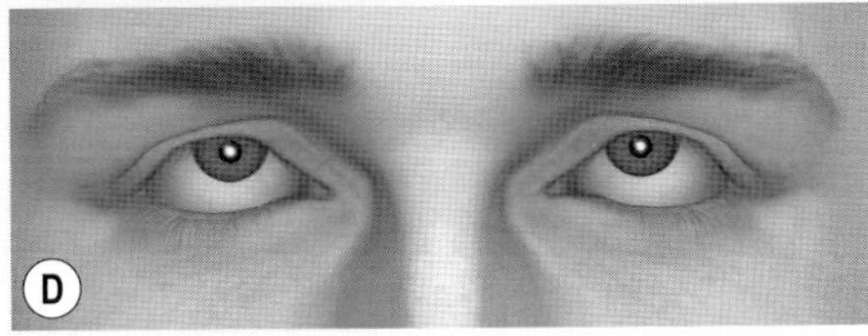

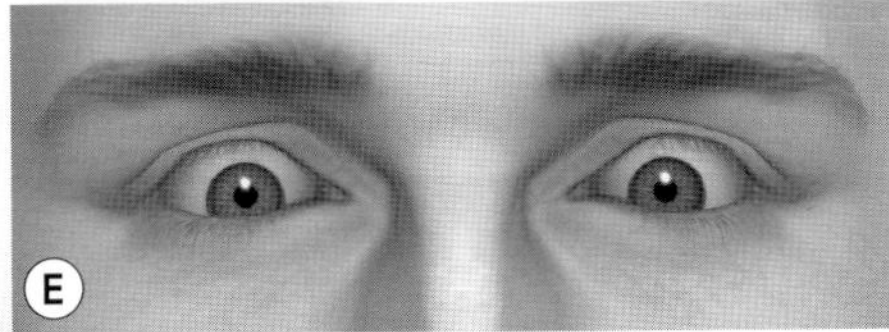

Figure 18.2

Eyes in action

Lateral movement

When you make these movements with your eyes remember we are focusing our awareness on our *eye* muscles, so we do not move our head at the same time.

Starting by looking straight ahead (Fig. 18.2A), inhale softly and then as you exhale look as far as you can (*without moving your head*) to the left (Fig. 18.2B). Inhale there, and then as you exhale, bring your eyes back to the centre (Fig. 18.2A). Inhale here, and on your exhalation look as far as you can to the right (Fig. 18.2C). Inhale, and then on your exhalation return to the centre (Fig. 18.2A). Always work slowly, without pushing, and in combination with your breath. Do this several times. I like to do it six times before moving on to the next piece. When you have practised this a few times you can create a gentle rhythm by making your breath last for the same count each way. I find four seconds is comfortable.

Lifting and lowering

Starting by looking straight ahead (Fig. 18.2A), inhale softly and then as you exhale look as far as you can (*without moving your head*) upwards (Fig. 18.2D). Inhale there, and then as you exhale bring your eyes back to the centre (Fig. 18.2A). Inhale softly and then as you exhale look as far as you can (*without moving your head*) downwards (Fig. 18.2E). Do this several times, and use a rhythmic breath if you find it helpful.

Encouraging fluid flow in the environment of your eyes

When you wash your face you might use cold water to help you wake up in the morning. That's fine for your face but your eyes love warmth, so perhaps start off with cold water, then soak a washcloth in warm water and hold it over your closed eyes for a few moments. It feels fabulous. If you don't have a cloth handy then just gather warm water in your palms and hold them over your closed eyes. Your eyes will really enjoy this. Any time your eyes feel really tired simply sit with your elbows on a table and cover your eyes with the palms of your hands. Give yourself as long as you can with this one.

So that's all about us – what next? 19

How do we move from knowing about all this to understanding it and embodying it?

You will realise by now that, despite my effort to tell a little of my story without plunging into anatomical detail about my surgery, I come from a strong background of studying and getting things 'right' in order to pass exams and to prove that I am competent and successful.

Certificates of competence are important; they give us credibility and allow us to work safely and under the protection of insurance. We don't need to plaster the walls with them to show how important we are, but we will carry a confidence within us that permeates our being and we will be proud to say we have well-recognised qualifications in what we do.

However, it's no coincidence that in my bodywork practice I have encountered two clients with their liver on the left, and others who are the proud owners of three kidneys. With my left-brain tendencies and need to get things accurate and correct, my inclination to believe the many anatomy texts and courses I studied whilst preparing myself to work as a hands-on therapist was very strong. It's so easy to think we know what a client needs as we take their history and make our first evaluations, and to lose sight of what their tissue shows us as we palpate.

It took a while for me to really get that 'the map is not the territory' and that, if I gave up the need to know and trusted what my hands were feeling, I could palpate subtle changes and tissue responses and not overrule my hands with the knowledge of my brain, of which I was so proud, and which I trusted so easily. This was my *paradigm shift*, a complete change of my point of view. In my hands-on practice I needed to trust that all the information was 'on the table' and that the client had all the answers. I needed to develop the presence that would enable me to tune into the client's natural healing ability – their inner wisdom – and not allow my knowledge and my ideas about what was needed for that client to get in the way.

A great deal of my time with clients is spent on a deep level, noticing and paying attention to my own body. I am always aware, at this deeper level, of my feet, pelvis and shoulders, not to mention my breathing and my jaw. If tensions are appearing then they could inhibit my ability to palpate. If I notice something persistent then it is a sign that I need to get treatment myself.

What do our clients need to feel when they meet us?

How many of us who are complementary or alternative practitioners are, in effect, the 'last resort' for our clients. They might have gone to many others first, just like I did. They appear disillusioned and probably short of money, after promises that were not fulfilled. Despite medical and other complementary approaches and attempts at helping them with their symptoms, the first question I am generally asked is 'How many sessions will I need? I want to know how much this will cost'. Even more worrying is the question 'Can you guarantee you will be able to relieve my pain and sort me out? My friend says you fixed her'.

The three most powerful words I have learned to say – and I admit it was initially with some difficulty – are 'I don't know'. I also ask if clients have ever asked their medical doctor for a guarantee. Have they looked at the reports on the efficacy of the prescription drugs given? No one can guarantee anything because everyone is unique! One person's migraine is not the same as another's, any more than two people's back pain is identical. If a therapist does give a guarantee then they are not being truthful. They might be speaking from an inflated self-belief that is greater than their common sense. My answer normally goes that some people find the work I do helpful but that it's not based on a protocol for everyone, it's based on palpation of the body, finding areas of restriction and then gently treating them. If a client insists on a guarantee then I explain I am not the therapist for them.

As therapists we develop our confidence and understanding that it is not our place to rescue our clients but to create an environment where they feel listened to and are safe to say what they really feel. Over time, and with no pressure or pushing, they find the best time to come to an empowered sense of self-realisation.

The desirable characteristics of successful therapists, managers, negotiators and anyone who works with people

From the initial meeting it should be apparent that you are calm, professional and empathetic. You demonstrate good listening skills and show you take a genuine interest in your client by taking care with body language so that the client feels they are the only thing you are interested in when they meet you. Early in the meeting it is clear that you are able to handle anything the client can bring up, are able to think on your feet, and they are in a safe and respectful space.

As you bring the session to a close you show you have clear professional and personal boundaries, and leave them feeling they have been empowered.

20 What's the catch?

Recognising ourselves and our motivation for working with people

From my own perspective, I needed to accept things the way they were, not fight to return to my past patterns and career. Somehow I had to be in a place where it was possible to see my restricted mobility and discomfort as a starting point from where I could begin to manage things differently, rather than the end of the world.

Naturally, I sought those who could help me on this new path that had no clear destination, and then came to recognise that, far from emptiness, it meant endless opportunities.

When we 'try and strive' we become tense and we are driven to see only what we think we know is there, or not there. When we hold a mirror ourselves then we tend to see what we want to. We need someone else who embodies neutrality to 'hold the mirror' and also to enter into respectful questioning with us about how we view ourselves. Then we get a different picture, insights can happen and choices open up. We might already have seen people who are not neutral and who tell us what is wrong and what to do about it, and who expect us to take on solutions they advise, based on their own experiences and their own wishes and ideas about what is best for us.

Despite their lack of neutrality, these people are generally well meaning. They can be natural carers and advice-givers, but they might not be suitably qualified to offer this service. They might well have a personal agenda, like the characters who need to be needed and who are acting out of some unhealed wound from their own past. They will not offer us an empowering experience; they may want us to be dependent on them. Then there is danger. The boundaries of a therapeutic relationship have been broken. When we, or our clients, are vulnerable and in pain, these folk can be difficult to recognise and to separate from the genuine article.

The first friend we need to meet is ourself. The calm environment is one we need to create for our own good. How can this happen? Where do we find the resources and the energy in the midst of the challenges in life? Is it possible to meet ourself with compassion, with a smile? Can we be a neutral listener to the messages from our own body? Can we be as gentle and respectful with our touch on our own body as we would be on someone else's? Be as interested and non-judgemental when we feel a restriction or an area of pain? Can we get to know and respect ourself in all the facets of who we are?

With work and time of course we can. Then we can embody the memory of stillness and work from it with neutrality.

How do we maintain neutrality?

My role as a craniosacral therapist is one of enabling clients to make their own decisions and gain their own insights about the best way to optimise their wellbeing. The power base in the relationship is with the client. They often use the therapeutic session to go much deeper in their process and my role is to assist them in their exploration of themselves so they can choose their course of action or even not to act at all. If my role is to enable and empower my clients to grow and evolve, then what are my own responsibilities in this?

I need to create a therapeutic environment to facilitate their growth, and to ensure that I am in the best possible space and health myself. My awareness of my own health needs is vital – ensuring enough sleep, nourishment for my body and stimulation for my brain. Receiving treatment is essential for my own journey to greater self-awareness so that I can remain grounded and neutral during my clients' processes.

My role is to create a therapeutic space in which there is the possibility of their processes leading them to insights and discoveries and enabling them to heal themselves. By undertaking more advanced training I have the possibility of using a wider range of therapeutic tools, such as imagery and dialogue, to facilitate their discovery of their own resources, strengths and depths. Through developing my therapeutic presence I can show my awareness of the need for confidentiality and for self-responsibility, and to let my clients know that they are always in charge and that their belief system is sacred. I have no attachment to a particular outcome – 'healing' or making 'better'.

There are no limits to the extent of the client's processes within an enabling and facilitating environment. They can enter whatever dimensions of self they need, explore and gain insights and awareness of their potential to grow and evolve. My role is to be totally present for them, a neutral witness, and to understand that if the client feels able to say 'No' then their 'Yes' can be trusted.

My clients are always teaching me. I don't believe – in fact I could not be more certain – that I could take on the learning they offer if I thought I 'knew' what they needed.

Working in my practice is a source of inspiration, never dull or repetitive. Every session challenges me to listen attentively to the tissue so I can facilitate the client's own treatment plan. I trust the process absolutely. If I were not aware of the work I need to do to remain neutral, grounded and non-judgemental, I don't believe that trust would be easy.

Dr John Upledger had a great way with words:

Therapists can either facilitate us along our own pathways or tell us what they think we should do and inhibit our healing and growth processes.

How can we empower our clients or co-workers?

In our role as therapists we need to maintain the power base as belonging to the client. When a client reports progress I listen carefully to their words. If they say something like 'You worked a miracle last session', I point out that it was their body that led the session and I needed to tune into their natural healing ability to facilitate the work. It is always good to thank them for the feedback, to tell them how well they are doing, and then to ask them how they are feeling right now and ask what they hope to get out of the session today.

As teachers, we are the authority figure, but we are primarily a facilitator of learning. If we have an authoritarian approach and fail to see our students as our clients then the relationship can become soured. The teacher who has forgotten what it is like to learn, to be a beginner, or fails to see that with every group there is learning for themselves as part of the experience, is generally pretty stale and miserable.

Feedback can be a thorny topic: without giving advice, can we help our colleagues and clients with their choice of words?

It is important to avoid making ourselves appear to be a 'victim' when we prepare to bring up an issue with a colleague, friend or family member. Consider the difference between 'When you do this you *make me* feel angry' and 'When you do this *then I feel* angry'.

If we keep silent, building up resentment and anger, we do not give the other person a chance to change and, most importantly, we judge them for that. We cannot be certain of the outcome. Sometimes a small change in our language can open a door rather than close it.

Melding – how we steer a safe course at the beginning and end of the therapeutic session

Alexander uses the term *melding*. Melding is, I believe, the single most important factor in the therapist–client relationship. I would define it as the combining of energy fields around everyone involved in a treatment session. This resonance and harmony creates a space – a safe 'container' – in which the client can process what they need to and the therapist can support that process most effectively.

I believe melding starts when a client sets an intention and calls me. The way I deal with their enquiry, my focus, tone of voice and the type of questions I ask will contribute to the way they feel safe (or not) when they arrive at my door. My role is then to create the environment in my office for uninterrupted, relaxed and open communication, and to enable clients of all ages to feel confident and safe. I must pay attention to verbal and non-verbal communication to help facilitate the therapeutic relationship from the first moments of our meeting. If I feel uncertain about the client or feel there is something 'off' at this point then it is important to recognise that we are not under any obligation to treat anyone. We need to know when to refer and to recognise that the modalities we work with will not suit everyone. If all seems well then we continue with the session.

As I begin my therapeutic evaluation techniques, my choice of language register, body positioning and style of communication help the client to feel that the session is about their process, not something imposed upon them. Whether they are 2 days old accompanied by their parents, or 92 years old, making my respect for them clear and allowing and encouraging them to 'just be themselves' helps to reassure them well before the treatment begins. The client should feel they are the most important thing in the room – that they have my total focus and attention at every session, not just on our first meeting.

After my evaluation, I talk to the client about where I am going to start and then settle my hands into position. I take care that my hands are in an energetically 'neutral' state to start with – no intention – just being with the client and starting to listen. I then bring my awareness to the tissues and listen with my hands for responses. By using my hands in this way, melding develops. The body's natural resistances and defences are not provoked. The client is able to engage fully in the session, allowing their body's natural healing responses to emerge and be supported.

What if my client is an active toddler? My intention is the same, but I may be sitting on the couch with the mother at the other end, with her also 'hands on'. I may be treating a baby whilst it is at her breast. I may be using my intention and treating through the mother's hands or body. I may be using any part of my body to meld with the child – my trunk, arms, legs and so on. I often sit astride the couch with a small child immediately in front of me, facing the mother, and a bag of toys between us. This is still melding. It is meeting the child, and the mother, where they are. The melding encompasses all those in the room who are involved in the session: other therapists, relatives and friends.

Melding can be destroyed or rendered impossible by the therapist's fix-it attitude, insensitivity and lack of listening to or following the tissues. If I sense a withdrawal or 'shutting down' of the melding space, I ease back, return to neutral and backtrack in case I missed something. I might re-evaluate and let the tissues show me restrictions that will guide where my hands should go next. Sometimes I get a clear sense of 'stay where you are – don't change – just wait'. Whatever comes, I follow it and trust the guidance from the evaluation.

When a client's session has ended I set an intention for the melding connection to fade as they withdraw. I then 'see' my office and myself become really clear and free of everything created in the last session. This helps me become refreshed and ready for the next client, and better able to create a new and appropriate environment for their process.

I believe attention to melding creates the space for the client to embrace the opportunity for treatment. Melding opens the door, lights the path, enables communication on many levels and is at once the simplest and most complex of concepts.

In order to meld, I need to know myself and to embody the inner power of stillness.

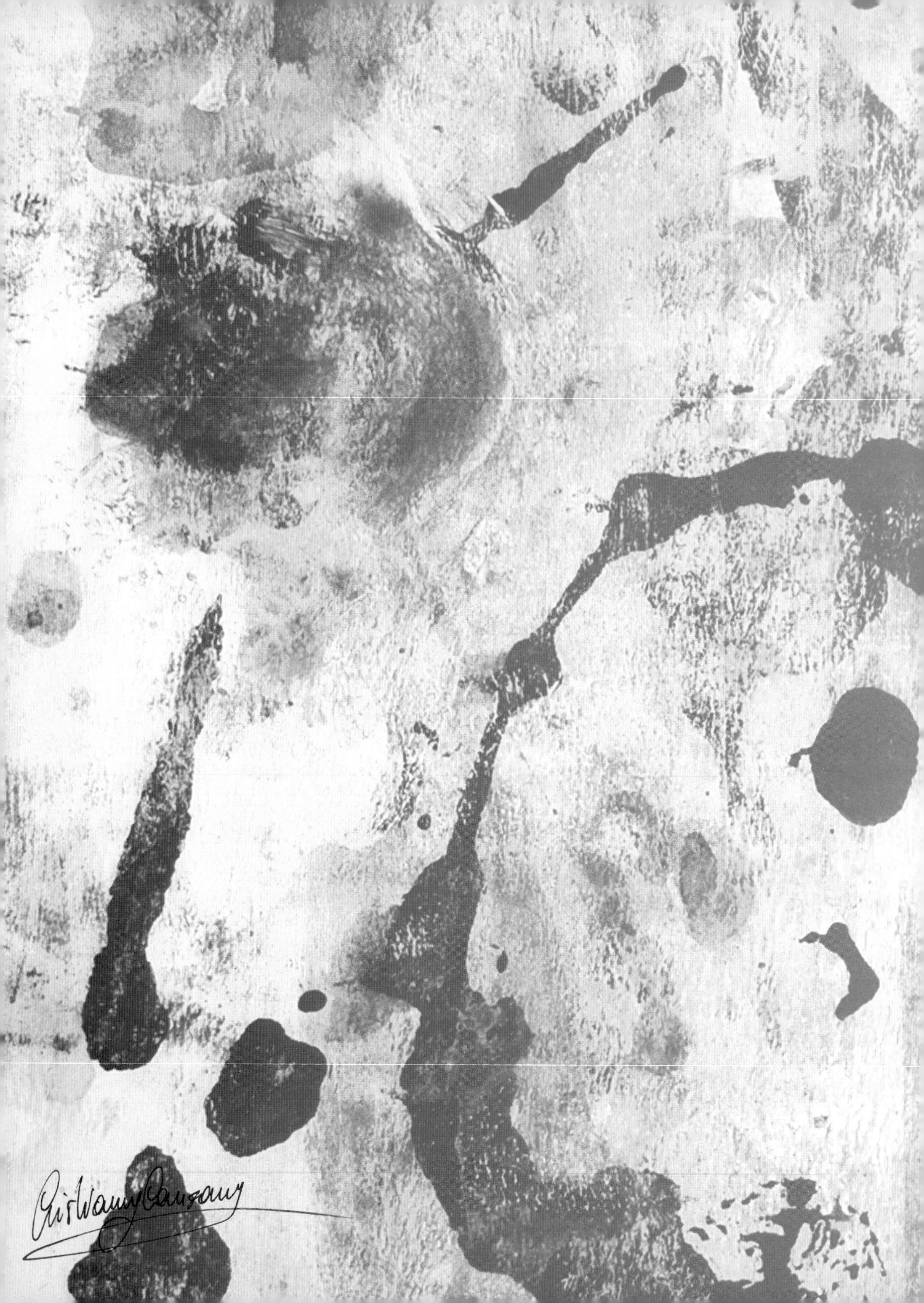

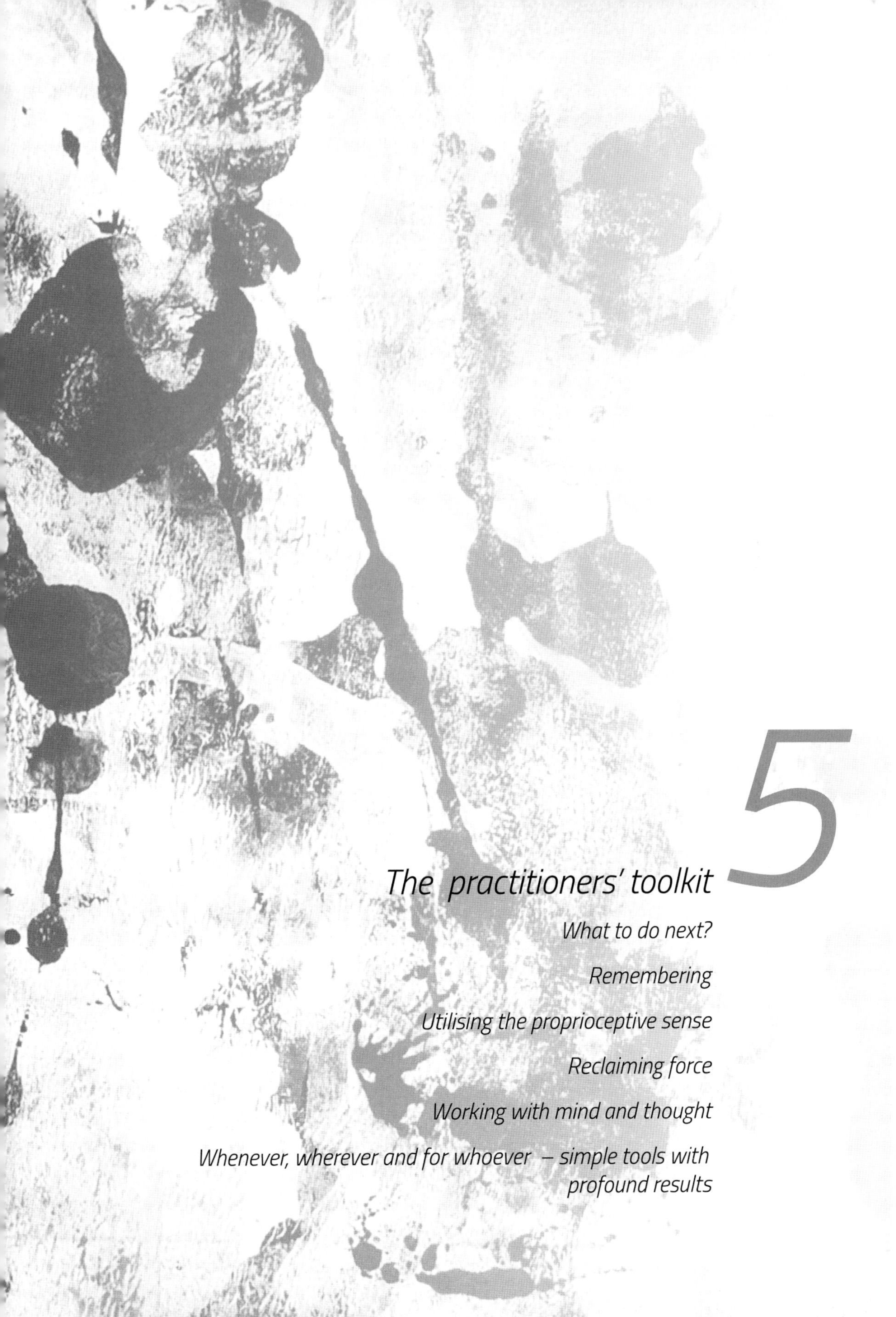

5

The practitioners' toolkit

What to do next?

Remembering

Utilising the proprioceptive sense

Reclaiming force

Working with mind and thought

Whenever, wherever and for whoever – simple tools with profound results

21 What to do next?

Less is more

Working with the inner power of stillness means less gives rise to more. That is, much *less* comes from us in the form of intentions and objectives, especially when we treat, facilitate, practise or teach, so that *more* can arise from the inner still-point, the middle place that is changing the way we work. If we work through intention, we are 'in tension', stemming from our will, even if it is the most subtle or subconscious action of will that is lurking underneath. Hence, getting to less means that the very first objective of our work is to gradually undo the default mechanism of doing and knowing, which takes us into allowing and being. We can't force ourselves to become still, but we can *allow* or give ourselves the permission to *be* still. That is, allowing is a process of undoing in itself, which is accompanied by an increasing sense of a natural inner stillness in our body and mind. Allowing, a quality that originates from a very high level of consciousness, is neither active nor passive. Something happens in allowing that is not driven by the force of our intentions, which might be biased.

Experiment

1. You have 30 seconds to become still, by means of your own will action and deliberate intention ...
2. This time simply *allow* yourself to settle into stillness ...

In the second experiment, things simply happen, evoking a sudden sense of relief in which we become at ease. However, in the first experiment, we might meet friction and struggle, and our attempt to make ourselves still does not go very far.

The above experiment demonstrates that the answer lies in our psychology. That is, allowing is an inner quality that acts on our psychology, giving rise to a process of undoing, which leads to inner stillness. Through allowing we seem to step out of 'our own way' by handing over our control and the will contained in our current 'I' and 'me' to something unknown that is connected to a higher purpose, aptitude and destiny. By simply allowing we suddenly cease to be the doer and knower, and can experience how things happen naturally through us, how our actions and the right knowledge spring from the 'insightful self', and how much congruency there is between us, the practitioners, teachers or therapists, the clients and the process within our clients, as well as how seamlessly the process seems to unfold.

You should apply the same 'less is more' underlying principle to the practice tips, techniques and exercises in this practitioner's toolkit. That is because the less you try to be good at all of this, the more you will experience (by truly not having to be good at this) how the profound shift in attitude throughout your whole psychology will make you truly good at this. It is at this point that we finally realise that 'we' or 'I' cannot do it, and, in the light of the teachings, the real work can begin.

Creating space

Nothing new can enter if we do not provide the space for it. In our adult life, contrary to our childhood, every bit of space in our psychology is occupied by everything we have learned and acquired emotionally, intellectually and through movement. The majority of what is occupying this so precious space within our psychological and mental makeup has turned into deeply engrained habits, which are not necessarily conducive to our work and the further evolution of our inner potential. In addition, every bit of space in our external life is usually occupied as well, forcing most of us to live in the fast lane. That's why there is never any room left for anything else to enter. So, how can we possibly achieve memory of stillness, and replace old 'in-formation' and knowledge that we no longer need with new information if all the space has been taken?

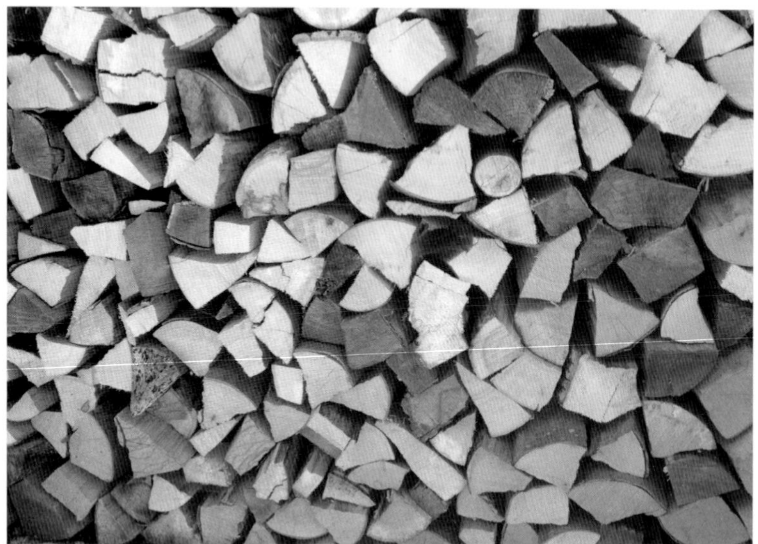

Figure 21.1

Allegorically speaking, our habitual life is like a pile of wood that has no space for something new to enter. Photography Alexander Filmer-Lorch

The answer is by simply sacrificing our subconscious resistance to change and new ideas, as well as our fear of the unknown. These occupy a tremendous amount of space within us, as well as in our lives.

Example 1

Some years ago, a student of mine worked in several different clinics, and two of them took an extraordinarily high percentage commission per client treated. For many years she complained that there was no chance for her to move forward in her work and life, because there was never time to make that happen as long as she had to work the extremely long hours she needed to do every week to make a decent living. In an inner work session, I asked her if she had ever considered the possibility that there was not enough space for anything else to enter, and if there was anything worth sacrificing to create more space, so that the unknown had a chance to fill it with something new that might change her life. Six weeks later she came back to tell me that the realisation my question evoked had given her the courage to leave the two clinics that paid so badly. Two days after she left, her daughter announced that she would soon be moving out to live with her boyfriend. The very same day she received an email with a special offer on an electronic massage table, which she bought, now that she had the space and time to work from home and turn it into her own clinic. Today she is running a successful business that has given her the freedom to study and acquire new knowledge and skills, as well as enjoying a stable work–life balance.

Example 2

Mr B struck me as an incredibly 'wired' person when we met before the start of our first session. He told me that his nervous energy kept him physically and mentally going all the time, and that he desperately needed some more space in his head, because it felt so full and overcrowded there. For years he had tried countless mindfulness and meditation techniques, but it had not given him any sense of stillness, and had actually made things worse. He stated that he would never want to go there again. I asked him in which situations he felt most centred and at ease. 'Oh, in water of course,' he answered, 'because water is the element where I feel most at home.' My suggestion to him was to utilise his frequent visits to the pool and, once he had completed his 30 lengths of swimming, to simply allow his body to float and be rocked by the water for not more than five minutes, and just watch how his breath settled after the physical exertion. In our weekly sessions I always finished his treatment with a five-minute rock and glide, where the client lies supine, his pelvis resting on one palm of my hand and his head on the other. He always said that this felt just like floating in water, and made him profoundly still and centred. After three months I asked him if he would like to give a breath exercise a go, where he would simply sit comfortably in an armchair, closing his eyes and connecting with the rocking motion he felt in the water whilst feeling the natural flow of his breath. After six months he mentioned that his head was not crowded any more, that he experienced prolonged times of deep inner stillness, and that if he had given in to his resistance to this simple practice of not doing, he would have forever remained a stressed-out person. Today his 'wiredness' has gone and he comes across as a calm and centred person.

These are only a couple of examples out of many that could be told. Both highlight the fact that, the moment we sacrifice our resistance to change and the fear of the unknown, by means of a conscious effort, which derives its strength from the force of meaning, the space it frees up will be filled with new possibilities that otherwise we can only dream of.

Replacing impressions

Our body and mind depend highly on specific nourishment. A vital body requires food and oxygen, and a healthy mind requires the nourishment of stimulus. The moment we are lacking either one of them, the homeostasis of both will be profoundly affected, ultimately resulting in ill health or even death. The public health sector, doctors and scientists all invest a lot of time and energy to encourage us to implement and sustain a healthy diet, and environmental organisations want to ensure that the air we breathe in remains clean. However, when it comes to nourishment of our minds, the vast increase in daily stimuli or impressions in our lives over the past 20 years is the equivalent of living on a permanent high-sugar and high-energy drink diet. The intensity and speed of the stimuli that act upon us on a daily basis mean that the majority of us live our life mainly in *attention*, leaving hardly any breathing space. That's why more than two-fifths of UK employers are still seeing an increase in reports of mental health issues at work (CIPD, 2015), and similar figures can be found when it comes to anxiety issues, burnout and chronic stress. It might not be possible to stop this flood of impressions altogether, without going into retreat and living in a cloister or ashram for a while, but we can work towards containing the flood and turning it into a more gentle stream by replacing many of the most common impressions we face on a daily basis with new ones.

New impressions open up new possibilities

1. Instead of watching TV before you go to sleep, which keeps your adrenaline going, you could read a book for 30 minutes (not on tablets, only e-readers and actual books). This can help your pineal gland to rebalance the circadian rhythm and the production of melatonin. Hence the possibility of a good night's sleep is not far away.

2. Instead of catching up with a good friend or colleague in a noisy coffee shop, grab a sandwich and go for a walk in the park or on the common. The change of scenery and fresh air can profoundly reduce your stress levels, and gives rise to the possibility that you will be back at work with renewed energy.

3. Take conscious action to open yourself up to stimuli that expand and extend your view of things. It upgrades and renews existing imprints of impressions within the grooves of your mind, leading to a new sense of purpose, as well as freeing up much more room to play with.

4. The most powerful impressions are those that inspire us and touch us on a deeper level, informing our being. They might reach us through inspirational people, places that make us remember, a group of people who selflessly work for the greater good, or regularly reconnecting with the influence of higher knowledge that we can derive from art, science, philosophy and psychology.

5. Eradicate as much as you can of the stimulus that is imposed on us by emails, text messages, social network platforms, mobile devices and to-do lists. From time to time we need to experience, even if it is only for a few hours a week, that the world is doing just fine without us, and our 24-hour availability.

6. Whilst you are driving or on a train or bus journey, don't listen to music or the radio but simply allow the world to pass by and be inspired by the beauty of the scenery and the world around you. When you are at home doing household duties or cooking a meal, keep the radio and TV switched off and allow the lack of constant stimulus to act upon you. You will soon enjoy the company of your very own inner stillness ...

Obviously, putting the different suggestions above into action requires energy and conscious effort. However, the moment we become creative with this, and start coming up with our own solutions that work for our own way of life, the initial conscious effort transforms into inspirational effort, through which we gain energy instead of losing it.

Using different reference points

Science writer Matthew Wright (2015) says that recent research shows that 'a "moment", to most people, is two or three seconds. Then that perception of "now" vanishes and is replaced by a new one'. This is a great basis to work from, because two to three seconds is a sufficient enough time span to access the now if our attention span can last that long. Wherever our thoughts, feelings and emotions might be, it is our body that is spending its whole lifespan in the now. We do not have to look elsewhere because, as long as we live, we will exist and be in our physical body, which is the most powerful reference point for the now. That is, we can't get any closer to it. We initially have to look for, find and connect with situations, places and manifestations that make the now more attractive than the past, the future or any of our habitual states, thoughts or momentary psychological manifestations, until the now has established itself as an easily realisable and powerful resource within us. Furthermore, being in the now does not mean not thinking. The greatest thoughts and ideas arise out of the now because the thought formations are highly conscious and opposed to compulsive or mechanical thoughts. So, what are the different options that connect us with the now?

1. Every exercise and movement method that has not become automatic or mechanical will keep us conscious and awake enough to stay connected with the present moment. That is, the same routine or exercise sequence repeated again and again is not going to do the job.

2. Different challenges exhilarate and inspire and can take us right into the present moment. Consider balancing on top of a tree trunk, or making your way hand over hand along a long rope stretched between two trees, or challenging yourself with a new recipe. Any kind of challenge that keeps you fully engaged!

3. Receiving treatment such as massage, reflexology, CranioSacral Therapy or aromatherapy, and pursuits such as sculpting, carving, dressmaking or any creative way to use our hands or stimulate our proprioceptive sense will keep us in the present moment.

4. Observational activities such as photography, filming, birdwatching, stargazing, diving, and all kinds of wildlife adventures, mountain trekking and coastal walks, where we continuously meet new views of outstanding beauty or encounter unexpected events in nature, will keep us emerged in the now.

5. Outstanding theatre and concert performances, beautiful spaces like galleries, museums, temples and holy places, and everything that touches us on a deeper level will be experienced in the now.

6. If none of the other options is available, we only need to look inwards, where we simply need to allow ourselves to rest and relax in the natural pause after the exhalation to gather precious moments of the present.

Please remember that the very moment your practice is infused by the meaning of its respective philosophical teaching and higher knowledge, its effect will profoundly increase. This is true for every exercise and experiment outlined in this book, and is simply done by remembering to remember the teachings and meaning of your exercise during your practice.

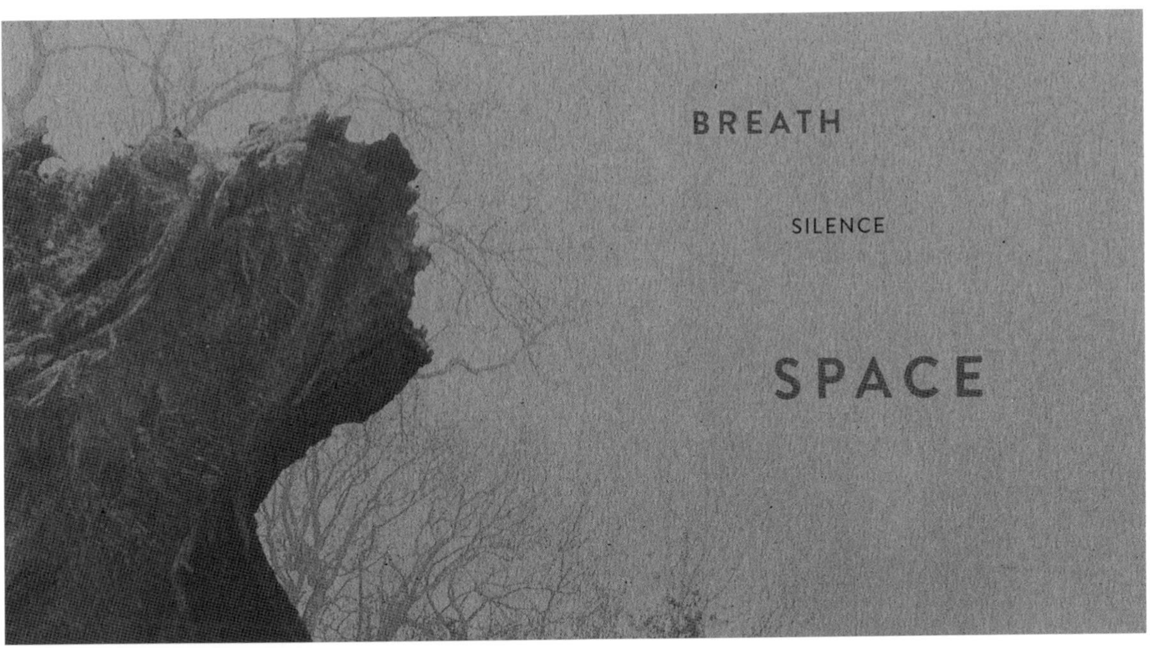

Figure 21.2

Artwork Victoria Dokas; photography Alexander Filmer-Lorch

All of the above, and so much more, evokes a deep sense of contentment and inner peace in us, as well as leaving us with a feeling that no time has passed, even when the whole event has lasted over two to three hours. Because in the now, where we finally totally forget ourselves, only the true self that can't perceive itself exists. Here, in this unencumbered and undivided pure state of perception, all the 'I's' and 'me's' have vanished for the time being, and what is left behind is a vital, undiluted living memory of an experience that took place beyond time.

References

CIPD (2015). *Absence Management. Annual survey report 2015*. CIPD, https://www.cipd.co.uk/binaries/absence-management_2015.pdf [accessed 4 Nov. 2015].

Wright, M. (2015). *How long is the 'now' moment we live in?* [blog], https://mjwrightnz.wordpress.com/2015/01/28/how-long-is-the-now-moment-we-live-in/ [accessed 5 Nov. 2015].

Remembering 22

> *Self-remembering is the experience of uncompromised concentrated centredness within an unmitigated moment of limitless spaciousness, through which the non-perceptual nature of the self is realised.*
>
> Alexander Filmer-Lorch

If we want to truly work from the insightful self, we first need to be able to access it so that we can genuinely feel it, and finally become it, otherwise everything we have learned so far in theory will remain a nice idea to which we can only pay lip service. The way we can access the insightful self is by applying the extraordinary but simple practice of self-remembering that leads to the realisation of this innermost self, which will ultimately determine and inform the way we work.

However, we have to remember what the Yoga Sutras taught us in Chapter 2. Sutra 3.9 states that we have to create *new latent impressions* that *prevent the activation of distractive stored ones,* so that *stillness begins to permeate the mind.* That is, we simply replace the memory impressions of what we have acquired by imitation and conditioning, and what we have been told, as well as what we think and believe is our personality right now, with impressions of what we truly are in essence. These new impressions will enable us ultimately to coalesce with our innermost self again, by means of self-remembering or self-realisation, through the four stages of cognition mentioned in sutra 1.17. That is, we first satisfy our intellect by thinking for ourselves about the technicalities, actualities and meaning of self-remembering, which ultimately leads to a sudden insight or realisation, giving rise to a state of bliss and finally the most authentic form of *feeling* of a unified, consistent and *coherent self.* Such is the process of remembering the self.

In this chapter we will explore possibilities and practices that will gradually take us towards this objective.

What it is

True work always requires a mission, and once this mission is put into action it will ultimately lead to the remembrance of the pure self. That is, the mission of all teachings about 'know thyself', self-study, self-enquiry, self-evolution, self-observation or inner work, you name it, is to discover, experience and maintain what we essentially are. Different schools of thought give different names to this complex idea, and terms such as self-realisation or self-remembering are regularly used to refer to this concept. Buddha remained silent when it came to answering this question, indicating that neither the notion of self nor of non-self does justice to the actual experience. However, everybody who experiences self-realisation or self-remembering will agree that it can't be put into words or be easily explained, and that it will only occur in the present tense. Nisargadatta said: 'At the moment of realisation the person ceases. Identity remains, but identity is not a person, it is inherent in the reality itself' (Prahlad.org, 2015). In other words, there is no such thing as a distinct and separate entity that we have to become, or that needs to be realised. Yet, in a state of self-remembering or self-realisation, a subtle substratum, a sense of individualisation in the form of transparent 'lucid cognition' will always remain. Even more to the point, self-realisation is nothing more than simply being oneself. That is, being what we simply are, have been and always will be at the core of our very existence. The closest we usually get to this experience is when we are in a state of deep inner stillness. In inner stillness, 'when you're not thinking yourself into existence, there really isn't a self' (Adyashanti, 2011). What remains is what we are. The state of self-remembering arises when our awareness of a distinct sense of 'I' or 'me' in relation to everything else disintegrates. But a true disintegration of all sense or condition of 'I' or 'me' is usually caused by totally unexpected circumstances, such as an adventure on holiday or a challenging competition, or by highly emotional states such as falling in love, a sudden unexpected surprise, news of the death of a loved one, or in times of great disillusionment. This means we have all experienced profound moments and times of self-remembering and self-realisation in which we become highly conscious, are fully present for a more prolonged period of time, undergoing an experience that is void of any sense of 'me' or 'I', and replaced by a pronounced state of being in the presence of a far greater truth and all-encompassing reality. In self-realisation or self-remembering, we shift from the 'I' that is subjective in its nature to the 'am', which comprises what we are in essence, experiencing itself as an undiluted expression of pure being.

Experiment

1. In a quiet moment, when you are on your own, say out loud 'I am' and simply stay with the feeling that arises after the word 'am'. Vocalise 'I am' again after a few moments.
2. Keep practising in moments when you need to regroup …

The experiment might leave you with an unexpected brief, but distinct, experience of a moment of self-remembering or self-realisation. The shift from perceiving the world through the 'I' state that we are so familiar with to pure perception, void of conditioning and experienced as an authentic and natural state of being, is so subtle and unspectacular that it is easily missed. The moment we try to grasp the quality and feeling that arise when we *listen* to the silence after saying 'am' is the moment we objectify it and lose it, finding ourselves back in the default state of 'I', which gives rise to the realisation that we can only feel it and be it, without ever being able to see it.

Now, consider the world without any mirrors. In such a world, we would never be able to see our face, and the same is true of our inner self. We can picture our personality with our mind's eye. However, the mind can't produce or project a form or shape of the actual self, so that we can grasp and see it. Our mind can't understand this paradox, because it sees and experiences itself, our personality and features, as well as everything else as *things* via thought, form, shape or substance. Hence, if it is not a shape, thought, form or substance, the mind

OUR FORMLESS SELF IS COMPRISED
OF A DEPTH OF SILENCE AND STILLNESS
THAT IS
TRANSCENDENTAL

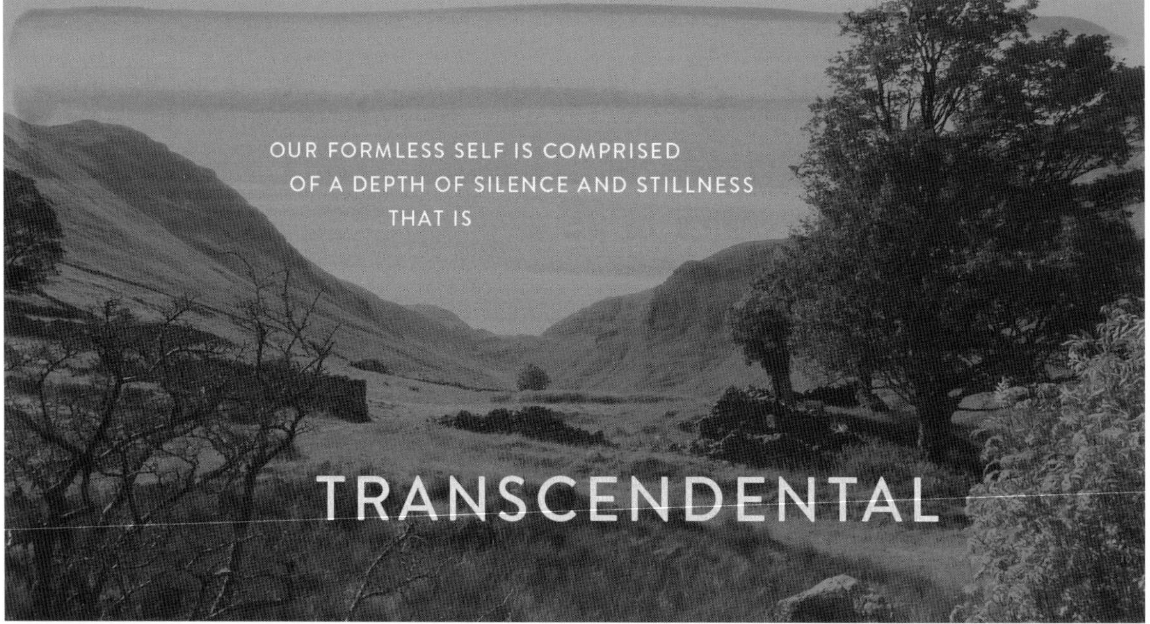

Figure 22.1

Artwork Victoria Dokas; photography Alexander Filmer-Lorch

will desperately try to turn it into such by means of imagination. Yet, when it comes to what we essentially are as pure beings, the mind gives up and goes blank. The moment it blanks it disintegrates, and the shock of change induced by the blank causes us to self-realise, which will be discussed in the next section.

Shocks of change

Once we have got our head around the paradox of self-remembering and self-realisation, we might come to the conclusion that waiting for life to give rise to unexpected experiences that lead to a glimpse of self-realisation does not really do the job. That's why the ancient teachings offer us simple solutions to take this matter into our own hands, so that we can gradually shift from our relative everyday state of consciousness – that of 'I' in relation to everything else – into one where we experience the world through the eyes of the insightful self that is not biased or exclusive. We become creative in seeking out situations throughout the day that wake us up from our default mode. This requires something that is more powerful than our default mode or routine itself, and Ouspensky calls this a 'positive shock' or 'conscious shock', which once implemented causes us to 'wake up'. Dewey describes this shift in consciousness as 'shocks of change due to interruption of a prior adjustment. They are signals to redirections of action' (Dewey, 1957). It still surprises me that this simple yet transformative tool of working with 'positive shocks' is so rarely mentioned in other schools of thought.

So, what exactly is a 'shock of change' or 'positive shock'? In our work as practitioners, this means everything that takes us out of our default responses in the way we treat, facilitate or teach, opening us up to different possibilities we would never consider worth pursuing otherwise. A positive shock gives rise to a heightened sense of awareness and alertness. It makes us think outside the box and connects us with the creative potential that arises from our insightful self in the form of inspiration and intuition.

For example, if we are working in a mode of *doing*, the shock of change could be to pause for a moment and shift into *allowing*. If our work is based on a deeply engrained protocol that we apply to every client alike, the positive shock could be to throw the protocol out of the window for a while and step into the unknown. If we are used to chatting along with our clients throughout the session, the shock of change could be to implement phases where we work in silence. To avoid repetitive strain injury, we regularly use a counterbalance and change sides and positions. Another powerful waking up method is to regularly attend complementary training (CPD) and become creative at integrating the newly acquired skills into our familiar ways of work, which will transform our practice. However, despite all of this, one of our main priorities should be to receive our own treatment, as well as to keep up the work on ourselves, which in our field of expertise is the most powerful shock of change of all.

All experiments and exercises in this book can be used as positive shocks to facilitate the necessary change to gradually become a more centred person and practitioner. Each exercise has the potential to help us remember and self-realise. However, without an active observing presence within us, shocks of change can't be implemented.

Experiment

For the next four months, put into practice one of the above suggestions, including some of the experiments described in this book. Feel free to start with the ones that most attract your attention.

States of awe

> *A state of awe is synonymous with a state of utter coherence.*
>
> Alexander Filmer-Lorch

We all know them, embrace them and cherish them, because the experiences and feelings that states of awe create in us cause us to hold our breath, keeping us in blank astonishment for a more prolonged moment in time. An awe-inspiring situation can truly touch us on the deepest level, which is an exhilarating experience. Sometimes, it might even take us into a transient moment of sheer bliss, a state of joy and happiness that lies beyond words. A state of awe does not only make us remember our self, it literally liberates the innermost self from everything that covers it and prevents it from its birthright of existing right here in the present moment. This is the reason why we feel so open, free, spacious and authentic when we are in a state of awe, and we sometimes wish that it could last forever. Hence, a state of awe is *coherence in action*. Philosophically speaking, states of awe cause us to experience the subtle inner quivering of our soul that is striving towards union, giving us a glimpse of the beyond, and might give rise to the sweetest inner longing, which has the power to transform and transcend.

However, we can't produce a state of awe by sheer willpower, which means we can only be ready to meet it; or, to be more precise, a state of awe usually meets us in the most unexpected circumstances. The moment we establish contact, it imperceptibly makes us forget ourselves, and we discover the pure being of our innermost self.

In our everyday life, it can take a very long time before we experience a state of awe, yet at no other time in history have we had such easy access to so many possibilities for awe-inspiring impressions. So, what kind of places do we have to seek out in order to expose and open ourselves to more awe-inspiring situations and experience this living imprint of true self?

The answer in this case is that the world is your oyster! We only need to enquire into the mystery of life to discover awe-inducing revelations. Cosmology, quantum physics, science and medicine are continually discovering new facts that can blow our mind and leave us speechless. Literature, theatre, movies, music and the arts can reach into the depth of our inner being, shifting us into unfathomable heights of our existence. But nothing can take us into a more exhilarating state than the wonders of the universe and the powerful impact of the outstanding beauty of nature that our planet earth has at its disposal.

Furthermore, there are countless places to be discovered that make us withdraw from the external world of experiences and turn us inwards. Places such as temples, mosques and churches, galleries and architectural buildings radiate a depth of tranquillity that instils the most soothing silence and peace within us that seems to reach into our very existence directly from somewhere beyond. Then there are the wonders of philosophy and the universal teachings that awaken the potential within us through experiencing higher emotions that carry the power to pull us through the work, and which ultimately transform us into what we were always supposed to be.

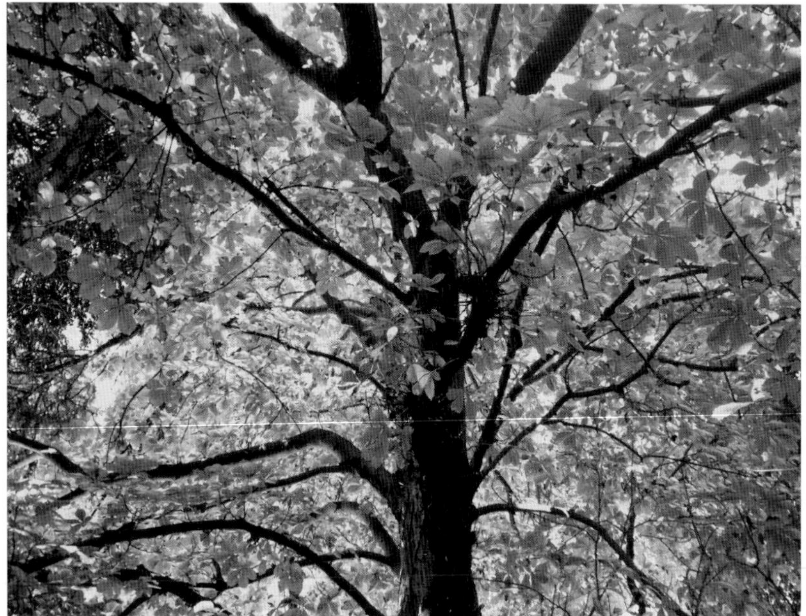

Figure 22.2

Nothing can replace the power of nature. Even the canopy of a tree, illuminated by the sun, can take us into a state of awe. Photography Alexander Filmer-Lorch

Lastly, there is our work as therapists and practitioners, through which so many of us are gifted with the astonishing awesomeness of the healing process, or sometimes miraculous changes taking place in our clients, which we can witness and become part of on a daily basis. What else do we need to make us wonder – and remember?

Experiment

Use the countless possibilities you have at your disposal to expose yourself to potential awe-inspiring impressions. Observe how this acts on your life and on the way you work.

'Trivided' attention

Once we have gathered more conscious memories of self, evoked by the unknown and different states of awe we meet in life, or by subtle shocks of change that we apply to ourselves, and are regularly connecting with the distinct sensation we feel after the reverberation of the sound 'am', we want to look at possibilities that help us to reinforce and consolidate a more permanent connection to the insightful self that we feel in inner stillness. In Part 3: Chapter 13 we discussed the dynamics of the state of divided attention that most schools of thought, including mindfulness and meditation, utilise to evoke a state of separation in order to establish a greater connection to self. However, we discovered that a state of divided attention can't be kept up for very long by our own will before we find ourselves within the swing of opposites again (bouncing between subject and object), which is the main reason why many people give up, because they realise that they can't possibly be the winner in this disproportionate arrangement. Yet the moment the neutralising element comes into the equation, all things fall into perfect balance.

Most of the time, especially at work, we are in what could be called an object/event state, where we identify with pretty much everything that is asking for our attention.

Experiment

1. Observe and recognise the moment when you come out of complete absorption and identification with an external happening.
2. Feel the change in quality and acknowledge when and how you regroup your sense of 'I' ...

In the object/event state we have completely lost connection with our sense of 'I', and our field of perception is pretty much restricted to only one dimension in which we lose ourselves in the object.

Fig. 22.3 illustrates that the moment we divide our attention between the seer and the seen – when we are aware of both subject and object simultaneously – our field of perception has slightly increased, yet is still more or less restricted to a more horizontal and two-dimensional view of life, in which the powerful swing of the pendulum reigns.

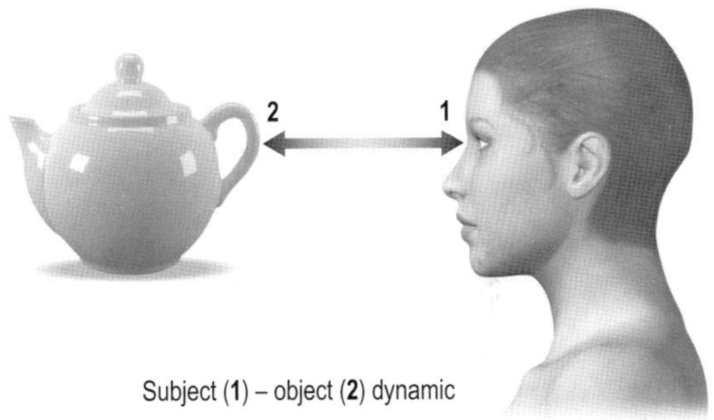

Figure 22.3

When we divide our attention, we are bouncing back and forth between subject (1) and object (2)

Experiment

Watch and recognise how much time you spend bouncing back and forth between the external and referencing it with a position, memory or knowledge in the internal.

We escape this linear dynamic the moment we include the space surrounding the seen, in which our field of perception increases, providing us with a much more three-dimensional view of life, as illustrated in Fig. 22.4. Here we see the world through the lenses of our 'I-believes' and personal philosophies, which are firmly rooted in a strong 'I' state and not the object/event state.

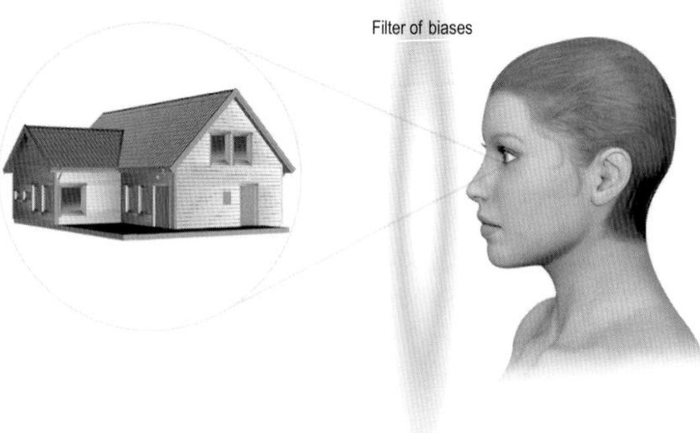

Figure 22.4

When our awareness is more spatial, we gain a more three-dimensional view on things, but perceive the world through the filter of our biases, I-believes and personal philosophies

Experiment

Acknowledge how often during the day the world is centred around you, your 'I-believes' and your personal philosophies.

The moment we settle into the fulcrum in the middle, the still-point within which we are truly neither this nor that (neti neti), the shock of change that action through non-reaction causes shifts us into a four-dimensional view, in which we experience and recognise the subject and the object, as well as the space surrounding both, as one undivided whole, held and effortlessly sustained by a perfectly balanced and frictionless triad of equal strengths or quantities of active (impressions/attention), passive (perception/awareness) and neutralising (place of no position/stillness) energies or forces, as illustrated in Fig. 22.5.

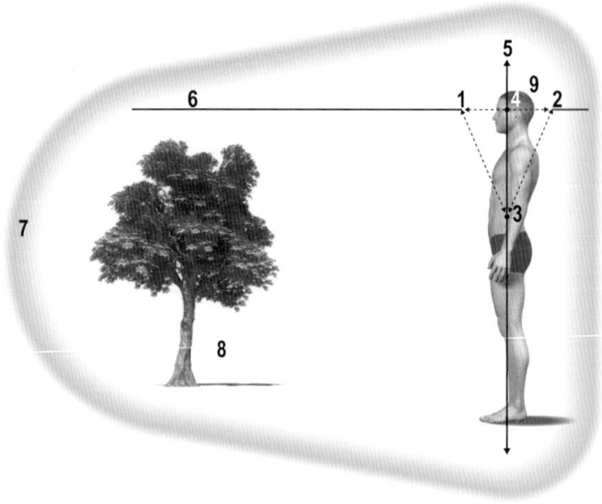

Figure 22.5

In a state of 'trivided' attention, symbolised by the triangle comprised of attention (1), awareness (2) and place of no position/stillness (3) that arises by means of action through non-reaction in the fulcrum in the middle (4). Our field of perception expands into four directions along the vertical (5) and horizontal (6) scales of life. Here we perceive the 'is-ness' of things including the space surrounding things (7) (including ourselves), subject (9) and object (8)

This profound leap of separation is accomplished by recruiting our proprioceptive sense or felt sense. That is, we want to become immersed in a place within us in which stillness-memory and the non-perceptible nature reside and can be felt, and we will explore this in the next chapter.

Experiment

Observe moments in which things are allowed to be as they are, and how that impacts upon your state of mind and state of being.

References

Adyashanti (2011). *Falling Into Grace*. Boulder, Colo.: Sounds True, Inc., p 36.

Dewey, J. (1957). *Reconstruction in Philosophy*. Boston: Beacon Press.

Prahlad.org (2015). *I Am That, chapter 13*, www.prahlad.org/gallery/nisargadatta/concordances/I_Am_That/html/IAT_013_1044_1229_.htm [accessed 10 Nov. 2015].

Softening back

A leap of separation is substantiated by what is known in ancient teachings as our inner sense. In today's language, the inner sense is known as our somatosensory or tactile system, registering sensations such as light, temperature, pressure, touch, joint and muscle activation, as well as bone and body positioning in space and gravity. The somatosensory pathway (primary, secondary and tertiary) comprises three neurons, with their respective cell bodies situated in the dorsal root ganglion, the spinal cord and the thalamus. Each of them performs a different task: temperature and pain, discrimination of touch, and proprioception. It is the proprioceptive sense, also called our sixth sense, that detects what is happening below the surface deep within the body, by engaging nerve receptors that are known as proprioceptors.

It is known that very many of our emotions are influenced by the nerves in our gut and, according to *Scientific American*, it looks like our 'everyday emotional well-being may rely on messages from the brain below to the brain above' (Hadhazy, 2010). This refers to our 'second brain' within our enteric nervous system (ENS), containing, according to neurogastroenterology expert Michael Gershon, 'some 100 million neurons, more than in either the spinal cord or the peripheral nervous system' (Hadhazy, 2010), with approximately 500 million neurons in total in our ENS. Commenting on recent scientific research, therapist Michael Sterling (2014) says: 'We now know that the ENS is not just capable of autonomy but also influences the brain. In fact, about 90 per cent of the signals passing along the vagus nerve come not from above, but from the ENS.'

The ENS is made up of different neurons and glial support cells producing 40 different neurotransmitters and a large number of hormones. The neurons here produce as much dopamine as the neurons in the brain, and the ENS also contains about 95 per cent of our serotonin (Azan et al., 2011). Serotonin is regarded by scientists as the balancing instrument of our moods and emotions and, as our so-called 'feel-good' molecule, it helps to regulate sleep and prevent depression. Hence, it is not surprising that research has shown that chronic depression can be treated by stimulating the vagus nerve, even where other treatments have failed (Corcoran et al., 2006).

You might have observed that our hands frequently point towards the solar plexus when we talk about ourselves, an indication that we reinforce our sense of self by pointing towards the 'home' of the self, which we subconsciously feel and sense in the solar plexus ENS. We also feel 'butterflies' in our tummy before we perform, the moment we have fallen in love or embark on a new adventure. We experience a big lump and contraction in our tummy when we are in fear. Then again, any deep sense of contentment and peace is also usually felt in our solar plexus, which is the physical location of our ENS. A sigh of relief might give rise to a sense of space and relaxation in this complex second brain, and if things are still and settled in the ENS, our state of mind and emotions are tranquil and calm. Based on feedback from my clients and students throughout the years, most of our stillness-memory will affect our ENS and, figuratively speaking, accumulate and be stored as an energetic/vibrational blueprint around this area, from where it acts on our whole physiology and emotions, as well as our mind.

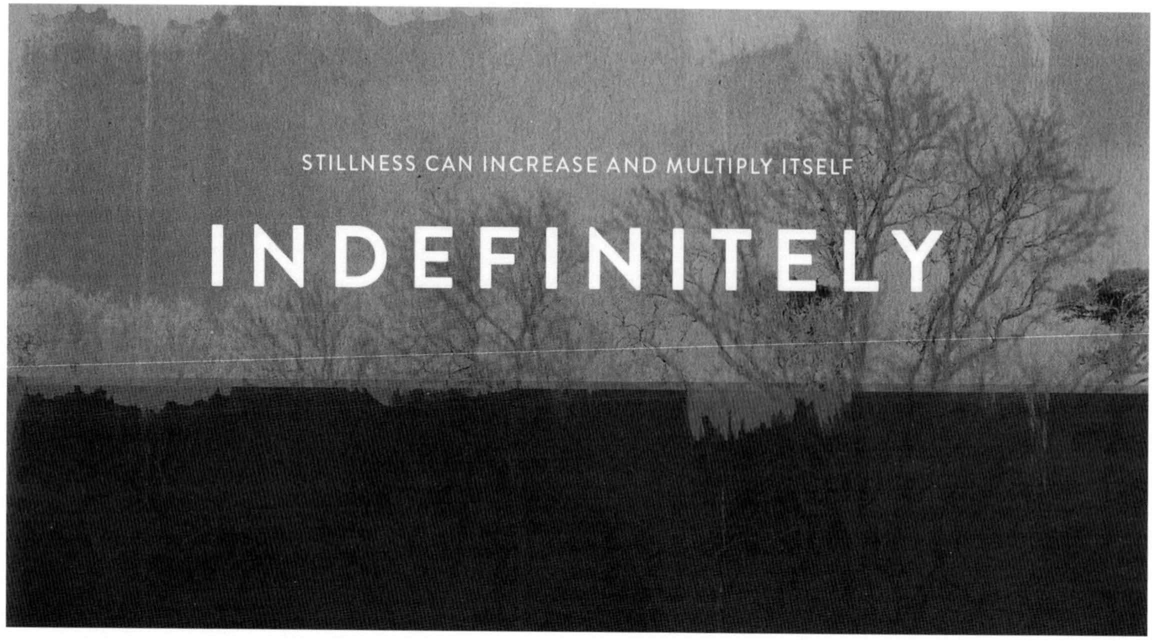

Figure 23.1

Artwork Victoria Dokas, Photography Alexander Filmer-Lorch

Experiment

During moments of deep inner stillness, acknowledge how profoundly you rest and settle in your solar plexus, a centre of gravity of dynamic stillness. You might feel that you have retreated back into your 'self', experienced as a subtle quality of inner stillness …

However, the leap of separation required to anchor us into our centre of gravity happens through our proprioceptive sense, which we can access at the fulcrum or still-point, in the middle between opposites comprised of our external world and our internal world of experiences. Here, in a short moment of inner attunement, we simply sense inwards, by softening or leaning further back into ourselves, as if we are resting into the back of our body.

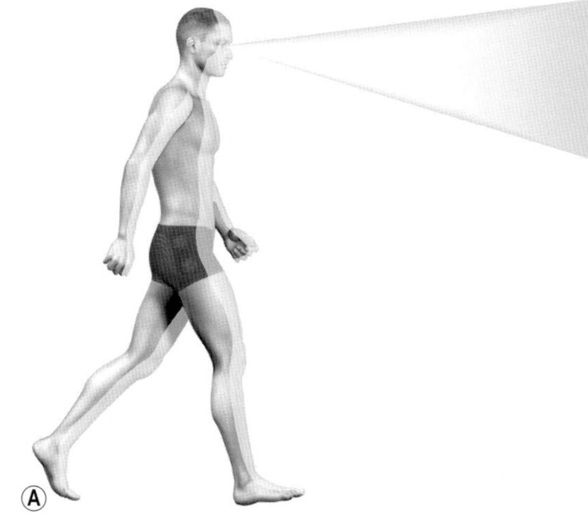

Figure 23.2

During the day our attention is focused outwards via our five senses, hence we mainly respond and approach life through the front of the body

Normally when we are in focused attention we very much move from and act through the front of our body, with concurrent full activation of our five senses. Our overall body tonus is heightened, and our breath has become shallow and flat. Everything is geared towards our objective, in which we have become fully emerged at this stage.

Experiment

Monitor what happens when you are pursuing a specific objective or in complete doing mode, like having to catch a bus or working towards a deadline, or in a period of multitasking …

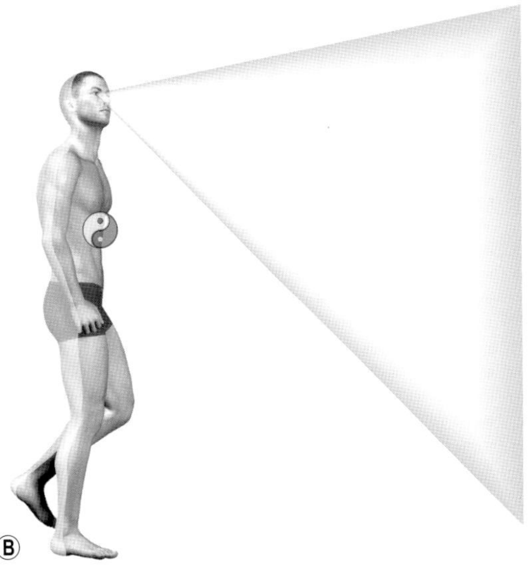

Figure 23.3

When we go through the day by remaining connected with the back of our body, we can sustain a sense of inwardness and centredness throughout the day

Here, unlike in our 'front of the body life', we can explore using the doing mode experiment. The moment we ease and connect with the back of our body, we instantly gain enough separation from our five outward-orientated senses and our highly alert attention. In the 'back of the body life', our body tonus relaxes, our breath calms and we gain more spatial awareness, as well as a sense of fluid centredness and inwardness.

Experiment

1. During the next couple of weeks, whenever you can, keep your senses and whole being connected with the back of your body, truly feeling the support you get, and allowing every movement to come through and from the back of the body.
2. Observe what changes when you shift from back to front, and what changes when you rest into the back of the body (yourself) again.
3. During sessions and classes treat, teach and facilitate using the support you get through this sense of inwardness of back of the body connection …

The experiment might make you question whether you are falling too much into awareness and passivity. Do not worry. Because we spend so much time using our external senses, which has become a deeply engrained habit, resting back into ourselves will, if we are lucky, get us just about into the middle, where possibilities lie. Remember: neti neti.

Experiment

Infinity breathing

1. Sit on a comfortable chair keeping your spine upright. Close your eyes and let them relax and soften, whilst easing back, softening towards the back of the body. You can do this exercise whilst lying down as well.
2. Place the palms of your hands on your tummy, and simply observe the rising and falling away of the flow of your natural breath through the palms of your hands (see Fig. 23.4A).
3. After a couple of minutes tune into the pause after the inhalation, as well as the pause after the exhalation, but not longer than a comfortable moment.
4. Then, whilst keeping your eyes soft, take a very subtle, gentle and slow inhalation, whilst you feel yourself expanding laterally. Stay in the pause after the inhalation (see Fig. 23.4B).
5. Gently exhale, and undo into the pause after the exhalation (1), when your diaphragm is relaxed, and whilst your proprioceptive sense and awareness (Fig. 23.4C) stay connected with the lateral expansion (2) throughout your body.
6. Keep repeating this breath cycle for as long as you feel comfortable. Then just rest in silence for a few more minutes letting go of all breathing ...

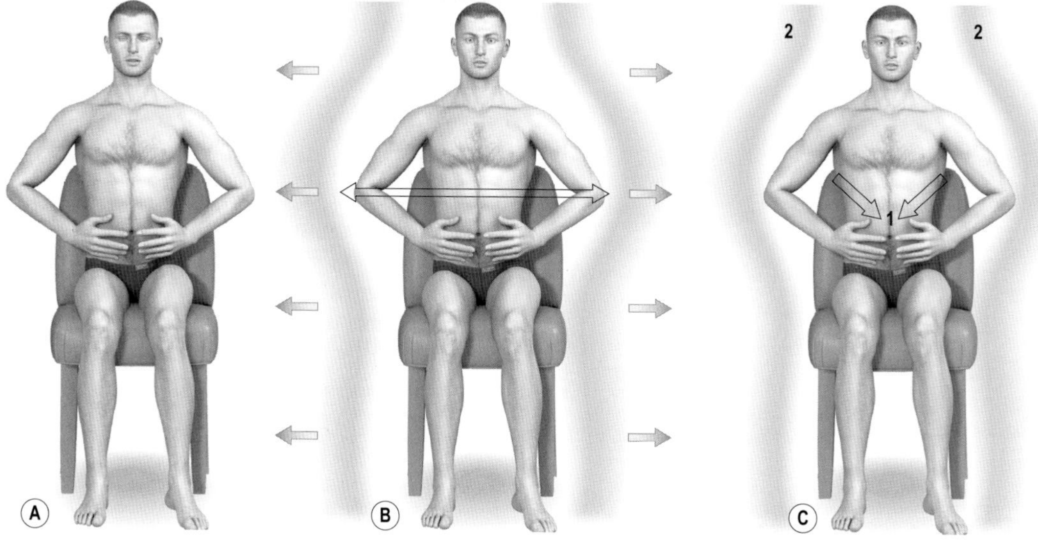

Figure 23.4

(A) The drawing illustrates steps 1, 2 and 3 of the exercise. Tune into the natural rising and falling away of your breath, through the palms of your hands. Acknowledge the natural pause after each inhalation and exhalation. (B) Execute step 4 with less doing and more allowing. Feel yourself expanding sideways, then rest in the pause after the inhalation. (C) In step 5, let the exhalation simply happen (1), whilst you feel the lateral expansion increasing (2), then follow step 6

Infinity breathing

Breathing has four stages: the inhalation, the full pause after the inhalation, the exhalation, and the empty pause after the exhalation. It is the autonomic nervous system that controls our breath, and it really knows best how to do that without requiring any interference on our behalf. This is the reason why all the exercises in this book that involve breathing should be approached and executed in the most respectful and non-invasive way possible. Please remember, less is more! That is, as we mentioned before, less doing and much more allowing.

On a physiological level, when we breathe in, our diaphragm contracts and moves downwards, freeing up space for the lungs to expand and sucking air into the lungs, from where it passes through the bronchial tubes to enter the alveoli, passing oxygen to the surrounding capillaries. When we breathe out, our diaphragm relaxes and moves further up into the chest cavity again, narrowing the space in the chest cavity, which forces air enriched with carbon dioxide out of our system.

Normally our breath does not require any effort on our behalf. However, most people these days spend the majority of their time in shallow breathing, which is a sign of tension and stress. We can well imagine how that impacts upon the ENS and our state of mind. When we are busy and task-driven, our breath is faster and our mind is agitated, possibly even running on overdrive. Yet in inner stillness, when we are relaxed, our breath is slow and our mind is calm. That means our breathing can influence our state of mind, and in return a busy mind will influence our breathing.

In this practice we aim to stay with the moment-to-moment experience with the help of our breath. Our inner sense should stay connected with the lateral expansion, which gives rise to an internal spatial perception that takes our awareness far beyond the physical confinement of the body. We almost touch upon or tap into something infinite that lies outside our ordinary sense of perception. Hence the name 'infinity breath'.

'I' is the inhalation, 'am' is ..., the 'pause' is ...

I am not that which thinks; I simply am! Enquiry into what we are is the basis of philosophy – an eternal quest into the true nature of the self. The ancient teachings highlight the possibility that there is something in us that can observe, witness and even listen to the continuous voice in our head that is verbalising each thought that arises.

The most common understanding of this process

Experiment

'I am' practice

1. Sit on a comfortable chair keeping your spine upright (Fig. 23.5). Close your eyes and let them relax and soften, whilst easing back to settle into the 'am' space.
2. Apply the same gentle breathing technique as practised in infinity breathing.

   During a gentle inhalation mentally pronounce 'I' (very slowly), truly feeling the 'I' expanding out from the 'am' space (solar plexus) beyond the confinement of your physical body. Then pause for a glimpse of a moment of stillness, feeling the 'I'.

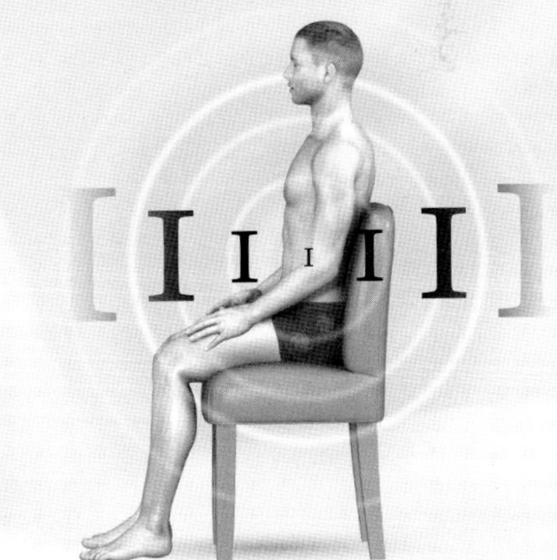

Figure 23.5

In steps 1 and 2, connect with the 'am' space

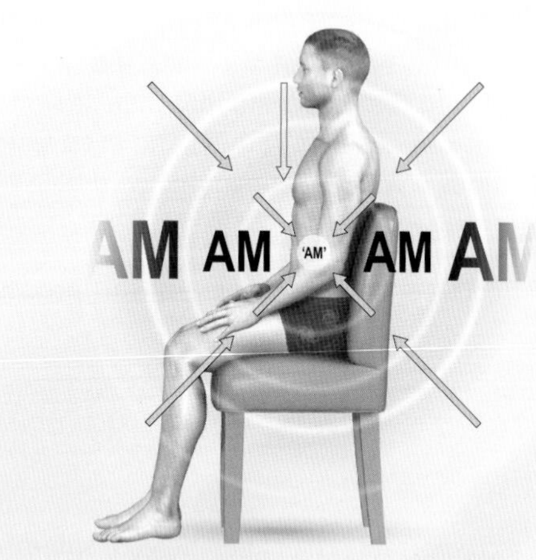

Figure 23.6

3. Exhale (Fig. 23.6) with a sigh-like sensation whilst mentally pronouncing 'am', and fully feeling the 'am'.
4. Truly immerse yourself in the feeling that arises in the stillness of the pause after the inner sound of 'am' has fallen away (Fig. 23.7).

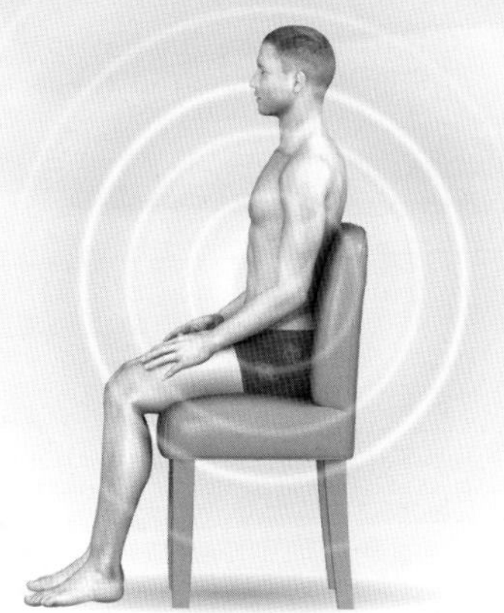

Figure 23.7

5. Slowly repeat the 'I am' for several minutes. Then just stay with the feeling of deep inwardness for another five minutes …

amongst neuroscientists is that the central part of the prefrontal cortex seems to play a role in this voice production by controlling two distinct neural loops, of which one activates regions near the visual cortex at the occipital lobe and the other uses the Broca's area of the left hemisphere of the frontal lobe as an inner voice producer that continuously repeats words and sounds. According to Scott (2013), this inner voice seems to be an internal copy of the external voice. Furthermore, he states that 'corollary discharge is a prediction of the sound of one's voice generated by the motor system … [and] provides the sensory content of inner speech'.

However, what neuroscientists don't know is to whom this inner voice arises. The ancient teachings hold an explanation that is not necessarily scientific, but is very plausible, saying that the answer can be found in the 'I am' or 'Aham' (Sanskrit). That is, the 'I' is the final thought that remains when all references to it have ceased to exist, being experienced as an inaudible echo of 'I' as identity. The 'am' is considered as the process of complete dissolution of the final 'I'. The pause after the 'am' gives rise to the emergence of pure being that genuinely understands, yet can't fully know itself, or ever be known. The following practice exercise helps lead to an initially subtle experience of the process of 'Aham'.

What we are aiming for in the 'I am' practice is to completely undo, or 'un-become', in the pause after the exhalation. In the first part we truly acknowledge the 'I'. In the pause after the exhalation, however, we can finally allow ourselves to not have to be anybody. We are allowed simply to be and reach a pure and natural state of being for a moment that simply 'is'.

Gaze of compassion

This is one of the most simple, yet most powerful, practices when it comes to creating a state of perception that manifests enough separation and spatial awareness, without shutting off the line of communication and connection with others, as well as whatever we are dealing with. Here, we interact from a much closer connection to the insightful self, in which everything that arises is met with unwavering authenticity, and handled with utter integrity, within the limitations of

Experiment

Gaze of compassion practice

1. Lean back into yourself by taking your inner sense into the back of your body.

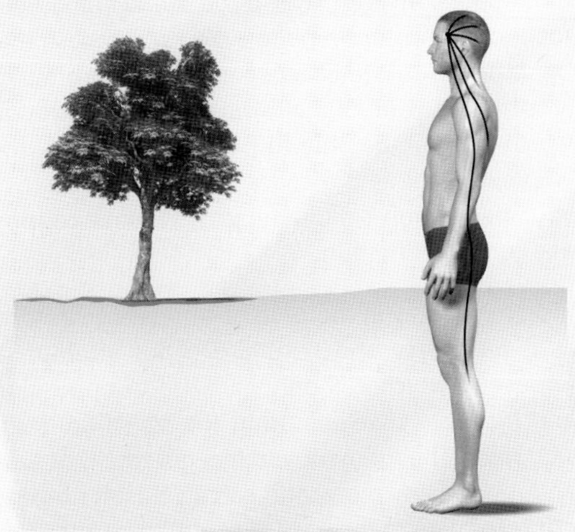

Figure 23.8

2. Once you have established a deeper sense of inwardness, settle into the gravitational pull of the 'am' space.

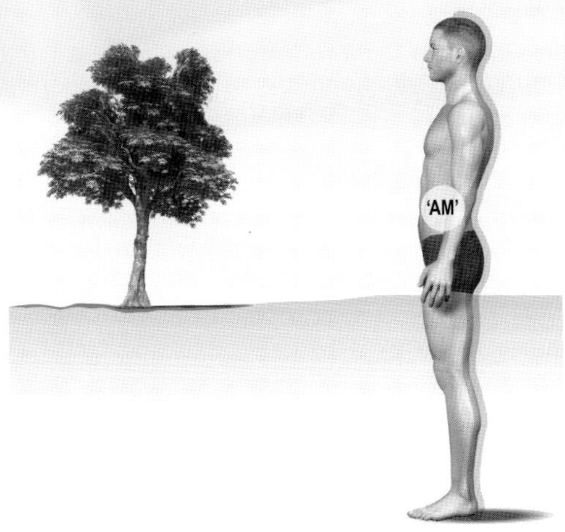

Figure 23.9

3. Allow your eyes to soften and relax, which takes you into soft gaze and gives rise to a greater spatial awareness.

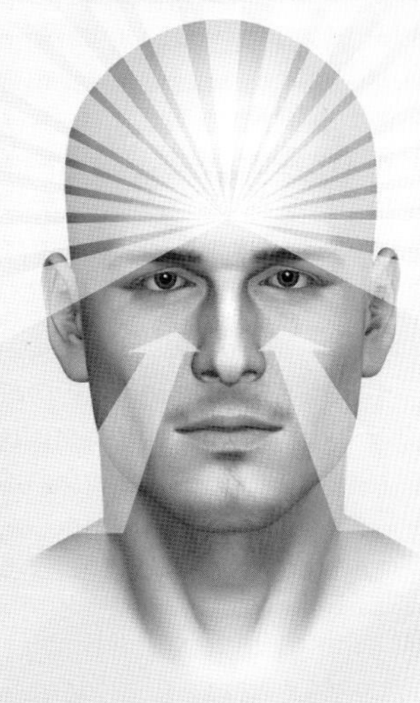

Figure 23.10

4. In soft gaze, whilst you stay centred in the 'am' space and keeping your inner sense connected with the back of your body, let your soft gaze wander.

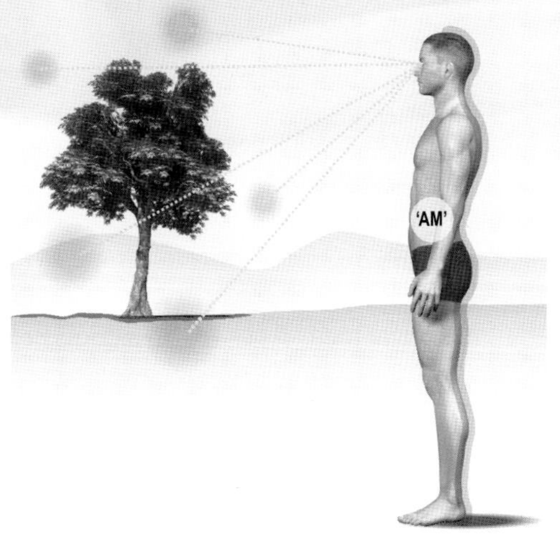

Figure 23.11

our human possibilities, of course. According to the Fourth Way philosophy, in everyday life we are under the law of the pendulum. The gaze of compassion will gradually neutralise and take us out of the law of the pendulum, as far as our psychology and inner states are concerned. However, experience shows that it will take quite some time to master this simple practice without giving rise to an imposed and artificially created state. There truly are so many subtle layers to it, and even more refined ones will be discovered throughout the years of our practice, which is the reason why it is important to be fully established and at ease with the softening back technique, the infinity breathing and the I am practice before we start practising the gaze of compassion. Even after three decades of daily practice, I am still discovering more refined layers in this simple, yet so profound, gaze of compassion practice.

The ancient teachings understand that it takes about 1.5 to 2 seconds until we have fully identified with an object, can label it and start adding a story to it, usually based on our associations, experience and history in relation to the object or event. The gaze of compassion allows us to keep perceiving things and the world for what they really are, which means from an inner place of no position. If we can turn the gaze of compassion into a conscious habit, which is another philosophical paradox (it can't be executed through default mode), it will transform us and transcend countless non-conducive habits, and our whole way of life will change for good because it will be lived from the middle, which is the true gateway to possibilities.

Tips and progression

- Please start this practice in open space, for example on a walk in the park, in nature or whilst you are sitting somewhere high up or strolling along a beach. Let your soft gaze wander without dwelling on any object longer than 1.5 seconds.

- Once that feels natural and effortless, 'trivide' your attention between the 'am' space, the back of the body sensation and a feeling as if you are looking through your physical eyes and perceiving the world from somewhere further and deeper within, all whilst your soft gaze wanders.

- Once that feels natural and effortless, use this technique in your work whilst listening to clients, during treatments and classes and even whilst you are having a discussion.

- The final stage of this practice is to stay in the gaze of compassion even whilst you are keeping your focus on things or on people. You accomplish that by shifting into lateral awareness, which profoundly increases your spatial awareness, and through which you will be able to perceive the parts, the whole, as well as the space around the object of your perception simultaneously, without causing any conflict or friction.

- Please only stay in the gaze of compassion as long as it feels easy and natural. Do not attempt to impose it, which will only give rise to opposition and friction, as well as using too much unnecessary force. The moment you feel not totally at ease and relaxed any more, and catch yourself exerting effort to keep up the gaze of compassion, then you have fallen into attention and will be under the law of the pendulum again.

References

Azan, G., Low, W.C., Wendelschafer-Crabb, G., Ikramuddin, S. and Kennedy, W.R. (2011). Evidence for neural progenitor cells in the human adult enteric nervous system. *Cell and Tissue Research*, 344(2): 217–225. doi: 10.1007/s00441-011-1130-9.

Corcoran, C., Thomas, P., Phillips, J. and O'Keane, V. (2006). Vagus nerve stimulation in chronic treatment-resistant depression: preliminary findings of an open-label study. *British Journal of Psychiatry*, 189(3): 282–283.

Hadhazy, A. (2010). Think twice: how the gut's 'second brain' influences mood and well-being. *Scientific American*, www.scientificamerican.com/article/gut-second-brain/ [accessed 18 Nov. 2015].

Scott, M. (2013). Corollary discharge provides the sensory content of inner speech. *Psychological Science*, 24(9): 1824–1830.

Sterling, M. (2014). The second brain, our enteric nervous system [blog]. MFIT, www.mfi-therapy.com/the-second-brain-our-enteric-nervous-system/ [accessed 18 Nov. 2015].

Reclaiming force 24

Our whole physiological and psychological being only works to its full potential when it can keep its natural equilibrium and sustain its homeostasis. A delicate and complex exchange of information, energies and forces makes this possible. If we lose force, we go off balance, and it is this precious energy that leaks through different non-conducive loopholes all the time. Using a symbolic picture from the ancient teachings, we can all draw from a massive reservoir of life force, which is subdivided into a reservoir we use on a daily basis and a powerful main reservoir we only access when it comes to emergency situations and our survival. Unfortunately, our modern way of life and its associated stresses seem to keep us on emergency alert all the time. That is, the subreservoir that is supposed to sustain us during the day, and in normal circumstances replenishes itself with new force and energy that is naturally generated during the deep sleep phase at night (delta brainwave activity), is in a condition of chronic depletion, continuously refilling itself by drawing force from our emergency reservoir. The consequences of this loss of force are wide-reaching. The following chapters provide some simple, yet incredibly effective, tools that will enable us and our clients to reclaim and maintain our life force balance.

Watching the pattern unfold

We all enjoy the beauty and complexity of patterns, such as the patterns of nature and the universe, and the patterns of the fabric of our life. These patterns of life are formed by occasions and events, and the patterns of events unfold on many different levels simultaneously. They take place locally as well as globally, and even on a universal level. We are usually absorbed in the events of our immediate local life, which keep us busy and engaged 24–7, without ever being aware of the pattern they create. We hardly ever experience an event as separate from us because we are in it, are part of it and literally have become it. In this condition we lose a tremendous amount of energy because we identify with every aspect of the current event.

It is only when we enjoy some leisure time or in tranquil moments that we suddenly become aware of the patterns created by light reflected on water, the patterns of the clouds formed by the turbulence of the wind, the patterns on fabrics and furniture that almost seem to move, or the patterns we see unfolding created by a crowd of people in the street below us. In these instances we perceive the parts as well as the whole, and are conscious of when the course of events is changing, giving rise to successive new events in a chain reaction. We are left with an imprint of a pattern we would not recognise if we were part of the crowd that is being moved and driven by invisible forces, a pattern nourished and fed by the energy of each respective part of the current event. Although we form part of the occasion, we are not losing force to the event because we are one step removed, which allows us to watch the pattern unfold. That is, we are conscious that this is simply one occasion out of many that will change and unfold, without depleting our energy, giving us the freedom to put this current local happening into the context of a far greater pattern that our event is part of. We even have the freedom of choice to participate in another event that might be of much greater relevance, simply because we are aware that other events exist.

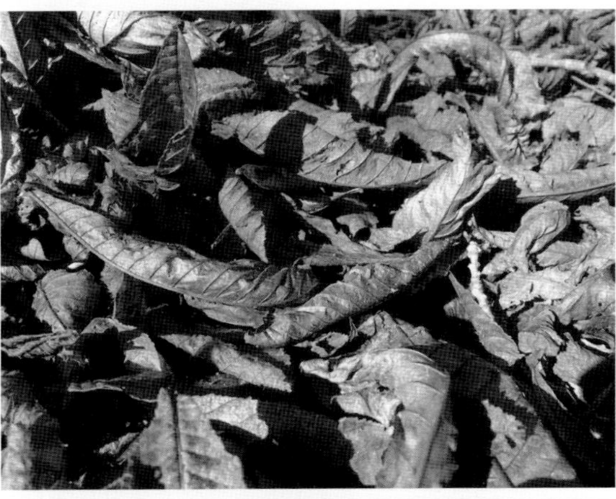

Figure 24.1

Autumn leaves symbolising the patterns of life

We can use this idea in our practice. Each treatment, session or class, from beginning to end, is a process comprising a succession of different events that take place on many different levels from local to global. The treatment, session or class is the exclusive event of our clients, who have the sole right and unspoken permission to fully immerse themselves in their event, because that's what they have come for. As therapists and practitioners, our role in the event is to simply watch the pattern unfold locally, as well as globally, which gives rise to a window of possibilities we can't access if we become part of, or get completely lost in, the event of our clients or students. Indeed, to do so would load the event for our clients with an invasive force, which of course would be totally counterproductive to the treatment, session or class.

Experiment

1. When you are out with your friends or family, or at any non-specific occasion, remind yourself: 'This is me, participating in a [name of the occasion] event.' Observe what has changed.
2. On your way to work, remind yourself: 'This is me, in my on my way to work event.' Then connect to a wider event that your 'on my way to work event' is part of.
3. During treatments, sessions or classes, simply watch the local and global patterns unfold. Observe what changes in the process, and if there are any changes in the response of your client to the treatment, session or class ...

This simple experiment teaches our mind to enjoy looking at things from a far greater perspective. You will soon realise how much freedom that implies, as well as how much energy is saved that would otherwise get caught or lost in the details of things, where it is of no benefit to the whole.

Neutralising psychological habits

There is a theory in psychosynthesis that whatever lies in the unconscious controls us, and whatever we consciously identify in the unconscious can gradually be controlled. Eastern psychology works with similar ideas, but takes this one step further, indicating that to be able to control something it will require energy, and once the energy is used up, things just go back to where they were. However, the moment whatever unconsciously controls us is made passive, it will stop acting on us and stop using up force. This is the real meaning of reaching peace with oneself, by neutralising whatever keeps us away from the middle, where real possibilities lie.

According to different schools of psychology, ancient and modern alike, there are various 'non-conducive' psychological manifestations we acquire in life that eat up a tremendous amount of force. All of them are of no use or benefit to anything in our life, so if we neutralise even a few of them and reclaim the force they hold, our whole state of being and outlook on life and work will have transformed. The Fourth Way philosophy calls those psychological manifestations mechanical states. A prime example is habitually worrying about things that haven't happened yet and usually never will. Another is called instant considering, which includes what other people might think of us, as well as considering whether what we think, do or haven't done is OK or not OK. Next is the non-conscious habit of thinking and speaking negatively about everyone and everything, including ourselves, which is the most limiting of all, because nothing can grow from it. Habitual imagining that replaces the actuality of a situation, such as thinking, 'But I imagined this would turn out to be different', is another example. Imagining a lot of unnecessary things, which only leads to disappointment if they don't materialise, also takes a lot of energy. Old habitual 'I-believes' and personal philosophies that prevent us from seeing things more neutrally and objectively are some of the most common non-conducive states that most people find difficult to let go of.

We can well imagine the pitfalls of the above habits during sessions or classes. For example, thinking whether what we just said to the client could lead to misunderstanding; imagining the final outcome of the session and how great the client will feel afterwards; worrying when things do not go according to our plan, or that the session or class was not good enough and the client might not come back; thinking negatively the moment the client points out that things don't feel comfortable; or at the end of the session telling your client that your personal 'I-believe' is

I EXPERIENCE THIS WORK AS A GATEWAY TO
POSSIBILITIES
THAT LIE FAR
BEYOND
THE IMAGINABLE

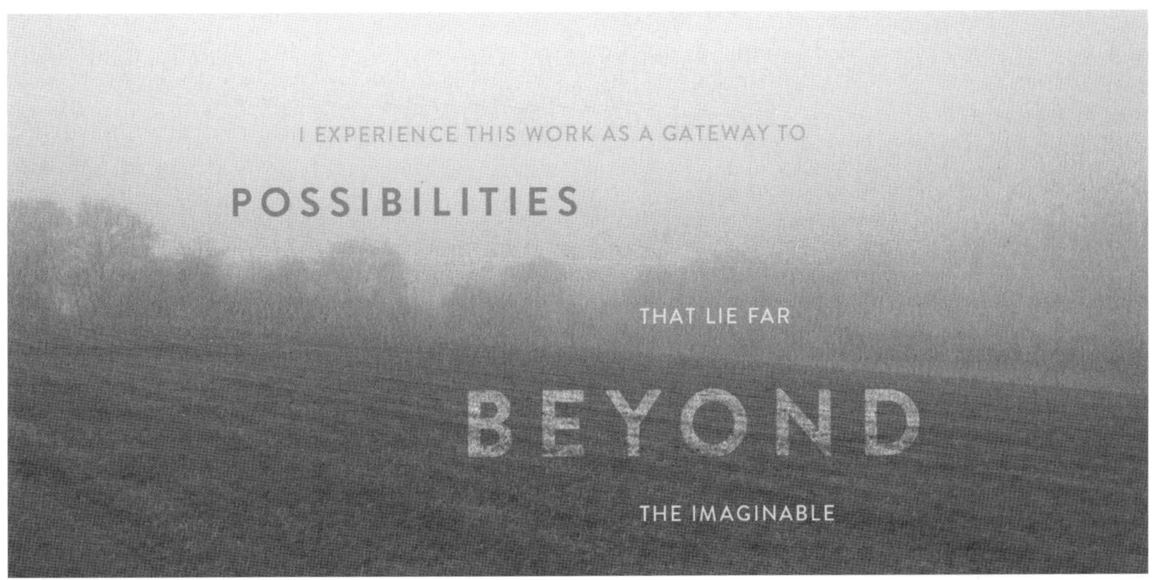

Figure 24.2

Artwork Victoria Dokas, photography Alexander Filmer-Lorch

such and such, which would need to be assessed in a specialist medical examination. I think you get how it works, and the best way to deal with it is to smile about it, because no one is free of these things; but that does not mean we can't do anything about them.

Experiment

1. Neutrally observe when you fall into any of the above habits, or any other you would like to make passive. Choose one habit to work with for a while.
2. The shock of change you need to apply the moment one of these habits is about to move into the foreground is to pause for a moment, smile and acknowledge it, mentally saying 'I am aware that this is only imagination', or 'I am aware that instant considering wants to take over'.
3. Then access your proprioceptive sense to regroup by connecting with the 'am' space, heave a sigh and stop giving the habit any further attention …

You might experience that, even if only one of these states has become passive, some of the remaining related habits that live in our unconsciousness might have become pretty quiet as well.

Please always remember that there is no place for judgement in this exercise, which should be approached in a very light-hearted and playful manner. It is good to be able to smile about things we have simply acquired by imitation and conditioning, which is all it really is.

Changing gear

Each of our functions, including thinking linked to our central nervous system, emotional function linked to our enteric nervous system, movement and physiological functions linked to our autonomic nervous system and its sympathetic and parasympathetic divisions, has a natural threshold beyond which it fails to work at full potential. If we override this limit our functions will deplete. When it comes to our intellect, it usually tires out after 45 minutes of working at full potential. The movement function will slow down when we run out of stamina, and when we over-exercise we are prone to injuries. However, it is our emotions and feelings that eat up the greatest amount of energy if they run on overdrive caused by specific emotional states, such as the breakdown of a relationship, in times of fear, or the loss of someone dear to us, as well as fallouts or upsets at work, with friends and with family.

Our intellect and emotions are usually kept busy in times of stress and, if they don't slow down, our physiological function will go into overdrive, producing more and more norepinephrine and other stress hormones. In other words, our functions will drain our energy and deplete us if they do not get a break. The following experiment will help to get things back to normal function and balance.

Experiment

1. After an hour of concentrated work that involves the whole focus of your intellect, simply shift to your physiological function with a simple breathing exercise for five minutes. Then fetch yourself a glass of water and stretch out your legs and arms. In this little amount of time your intellect has a chance to recharge and can go back to work at its full potential.
2. If you find yourself in an emotional state caused by an upset, go for a run or brisk walk in the park, so utilising your movement function.
3. If you have completely exhausted your physical capacity, for example through a trekking exertion, completing a building project, or caused after too many treatments back to back, take time every 50 minutes to hydrate and rest your body for 10 minutes by simply lying down …

Most of our non-conducive states can be neutralised by a proper workout or exercise regime, or by shifting into one of the other functions. A massive amount of energy can be saved, contained and reclaimed by simply changing gear at the appropriate time.

Back to balance

The following exercise (see Fig 23.2), known as alternate nostril breathing or nadi shodhana, is a simple yet effective breathing technique (pranayama) that has a profound calming and centring effect on our body, mind and emotions. Nadi, a Sanskrit word, means channel and shodhana means purification, which relates to the purification of the nervous system. I practise this wonderful technique on an almost daily basis, cherishing the scope of its impact, which initially, at the preliminary stages, might not be very obvious. However, after a few weeks of practice, you might be surprised how much it will refine your ways of perception. In the classic nadi shodhana practice, one finger closes one of the nostrils, switching to the other once you go into alternate nostril breathing. I personally prefer to do this by mentally focusing on the respective nostril, and shifting my attention from one nostril to the other throughout alternate nostril breathing.

If three counts on the inhalation and four counts on the exhalation is too long for you to sustain, inhale for two and exhale for three counts instead. Do not impose too much effort on your breathing but keep it gentle, and do not forget to keep your eyes soft. When you feel out of breath just stop for a moment, allowing the breath to settle before you go back to your practice. Nadi shodhana is a perfect exercise to rebalance and shift back to your centre.

The sound of stillness

Stillness is audible, and the sound of stillness can be perceived by our inner sense. In ancient teachings this subtle sound is known as naad, which is a Sanskrit term that means universal sound. It is also known as the sound current or shabad that emanates from somewhere deep within. The music it produces is so soothing that it has the capacity to transcend all thought formations and mind activity. The ancient mystics reiterated often that the only thing required is to listen to the music of stillness. That is, it starts with stilling and it ends in the all-encompassing sound of stillness.

Experiment

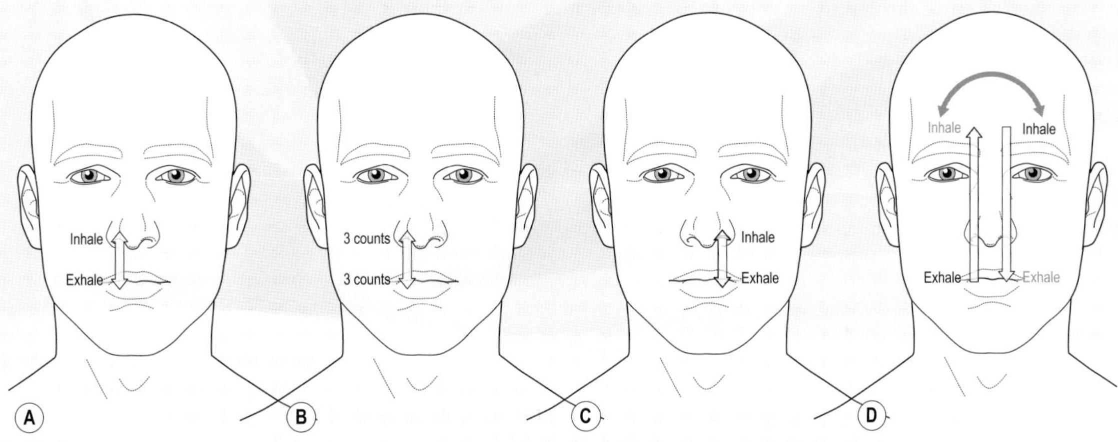

Figure 24.3

(A) Focusing on inhalation and exhalation in the right nostril. (B) Gently inhale for three counts and exhale for three counts. (C) Apply steps 1 and 2 on the left nostril. (D) Inhale for three counts through the right nostril, pause, and exhale for four counts on the left nostril, pause. Then keep alternating

Experiment

1. Make yourself comfortable on a chair, close your eyes and rest back into yourself. Place your hands comfortably on your thighs. Soften your eyes, and take your attention towards your right nostril. Feel the inhalation and exhalation predominantly in the right nostril for a while as illustrated in Fig. 24.3A.
2. Gently inhale through the right nostril for a count of three, and exhale for three counts. Keep inhaling and exhaling three counts through the right nostril at your own pace. Then let go of all conscious breathing and absorb the experience. See Fig. 24.3B.
3. Repeat steps 1 and 2 using the left nostril, then absorb the process again (see Fig. 24.3C).
4. Next inhale for three counts through the right nostril, pause for a brief moment, exhale for four counts on the left, inhale for three counts on the left, pause and exhale for four counts on the right, as illustrated in Fig 24.3D. Keep alternating for several minutes, then let go of all conscious breathing and rest within yourself …

Experiment

1. On your next walk in nature, find a tranquil place and open yourself up to the music of stillness, not by focusing or following a particular sound around you, but more by relaxing back and passively listening from within.
2. Finish every breath exercise, deep relaxation, meditation or any other stilling practice you enjoy by tuning into the vibration of stillness within and around you for several minutes. Observe how that impacts upon your body and your mind …

The exercises need to be approached through *allowing* and *undoing*, because the moment you try to grasp or look out for this sound of stillness it will vanish. If you surrender and give up listening, it will appear. Initially, it will be subtle and almost inaudible, taking the form of a soothing current of sound that can't be easily distinguished from the interference of other sounds. Later on, with more practice and less doing and trying, your level of concentration will naturally increase and stop fluctuating. However, in this matter, concentration should not be mistaken for focus. It is more a gathering and settling of distractions and forces that merge into an unfluctuating concentration of receptiveness that is void of any expectations. It is at this point that the soothing sound of stillness gives rise to the Urklang, a German term that means elemental or original sound, which becomes all-encompassing until nothing else remains – a state of pure bliss.

Working with mind and thought 25

Thought

Most of us subconsciously derive our sense of self from the existence of our physical body and the fact that we think, as well as from what we do and what we have achieved. According to Ouspensky's *In Search of the Miraculous,* our sense of self is also reinforced by the fact that we were given a name we hear all the time, which usually does not change throughout our lifetime. That is, I am my body, I have a past comprising my history, and I am what I do in life, for which I am recognised by others. It is our thinking that tells us what we know, that speaks to us in past tense and future tense, illuminating our history and possible future. At most times, however, our thoughts are unguardedly and randomly rolling along evoking different states of mind, feelings and emotions in us. If we look at our thinking from a wider perspective, we will recognise that we have three different kinds of thoughts, which are known as mechanical thoughts, conscious thoughts and higher thoughts. We can well imagine that absolutely nothing can grow out of mechanical thoughts, and because of their non-conscious nature we can't even remember them. Most of us have been in situations where we sat next to a group of friends involuntarily listening to the flow of their conversations. Imagine each of them continuously talking, changing theme in mid sentence and verbalising what is going on in their heads produced by their thought processes. Surprisingly, they even do not recognise that they are talking over each other all the time, and no one will remember in detail afterwards what anyone has said. But what each one of them will remember is that they spent an evening together that felt very pleasurable and enjoyable. This is a perfect example of mechanical thinking, and unconsciously verbalising it.

In contrast, we need our conscious thoughts when we are problem-solving, writing an essay, preparing a speech, or during an interview or a meeting. We usually apply conscious thinking when we are creative, whether that means being a designer, artist, scientist, project manager, engineer, teacher, academic, therapist, craftsman or the like. Whilst we are in a phase of conscious thinking, we are clear, focused and present to every stage that evolves during this creative process. Higher thoughts are created by higher knowledge, and are required when it comes to working with ideas that lie above the limitations of the mind. In ordinary life, they usually arise out of 'aha' moments and deep insights. However, the great patience of our conscious thoughts, which enables us to not give up the moment things become difficult or seemingly unsolvable, because they reveal that we are onto something ground-breaking or life-changing, can lead to higher thinking that is strongly linked to our 'in-tuition' and inspiration. In fact, higher thoughts are 'given', and can't be produced by our different 'I's' and 'me's' found, according to Roberto Assagioli's 'egg of being', in our limited and ever-changing field of awareness and the unconscious.

Most of the time we are not bothered by our thoughts and find them rather useful. Yet, the moment we try to sleep, become still or sit to contemplate and meditate, it is our thoughts and the emotions they produce that interfere and disturb us most. We are so used to being our thoughts and are so identified with them that the moment we don't really need them, or would like to have a break and be without any thoughts for a while, we can't free ourselves from them. This realisation of not being able to detach ourselves from our thought creation leaves us feeling utterly helpless.

We should not live under the illusion that we can eliminate or eradicate our thoughts altogether. However, the following exercises offer us possibilities that might make our thoughts and thought formation passive, so that in time they will move further into the background where we can't hear them any more. This will give rise to a state of absence of thought in which the inner power of stillness will prevail.

Experiment

This particular exercise forms the basis of the teachings on advaita of one of the greatest saints, Sri Ramana Maharshi, and enquiry into the self. He encouraged people to ask themselves this one simple question: 'To whom does this thought arise?' This leads to only one plausible answer, which is 'To me', hence 'I am'. That is, the 'I' or 'me' that we actually are at the core of our very being exists and experiences itself solely as a formless pure state of being.

1. In times when you want to make your thoughts more passive, mentally ask yourself 'To whom does this thought arise?'
2. Stay put and *allow* yourself to become completely immersed in the feeling that arises within you caused by this internal question and what is left as a reverberation the question gave rise to.
3. Before the next thought forms, stay put in the moment-to-moment experience of the rising and falling away of your breath. Relax and undo into this soothing flow of your breathing.
4. If thoughts re-enter, ask yourself again, 'To whom does this thought arise?'

Minimising editing

To genuinely listen to a client or student is one of the greatest virtues a therapist or practitioner can possess. True listening, a fundamental requirement in our field of expertise, might not be fully established or familiar to us at the beginning of our career. However, with a bit of work and focus, our listening skills can be gradually developed. We all carry the listening faculty within us as a dormant seed, and under the right conditions and with the proper respective nourishment this seed will undoubtedly flourish and grow. Yet, it is our responsibility to create the right conditions and feed it with the proper food it requires. We all know that a seed can't grow on barren ground, and the dormant seed of listening within the majority of people is buried in the ground of habitual editing and referencing, in which it has no chance of evolving and flourishing. To provide the right conditions, we have to plant this crucial seed in the ground of mental stillness, which arises when we contain this inner editing to a minimum whilst we are listening to our clients and students. The same is true when we are palpating and applying any kind of hands-on work, which is simply another form of listening.

So, how do we contain and minimise our inner editing and referencing?

Experiment

1. You shift into spatial awareness and a place of no position by leaning back into the self (connect with the back of your body and rest in your solar plexus, the 'am space'), whilst being open to every word the client says.
2. Whilst you are listening to the client, instead of going into habitual editing and instant formulations of your answers, make use of your conscious thinking to create different sticky notes in your mind of everything truly relevant to what the client says.
3. Then, kindly interrupt the client before too much information is given, possibly by saying 'Sorry to interrupt you, but just to get this right, and to avoid any misunderstanding ...', then repeat your sticky notes to the client, and create a pause in stillness in which you formulate your answers and questions, before you actually answer.
4. Ask your client if there is anything else that is important to know or mention, and when they start speaking go back to genuine listening again ...

The listening experiment brings space and quietness into the conversation. By applying this simple technique, we prevent ourselves from missing the really important details, because our inner editing and referencing creates too much noise. Clients may instead feel that the focus is really on them, and that they are being truly listened to, heard and genuinely understood. Try to avoid referencing yourself if it is not relevant to the conversation.

THROUGH MEDITATION ONE GRADUALLY
BECOMES PRESENT TO ONE'S OWN
PRESENCE

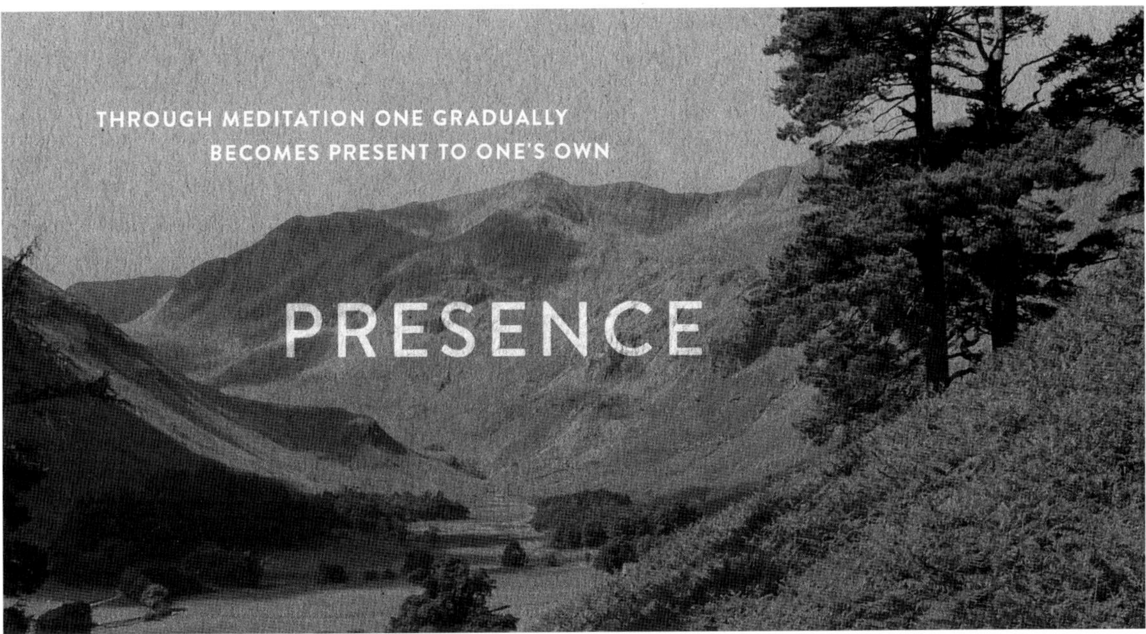

Figure 25.1

Thought space

We have all experienced how liberating it is when our thoughts are a bit more spacious and leave us in peace. This usually happens when we have had a proper workout through which our mental energies are channelled into dynamic movement and dissipate from the mind–body system through this physical activity, leaving us with a feeling of calm and relaxed satisfaction. But exercising is not the only way to establish more space in our thoughts.

We can actively extend the space between our thoughts using conscious thinking. In certain religions and ancient systems this idea is applied during the repetition of a mantra, a word or series of words repeated internally or verbalised to develop concentration. That is, the conscious repetition of word sounds simply replaces the stream of mechanical thoughts that the mind is producing all the time. The former is conducive to a state of peace of mind, whilst the latter is continuously taking force.

The following approach does not include the use of mantras, but highlights prolonged pauses between thoughts, leading to the experience that we can exist and function just fine without constant thinking when we don't need to. It is important to mention that the following experiment is based on an alternation between *allowing* and *doing* and will require conscious effort.

In the pause experiment we aim to relax and undo more and more into each pause after each repeated word that forms part of the sentence. Be creative and come up with your own sentences. Do not use the same sentence all the time. It is actually quite nice to apply this technique to certain affirmations you might find useful on certain days.

Tiring the mind out

The heading already explains the purpose of the following practice. The technique is derived from the ancient system of spanda yoga. Spanda means vitality

Experiment

Before each session, you might like to practise this simple technique.

1. Sit comfortably and take your attention to the tip of your nose.
2. Gently inhale, up to a point high above your head (1).
3. Slowly exhale down into your solar plexus (the 'am' space) through the centre of your spine (2). See steps 1 to 3 illustrated in Fig. 25.2A.
4. Whilst you slowly inhale again, feel your solar plexus expanding beyond the physical confinements of your body.
5. Then exhale and relax. See steps 4 and 5 illustrated in Fig. 25.2B).
6. Start with an inhalation at the tip of the nose again and repeat this whole cycle five to seven times.
7. Then just rest within yourself for a couple of minutes before you welcome your client into this open place of listening that you have established.

Experiment

1. Consciously read each word of the following sentence mentally a couple of times: 'I am not my thoughts, I simply am.'
2. Then very consciously repeat mentally the first word 'I', then allow a silent pause to enter, and the moment the next word of the sentence, which is 'am', is just about to rise up as a thought, consciously repeat 'am', then *allow* a silent pause to enter, and the moment the next word of the sentence, which is 'not', is just about to rise up as a thought, consciously repeat 'not' ...
3. Continue until you have reached the end of the sentence.
4. Then, just rest for a few minutes before you repeat the whole process again, which you can do a third time, but always having a nice break between each round ...

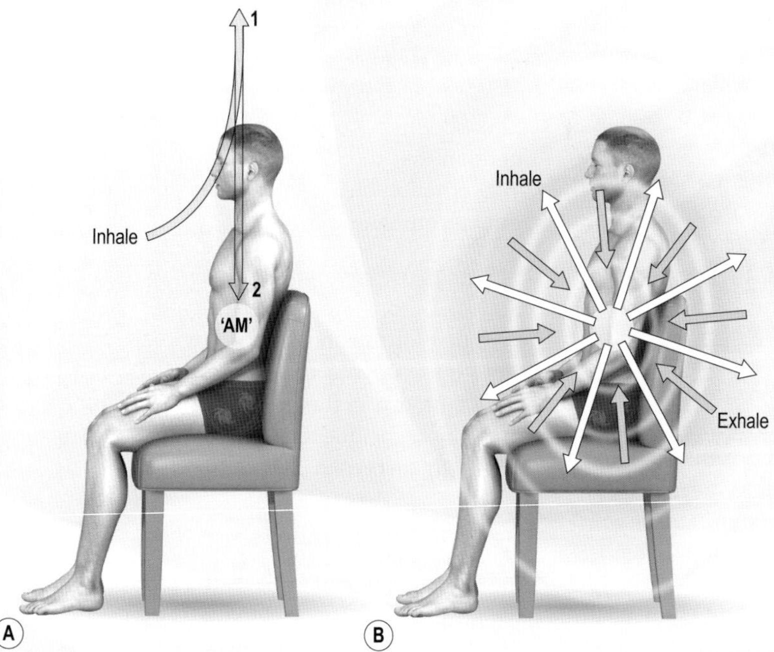

Figure 25.2

(A) Steps 1 to 3. (B) Steps 4 and 5

Experiment

1. Make yourself comfortable on a chair, keep your spine upright and lean back into yourself as described in previous exercises.
2. Close your eyes and let them soften, whilst resting your hands on your thighs.
3. Take your attention towards the tip of the nose and gently inhale up to a point high above your head (1).
4. Stay for a moment in the full pause, and acknowledge a further internal rising (2).
5. Slowly exhale down to the coccyx through the core of your spine (3). See steps 1 to 5 illustrated in Fig. 25.3A.
6. Take a gentle long inhalation all the way up behind your eyes.
7. Stay for a moment in the full pause.
8. Exhale, and let your awareness expand laterally to both sides simultaneously. See steps 6 to 8 illustrated in Fig. 25.3B.
9. Repeat the whole cycle until you gain a sense and real longing that you simply want to rest behind your eyes, then finish the last cycle and let go of all breathing.
10. Stay in that sense of spaciousness for as long as you enjoy it. See steps 9 to 10 illustrated in Fig. 25.3C …

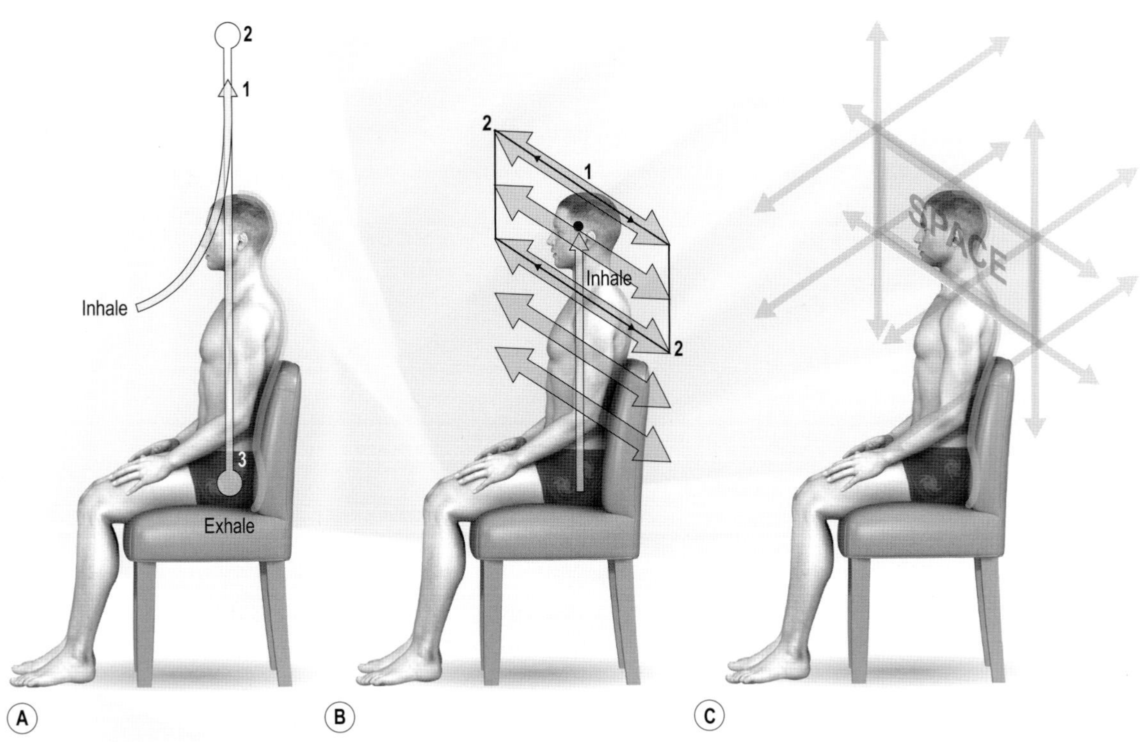

Figure 25.3

(A) Steps 1 to 5. (B) Steps 6 to 8. (C) Steps 9 to 10

or vibration. This describes the universal pulse of consciousness that, according to Kashmiri Shaivism, resides at the heart of our awareness. Spanda yoga is a very complex system but can be explained in the following simple words. Spanda induces our consciousness to expand based on the fact that the very nature of consciousness is to expand, and this natural expansion is utilised in spanda practice. The only thing that prohibits the expansion of consciousness, and in fact diminishes it and narrows it down, is our mind. However, the underlying vibration that is generated during our spanda practice unfailingly tires the mind out. This is the reason why this very simple exercise we are about to introduce is so powerful. Despite having taught and worked with many different approaches and techniques for mind and thought, it always surprises me how the practice of spanda cuts right to the point.

In this practice we aim to allow our breath to become more and more subtle. Our attention stays with the moment-to-moment experience, following the energetic pathway of the breath. Keep your eyes disengaged throughout. Your main priority is less doing and much more allowing. Cherish every pause after the inhalation and this wonderful sense of an inner rising.

Observe how this practice impacts upon your mind and how it acts on your day.

26 Whenever, wherever and for whoever – simple tools with profound results

There are so many exercises and experiments to try on our quest to create our own stillness-memory. As we practise we find more space and freedom in our bodies and enjoy a sense of improved circulation of fluids and energy. Then, as we move, especially in walking and breathing, we experience the empowering and energising sense of lightness that comes when we have a good connection to the ground.

What can we take right now into our working practice? How can we embody them and make them work for us? Here are some suggestions for taking forward the exercises in Part 4.

Experiment

Gaining ground – rediscovering your toes and appreciating your arches

As you walk, remember the three load-bearing points on your feet, and as you connect with them, whatever your pace and whatever you are doing, you will automatically 'grow lighter' and feel stronger. Remember to incorporate a soft breath as you walk and really work your toes. If your feet start to ache then that is a great reminder that they are opening up and will be stronger. It is so much better to feel your feet aching now than to feel your back aching in a few years' time due to postural weakness. If you are standing as you work, with your client on a massage table, then always wear shoes or sandals that allow your toes to move. You will probably find, as I did, that your toes naturally scrunch the carpet or wiggle around on the floor. You will not even have to think about it!

Experiment

Using a grounded pelvis to find lightness in your upper body and neck

Whenever you are seated, really connect with your sitting bones and feel your spine naturally stack up. Engage your tummy muscles if you feel you begin to roll forward, then you will find a place of balance where your spine is comfortable and you feel supported and are breathing easily. Your shoulders will feel easier if your pelvis is balanced, as will your neck and jaw.

Experiment

Keep your jaw soft and remember the muscles in the floor of your mouth

Whatever you are doing, if it involves speaking, then attention to creating softness in your throat and face will enable you to speak without pushing energy into your voice and feeling tired. Smile, smile, breathe and smile again. As you smile, connect to the levels of your breath and the action of your respiratory diaphragm. If you are nervous then try taking a breath in through the back of your body.

Experiment

Keep your eyes moving

Cherish and support your eyes. Remember to change your focal length if you are using your computer. If you are presenting or teaching, help your audience feel you are engaging with them by focusing on students in different parts of the room. Smile directly at them too. They will feel involved and will listen to what you have to say and the points you are making.

Experiment

Refresh and renew: a change of energy – brushing off and reconnecting

I am often asked by other therapists what I do to conserve my energy and how I manage to demonstrate on 10 or more clients if I am at an exhibition without looking exhausted at the end of the day.

So, here is my speedy, effective and easy-to-remember way of keeping clear and bright. I call it brushing off and renewing. I always wash my hands after treating a client or taking a class, then have a good-sized glass of water before and after doing this exercise.

Figure 26.1

Brushing off across the body – there are four steps

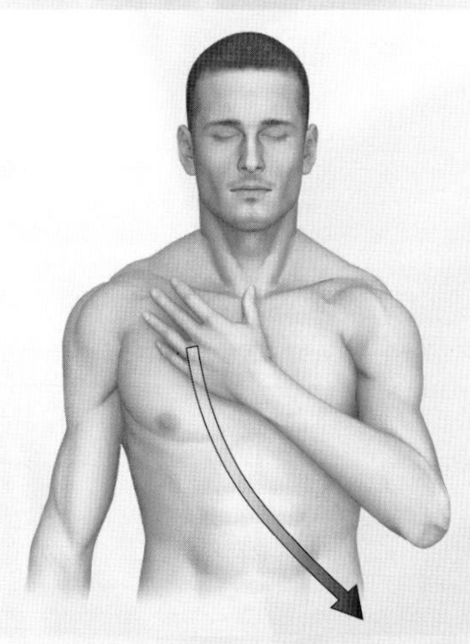

Step one: Take your right hand to your left shoulder. Take a breath in, and on the exhalation sweep your hand across your body as far as your right hip.

Step two: Take your left hand to your right shoulder. Take a breath in, and on the exhalation sweep your hand across your body as far as your left hip.

Steps three and four: Repeat once more each side.

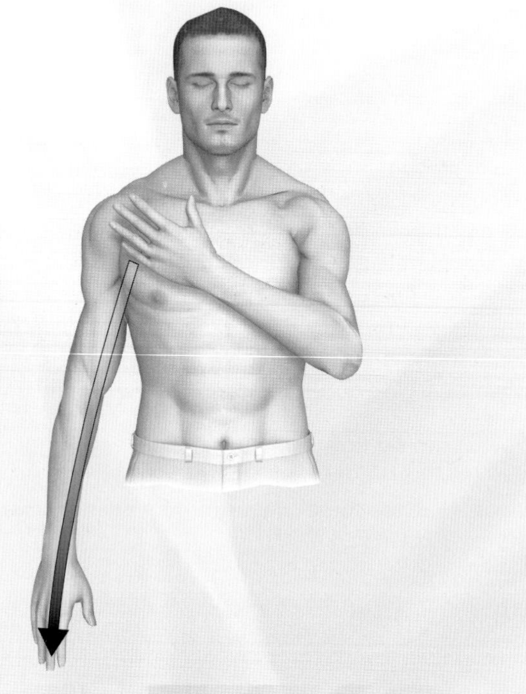

Figure 26.2

Brushing off from shoulder to fingers – there are four steps

Step one: Take your right hand to your left shoulder. Take a breath in, and on the exhalation sweep your hand down your left arm all the way to your fingertips.

Step two: Take your left hand to your right shoulder. Take a breath in, and on the exhalation sweep your hand down your right arm all the way to your fingertips.

Steps three and four: Repeat once more each side.

The Renewal

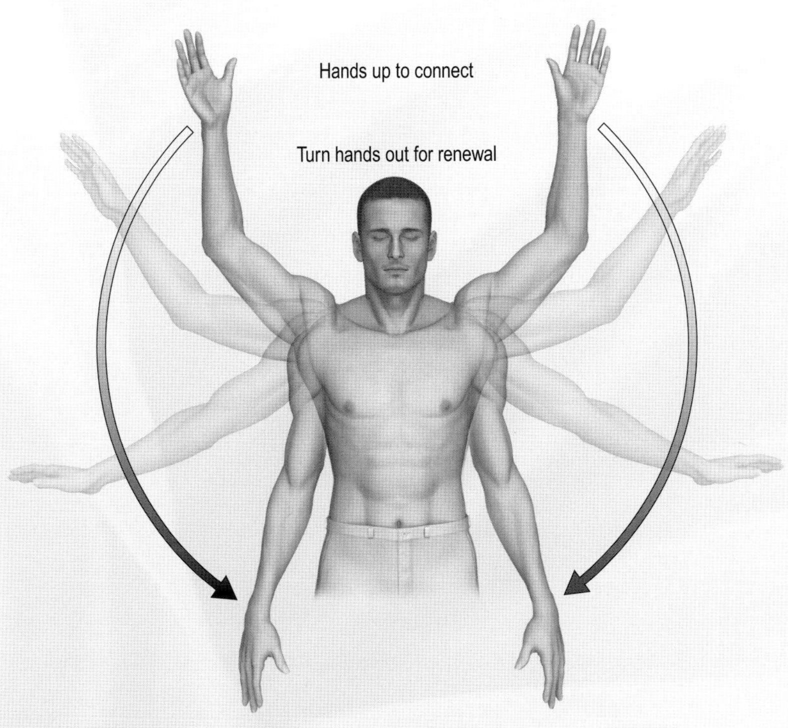

Figure 26.3

Renewing and refreshing

On an inhalation, raise both your arms above your head with your fingers straight up and pointed, palms facing one another. Intend new energy, clear brightness, to fill and refresh you. As you exhale, turn your palms outwards, away from one another, and bring your arms slowly all the way back down by your sides. You might like to repeat this part of the process, so simply do it as many times as you wish.

Experiment

Move your body as you are teaching or presenting; don't just wave your arms!

Walking around the room, and deliberately changing the place you are speaking from, serves to keep your breath and body more open and relaxed and keeps the audience engaged.

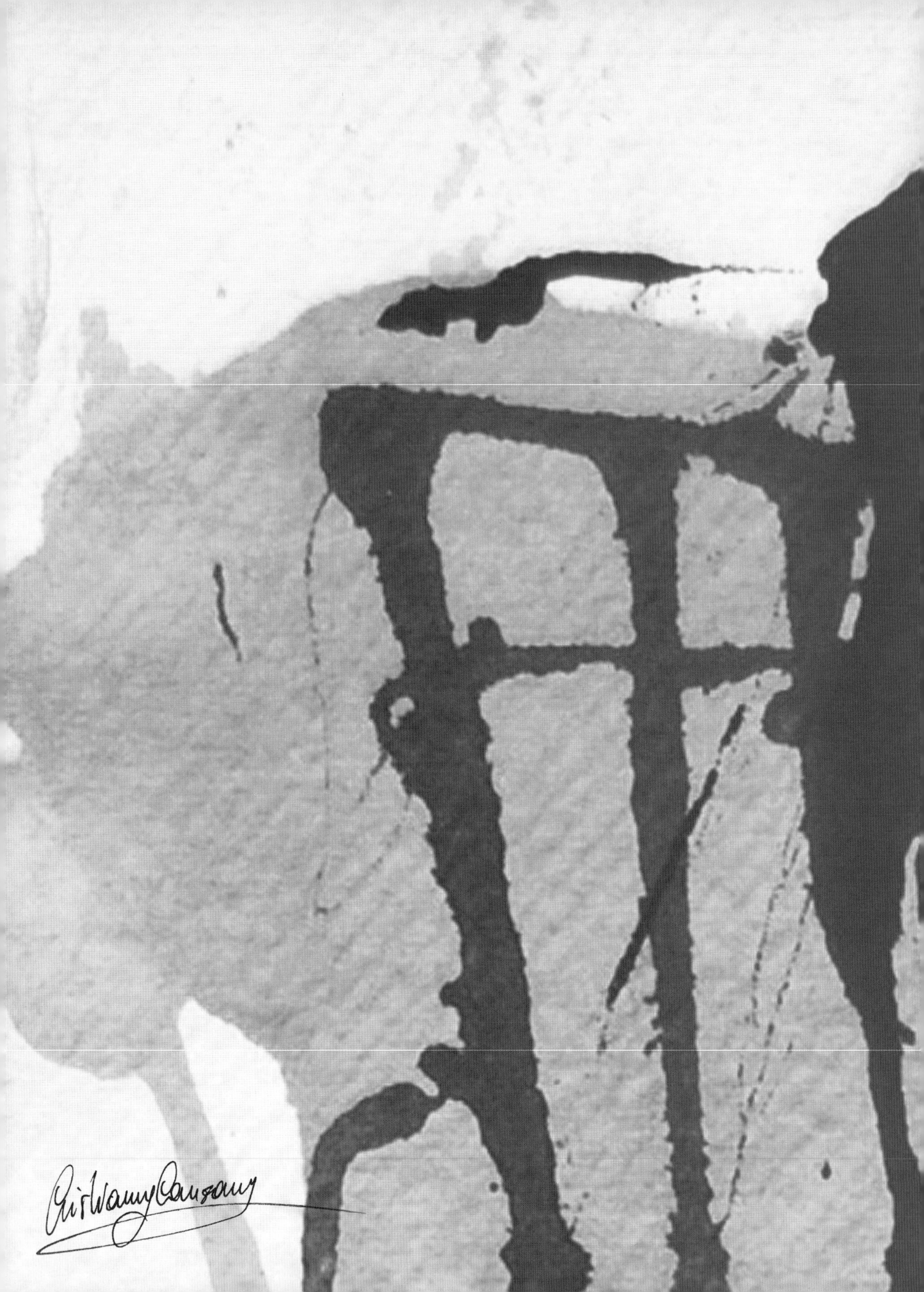

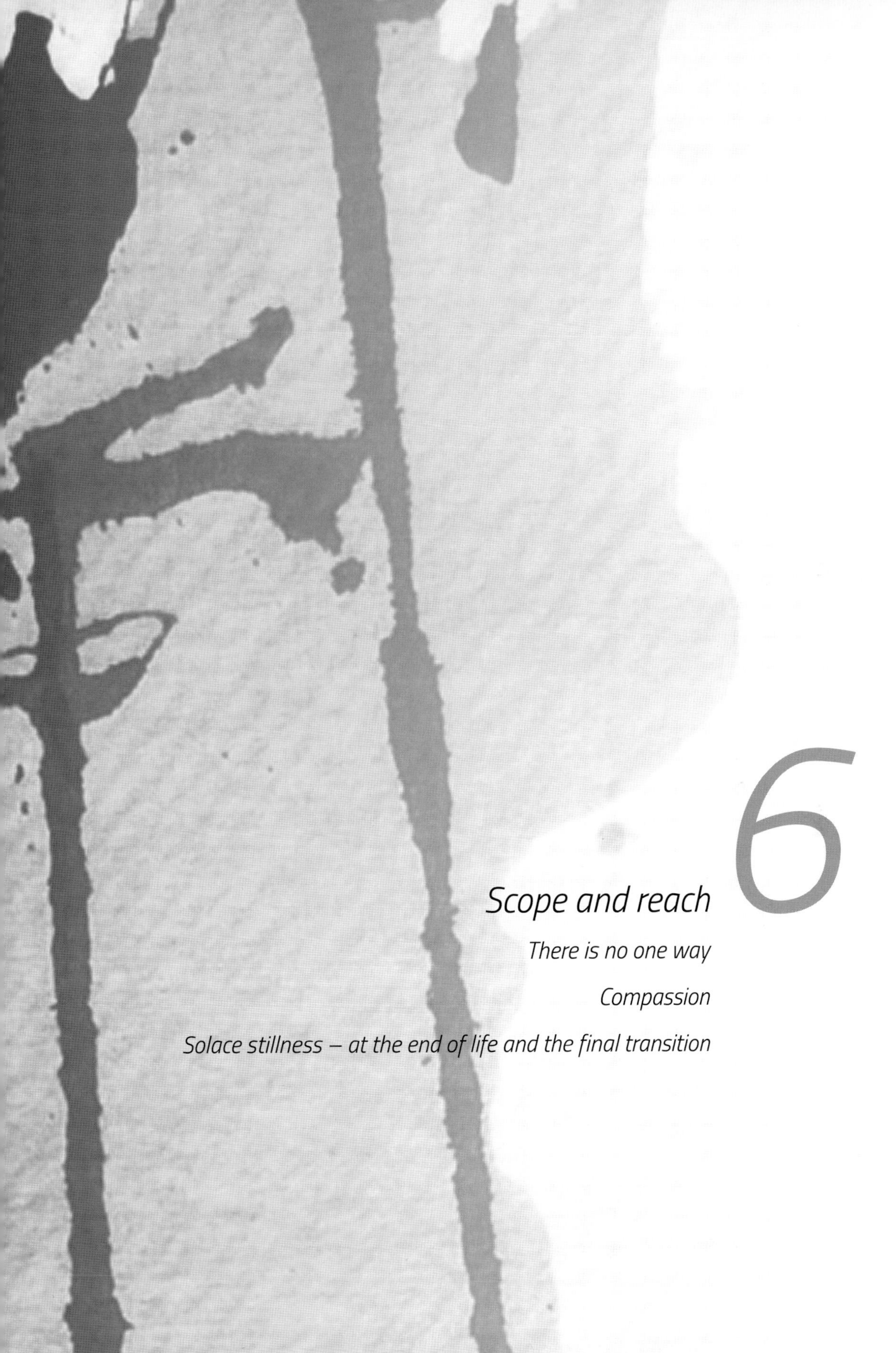

6

Scope and reach

There is no one way

Compassion

Solace stillness – at the end of life and the final transition

There is no one way 27

Mindfulness

The practice of mindfulness has conquered the world, and there is no doubt that it is a wonderful tool that helps millions of people to manage and work with a whole scale of issues in life. Due to the public interest it receives, its current hype, as well as the potential wealth it can generate, mindfulness has become a thriving business for many people. For some of them, it has become a business on a very large scale. Global companies like Google are running courses in mindfulness, and the well-known Headspace app, according to an article on 23 May 2015 in *The Telegraph* by Glenda Cooper, is considered to be worth more than £25 million. Fuelled by scientific research and associated press coverage, mindfulness now seems to have become the be-all and end-all, offering the ultimate solution to all things unsolved on a psychological or physiological level, as well as life in general. Alas, its actual place within the scope of work on consciousness and meditation has got lost in the hype.

When I started immersing myself in the studies and practice of ancient teachings and philosophy 38 years ago, the practice of mindfulness, which at that time was an essential part of Buddhist teachings before it was later converted into a secular approach, formed only one small part of a greater whole – a body of work that usually takes decades of study and practice to truly fathom out its whole scale and actual depth.

In the universal teachings, there simply is no 'one way'. Each way or method might, however, be a stepping-stone that leads to another. Based on my personal experience and observations, as well as feedback from colleagues, students and clients, each way, system or technique has a 'shelf life', a time and day when it will have fulfilled its purpose for us. Then it is up to us whether to say goodbye to it or not, and that comes down to our own openness and willingness to embrace the unknown again, before the current practice starts becoming habitual and mechanical. As mentioned in Part 3: Chapter 11, this letting go is not an easy undertaking, considering how safe we usually feel within the known.

Just recently, several articles based on the newest research were published that caught the public eye, criticising the scientific world for mainly outlining the positive effects of mindfulness without highlighting the dangers or mentioning its well-known side effects.

Looking at it from a wider perspective, this criticism is to be expected (the pendulum moving to the negative side), and it becomes obvious that, in a world under the law of opposites, there will always be shadow at one moment and light at another. Just as this is true of any other practice, so it is true of mindfulness. In the end, the experience of mindfulness as positive or negative is down to the depth of experience and qualifications of the therapist or teacher. That is, to equip a mindfulness trainee within a four-day training course with all the required skills and knowledge, which in reality take years to learn and turn into personal experience, is highly questionable.

Regardless of all the hype, we must not forget that mindfulness practice is a proven and powerful tool for self-observation and self-study, with the aim of bringing more light of consciousness into the field of our awareness. However, the moment we become mindful about our thoughts and behaviours we will be faced with our psychology, and it is at this point at which especially vulnerable people, or people with a specific condition or illness, require the support and guidance of an experienced therapist or mindfulness teacher. What is often lacking is consideration of the fact that most of the time our mindfulness practice is executed by the mind itself, because we haven't yet established any other faculty within us to be mindful. Furthermore, due to its divided nature, everything in the mind is continuously changing, which makes it very difficult for us to keep it in the present moment. Hence, our practice is initially based on will and doing, a deeply conditioned default mode we all have acquired, instead of allowing. As a consequence

THERE IS NO 'ONE WAY' THAT LEADS TO ONE'S
OBJECTIVES

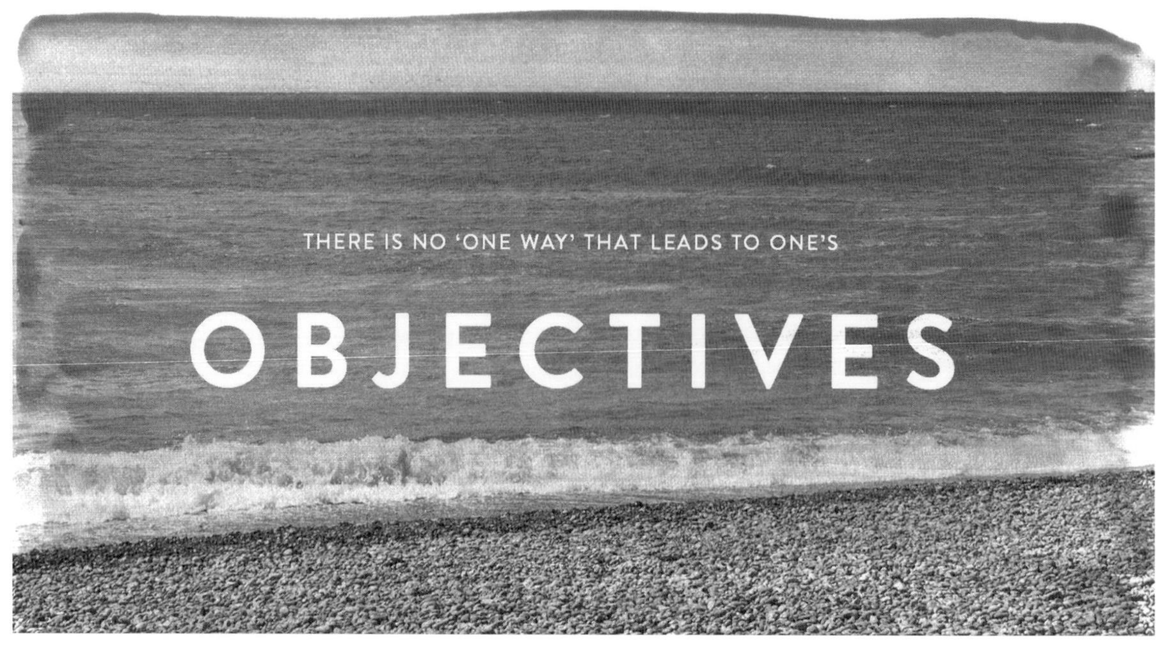

Figure 27.1

Artwork Victoria Dokas; photography Alexander Filmer-Lorch

we lose a great amount of force. That's why an experienced mindfulness teacher is required who knows how to facilitate our moving from doing to allowing, so that a natural state of mindfulness can arise. Here it is important to say that mindfulness practice is only one way amongst many others that lead to the same objective, which is natural presence. Yet, the current popularity of mindfulness obscures the significance of all other ways, regardless of their effectiveness or the unquestionable wealth of knowledge they contain.

From a universal teaching perspective (and this applies to any other school of thought that acts on our psychology and facilitates change), actual mindfulness practice should always comprise three different directions of work: mindfulness techniques and practice, the philosophical teachings of mindfulness, and the psychological teachings of mindfulness. Together they form a balanced triad, in which the philosophy gives meaning and depth to the practice by transmitting knowledge and keeping us inspired. The psychology illuminates what, and in which order, we need to be able to work within our psychology, which ensures that we do not get lost in the shadow. The mindfulness techniques and practice put the philosophy and psychology into action, and this gradually leads to change and the manifestation of a new proposition we can work from. The truly dedicated mindfulness practitioner works on all three aspects simultaneously. If only one of them is abandoned, the other two will cancel each other out.

There is something else that is important for us to know. Whether originating from a Buddhist, Hindu, Advaita, Christian, Islamic or secular background, at the core of any serious system, practice or philosophy lies the idea of the diminishment of 'I', as well as the awakening of higher emotions, so that the 'true self' can be experienced and realised. In mindfulness this means that, as long as I am conscious or aware that I am mindful or I practise mindfulness, 'I' will occupy a position that is not neutral ('I' as subject being mindful of everything else as object). However, the moment the last traces of this feeling, condition or sense of 'I am mindful' have been made passive, a natural state of presence arises, and the initial practice of mindfulness has fulfilled its purpose and needs to be replaced by work with others. This is partly based on the teachings and practice of compassion and empathy, as well as external deliberation (see Part 6: Chapter 28). Hence, our work is less about 'I' and 'me' and much more about 'be' and 'ye'.

Possible non-conducive occurrences of mindfulness practice

We all know the amazing benefits of mindfulness practice, but very little is said about the potentially less conducive outcomes. I can only speak from a universal teaching point of view, which includes all teachings that facilitate change.

- My teachers and mentors always stressed there is a danger that any kind of practice focused on self-evolution can easily turn into self-centredness in which the world starts turning exclusively around us. This is usually due to wrong interpretation of the teachings, the inexperience of the teacher or school, or misguided work that has been watered down by our own personal philosophy and 'I-believes', or by only working in one or two directions.

- For people who are vulnerable, or with mental health issues, there is a slight possibility that they might slide into another episode, or in some pathologies, according to the ancient teachings, even a possible danger of a person splitting into two personalities. This might be caused by the observing nature of mindfulness and meditation practice in which people learn how to divide their attention, and this can be confused with having to become two persons in which one observes the other. That's why a thorough training that focuses on all three aspects – the philosophy, psychology, as well as the practice – is so vital. Furthermore, as practitioners we need to know our limits, and have the courage to refer clients to another practitioner if anything arises that we have not been trained in or are not qualified to work with.

- For certain types of people, mindfulness is not the right practice because it causes them to fall even further into awareness, which makes it very difficult for them to deal with the responsibilities of life.

- Because the state of mindfulness or meditation can't be explained but needs to be experienced, people's acquired or preconceived ideas are the only reference points they have, and that is what they may look for in their practice. Deeply engrained preconceived ideas or misunderstandings can give rise to an artificial state of mindfulness or meditation that can easily turn into a habit, and this takes a significant amount of time and effort to replace with the true experience.

- Due to their conviction and enthusiasm, I have seen followers of the different systems and practices trying to impose their beliefs on their loved ones and friends, which can give rise to many problems and frictions. From the view of the universal teachings, just because one person has decided to become mindful does not mean that everybody else should. The teachings say that we are all struggling along the way, and there are as many techniques, paths and ways as there are human beings. Yours fits you but might not work for anyone else.

- People underestimate the importance of 'neutral' that should be the basis of every practice, whether it is mindfulness, meditation or self-observation. That is, mindfulness that is not practised in a genuine neutral state of mind is a totally different practice. However, for most people, it takes a long time to truly feel and understand that what they meet within their psychological world is what they are not. That is, most of what we observe was simply acquired and learned through our conditioning during our upbringing by means of repetition and imitation.

So which way?

Despite their popularity, ever since ancient meditative practices (including mindfulness) became mainstream and deeply rooted in our cultural and philosophical practices, concerns have been raised about how they are used. Williams and Kabat-Zinn (2011) say that 'the very essence of such practices and perspectives might be unwittingly denatured … and potentially exploited in inappropriate and ultimately unwise ways' and that 'this is a point in the development of this new field … where it may be particularly fruitful to pause and take stock'. My personal conclusion, after decades of practice and working with others, is that once you have gained a thorough understanding of the stilling process, why follow only one kind of system, philosophy or teaching, which satisfies our mind, intellect, deeds and habits, when all that is really required is to *be still*, which can be accomplished in any number of ways.

Inner work

Originating from 'know thyself', or in more contemporary terms self-study, inner work ensures that, before we start facilitating, teaching or treating other people, we *understand* enough about our own body–mind unit. By more fully understanding ourselves and how we tick and function, we gain a much better understanding of others, realising that we are in no way any different to anybody else when it comes to a purely functional view. We all comprise a physiological body that moves about and has countless internal movement functions that keep us alive, and if the body is trained accordingly it can move in extraordinary ways. All of us have feelings and emotions, as well as the ability to think and analyse. Additionally – and this can't be scientifically measured – we have intuition and a consciousness that we can further develop, increase and evolve. The incentive for the inner work required in our field of expertise is to ensure that we facilitate, treat and teach from the middle or neutral, through which a natural equilibrium as a balanced therapist or practitioner can be sustained. In the fields of counselling and psychology, ongoing inner work is ensured by regular supervision, debriefing and repeated therapy sessions. However, this is very often approached through the intellect only, and does not include any tissue work or movement. However, the ancient teachings show us that emotions can't be controlled or changed by the intellect only. The intellect can acknowledge them, gain knowledge about them, analyse and understand them, but we can only transform and change them in conjunction with consciousness, as well as through tissue work, movement and specific means that render our emotions passive. Consequently, we first need to establish something more permanent that is less subject to change to be able to deal with the speed of emotions. This something starts with inner stillness.

In the field of manual therapy, such as massage, osteopathy and physiotherapy, further development for practitioners usually focuses on new manual techniques, a deeper understanding of anatomy and physiology, including the latest research, and postural integration. The psychology, including feelings and emotions, as well as our different states of mind and levels of consciousness, is often treated as secondary, or in some approaches and training is not covered or mentioned at all.

Hence, in an ideal world, when we treat, teach or facilitate, we should not lose sight of the whole person whilst we are working on the parts. However, we will only be able to do that when we keep our own inner work going and focus on working not just on one aspect of ourselves, but all the different parts of us, so that we are able to integrate them into one unified and centred whole. Truly knowing how we tick and function emotionally, intellectually and physically, including our strengths and weaknesses, can be a humbling process; yet rest assured, once we start working on them respectfully and non-invasively, it will take our work with others to a totally new level that is built on empathy and neutral understanding.

Meditation

Inner stillness gives rise to a true state of meditation, and the practice of meditation is one possibility out of many for finding inner stillness. This means that meditation practice itself does not necessarily lead to a deep meditative state. The actual purpose of meditation practice is to tire the mind out, which gradually gives rise to a meditative state. Whether this is achieved through mindfulness practice, vipassana, the use of mantras, chi gong or any of the countless other practices is irrelevant. Once a meditative state has been established, the actual practice has fulfilled its purpose and needs to be dropped. We are all creatures of habit, so the moment our favourite meditation technique becomes mechanical and habitual, it needs to be replaced by a different one. That's why so many practices have been developed throughout the millennia, but what all of them have in common is the means to achieve a meditative state and a deep sense of peace, contentment and inner stillness, as well as the diminishment of 'I' that gives rise to greater empathy and compassion (see Part 6: Chapter 28). Depending on our psychological makeup and our physiological state, and our circumstances in life, some of the mainstream meditation techniques might not fulfil their purpose or work for us, but others will. Those of us more attuned to movement may find it very difficult to start with vipassana, and the intellectuals amongst us may struggle with chanting. However, once we have explored the whole scale of different practices, we can start becoming creative, because we know that today we might be better off with a movement meditation, whilst a few days later a deep relaxation technique that gives rise to alpha brainwave activity will do a much better job.

Once we have acquired enough living memory of stillness, technique becomes much less important. At this stage, regular practice and repeated stimulus has led to neurogenesis and neuroplasticity in the brain, which means the actual meditation technique might only be required for a few minutes before a natural state of meditation arises in which the practice can be dropped, so that we can enjoy simply being in meditation, instead of practising it.

Long-term practitioners who have acquired a permanent centre of gravity of inner stillness can consciously access it, which gives rise to a meditative state and a state of genuine presence that persists even when they go about normal daily life. This was confirmed by neuroscientist Richard Davidson, who was surprised that gamma brainwave activity (activated in deep states of meditation and inner stillness) is active in Tibetan monks who have been practising for decades, even when they are just out and about on busy roads, as well as whilst engaging with other people. Here again, it is all down to the inner power of stillness.

Developing the insightful self as a practitioner, therapist and teacher

Certain things can't be learned from a book, especially when it comes to studying a new method that is based on practical skills and ideas that are supposed to be applied in a treatment, counselling or teaching environment. First of all, a book can't answer every question, and second it can't demonstrate how to put theory into action or show us little tricks, adjustments and shortcuts that lead us to true understanding and the actual experience of the technique or practice we are learning. However, if we listen to the ancient teachings, knowledge is not only transmitted through the spoken or written word, or by teaching people a protocol that has been learned and understood intel-

WE NEED TO REALISE THAT THERE IS NO AIM
IN MEDITATION APART FROM
JUST TO 'BE'
IN MEDITATION

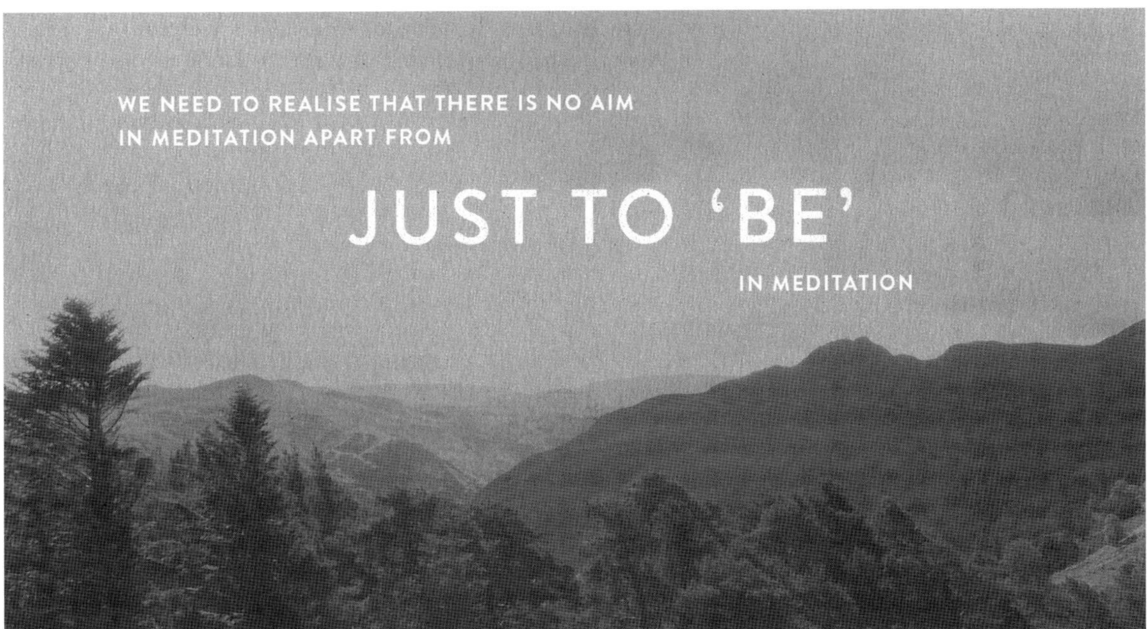

Figure 27.2

Artwork Victoria Dokas; photography Alexander Filmer-Lorch

lectually and technically. The actual essence of the knowledge is transmitted in silence through the presence of the teacher, within whom the knowledge has become part of their being. That is, the knowledge has turned into second nature through decades of dedicated work and practice nourished by the force of meaning. The inspiration and benefit we can gain from that is invaluable. In other words, the knowledge and insight of the written word becomes even more accessible, meaningful and of great value once it is taught and experienced in a live teaching environment by an experienced teacher or facilitator.

Putting things into action

To complement this book, and to be able to offer you a first-hand experience of this work, we have developed a series of training modules that cover all aspects of working from the inner power of stillness in a treatment, therapy and teaching environment, as well as how to sustain your own health and wellbeing during sessions and classes. Other important themes that you will study are how to make the most of the practitioner's toolkit, and simple stillness exercises that your clients can practise between treatments, sessions and classes. And of course there are lots of other themes that can't be covered by a book.

If you are inspired by this book, and would like to train in working from the inner power of stillness, then come and study with us. If you are a training provider and would like to add any of our training modules to your own curriculum, we are happy to teach them for you.

But enough of promoting the work we love so much, because there are two more chapters to come, on subjects I find essential, and without which this book would not be complete.

References

Williams, J. and Kabat-Zinn, J. (2011). Mindfulness: diverse perspectives on its meaning, origins, and multiple applications at the intersection of science and dharma. *Contemporary Buddhism*, 12(1): 1–18.

Compassion 28

Origins

The first evidence for altruistic behaviour by humans comes from examination of the skeletons of a female *Homo ergaster* from Kenya dating to around 1.5 million years ago and an even earlier hominin from Dmanisi in Georgia 1.77 million years old (Spikins, Rutherford and Needham, 2010), which both showed evidence of disease that would have required care by others in order for the individuals to survive. Based on historic discoveries that date back 530,000 years, long-term care was not only given to the older generation, but to toddlers as well, and with the arrival of the Neanderthal caring for others was already part of everyday living. Spikins and team also explain that, whatever caused the differences between modern humans, originating in Africa approximately 150,000 years ago, and our more primitive ancestors is still a mystery, but changes in our emotional makeup and the role of compassion within the dynamics of communal relationships might have played a part in it.

Not all thought systems see compassion as a virtue: 'Greek and Roman philosophers distrusted compassion. In their view, reason alone was the proper guide to conduct. They regarded compassion as an affect, neither admirable nor contemptible' (Szasz, 1994).

However, compassion has become a common theme in all major world religions. According to Federman (1999), in the monotheistic traditions universal love is often upheld by the idea that we are all 'God's children'. In pantheistic traditions universal love is rooted in the idea of unity, and that we are all one with everything else.

In Hinduism, Jainism and Buddhism, the idea of compassion is based on the concept of ahimsa, which means refraining from harmfulness. Mahatma Gandhi's whole teaching was based on the idea of ahimsa, which is that of love and non-violence.

The idea of compassion has evolved into the 'golden rule', which is expressed in the Torah of the Jewish tradition as 'love thy neighbour as thyself'. This means having to evolve or display the character traits of a mensch, a person who is full of compassion, love and kindness, and who genuinely follows each mitzvah (commandment). Compassion is the centrepoint of the doctrines in the Christian traditions, also expressed as 'thou shalt love thy neighbour as thyself'. According to Federman, 'Saint Paul, the founder of Christianity as a formal religion, claimed universal love to be the crucial defining attribute of a true Christian.' Talking about compassion and Islam, Federman continues: 'According to the Qur'an, the merit of a person is determined by their "righteousness," which involves extending oneself altruistically toward all those in need, as well as keeping faith with God' (Federman, 1999).

Federman's research reveals that, in today's world of increasing ethnic conflicts, we can see different movements arising in every part of the world that are working towards a greater common identity and universal values that we can all share.

How it works physiologically and psychologically

> *Compassion in its strict definition involves both feeling an emotion appropriate to another's emotion, empathising, and being motivated to help.*
>
> (Spikins, Rutherford and Needham, 2010)

Spikins and team (2010) state that certain emotional responses follow universal patterns, which in turn draw on specific patterns in the brain. According to their research, these patterns give rise to emotions such as compassion, love, remorse and guilt that we all have in common, known as 'sociomoral emotions', and these can now be scientifically explained.

Furthermore, they show that, from a biological perspective, the moment we execute a selfless deed, or actions that are based on love and kindness or that convey a caring nature, the well-known 'feel-good' hormone oxytocin is released into the brain. This means that compassion-based actions are not entirely altruistic, nor solely built on higher moral values, but also stem from a caring response that has evolved in our biology and which makes us feel good as well. Within a community, being inspired and motivated to care for each other is of great benefit, and likewise, from an evolutionary point of view, the combined strength of a couple genuinely caring for each other is of great advantage, so that the bond of love overrides our so-called 'selfish gene'. However, compassion for other human beings, as well as for animals, is not always without conflict, and most compassionate people have experienced situations of exploitation. Furthermore, many people have become immune to other people's suffering, and some people even respond to suffering 'with indifference, aversion, or even gloating' (Ashar et al., in press).

From a psychological point of view, our response to other people's suffering is a very complex process in which we usually weigh the pros and cons, which determine if we simply distance ourselves from the situation or offer help. Whether our response is compassionate or indifferent depends on the underlying emotional meaning in the situation. For example, our thought–feeling process might be, 'This person looks so vulnerable and helpless, I really should carry her shopping bags to the car', which is a positive response that might lead to an act of compassion. Another example could be that we experience a thought–feeling process such as, 'This woman looks like she needs some help', then we see the face of the woman and think, 'Oh, she looks far too hostile, and probably does not want any help from anybody', which might lead to an action in which we distance ourselves.

Ashar and colleagues (in press) describe two different neural networks. One supports sharing and understanding another person's suffering, and the other supports valuing and the pro-social motivation to help other people. 'We posit that compassion is supported by a medial prefrontal-striatal network constructing (potentially compassionate) emotional meanings.' They point towards further potential research, including a focus on compassion training, which may be linked with cognitive neuroscience, highlighting 'its potential for large-scale use and its clear societal implications'.

The more that scientific backup becomes evident for humanity, the higher the chances are that we are moving towards a more compassion-focused society and possibly a better world to live in. Besides the dedicated work of scientists who believe in the possibility of the evolution of humanity, there are other promising developments in the fields of therapy, medical care and alternative therapy that work towards the same objective. Professor Paul Gilbert has revolutionised compassion-focused therapy, an integrated approach that draws from developmental, social, Buddhist and evolutionary psychology, as well as neuroscience. Furthermore, the dedicated work of Professor H.M. Chochinov, Dr Atul Gawande and Professor Philip J. Larkin, to name just a few, has posed many questions and given rise to a continuously increasing compassion-centred approach in palliative end-of-life care.

A universal view on compassion

One of the greatest strengths or virtues we can develop in ourselves is real understanding. We can't use other people's understanding, because what others have gained from their own enquiries is individual to them and would not get us very far. If we simply copy other people's understanding, we will only have an artificial understanding that is lacking in substance. However, we can apply to ourselves and our being the knowledge that other people have derived from their own understanding and which they are happy to share with us, and this increases our own understanding, but it will of course be different to anybody else's understanding.

The Fourth Way philosophy says that knowledge and our state of being have to grow together, and that we can only grow our understanding when we apply knowledge to our being, because knowledge and being together comprise our understanding.

This means that true understanding changes the way we think, and a different way of thinking about ourselves, the world and others alters our mind, our attitudes and ultimately our being. Knowing about compassion and truly being compassionate, which

IF WE START WORKING ON BOTH (KNOWLEDGE AND SELF-KNOWLEDGE)
AND GRADUALLY SHIFT IT FROM THE PARTICULAR TO THE GREATER WHOLE,
THE GREAT DIVIDE BETWEEN KNOWLEDGE AND TRULY KNOWING HOW TO 'BE'
WILL FINALLY FALL
BACK INTO BALANCE

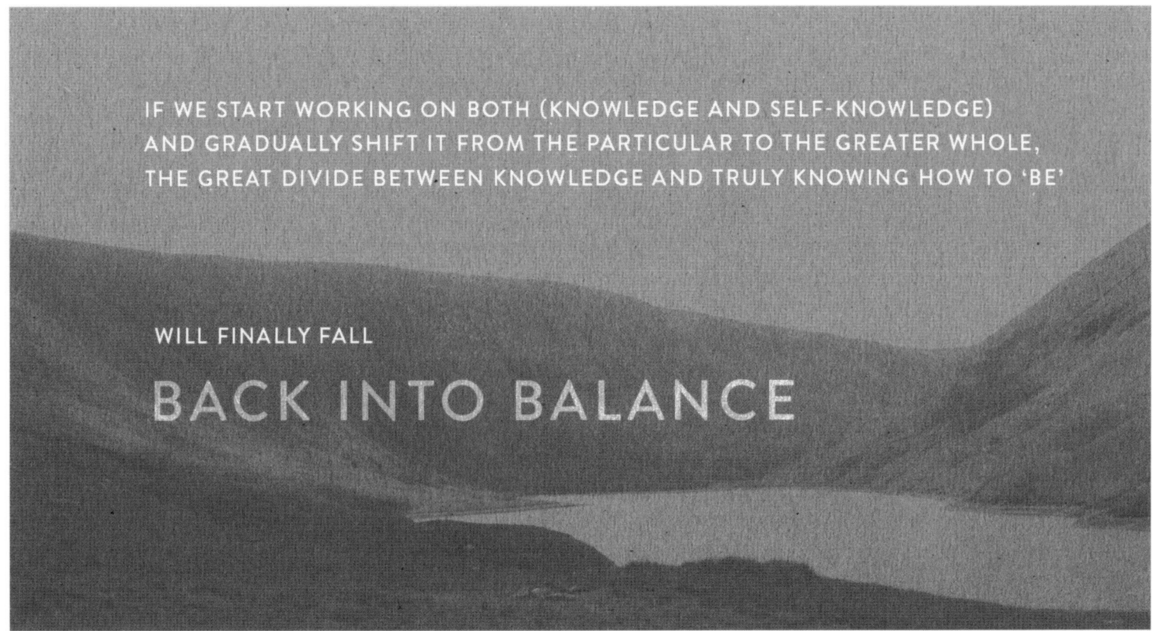

Figure 28.1

Artwork Victoria Dokas; photography Alexander Filmer-Lorch

gives rise to understanding of what compassion really is, are two different things. Compassion is a higher emotion and state that we usually meet in life in the form of a concept or philosophical idea. In today's world we are repeatedly reminded about the importance of compassion and, as we already know, science has given us enough evidence about its great benefits. A more compassion-centred intervention and interaction with clients improves their healing process and wellbeing, as well as the wellbeing of the practitioner. It is not surprising therefore that most people have very little insight into or real understanding of the actual state of compassion, nor how it feels to be in a genuine state of compassion that we can use as the basis to work from. Like love, we all carry the potential of real compassion within us in the form of a seed, and the degree of compassion at any given moment is inversely proportional to the diminishment of our 'I's' and our little 'me's', as well as our 'I-believes' and personal philosophies. In all schools of thought we come across the idea of transforming or sacrificing our personal suffering, which is a state that only concerns the so-called 'smaller parts' in us (our little 'me's'), which occupy a strong position opposing everything that does not feed their wants and needs, as well as all that goes against their personal philosophies. This is the real cause of our suffering. However, there is no place for bias and prejudice in compassion, because compassion is a path of *self-less* action that is deeply embedded in a highly developed conscience. Nicoll (1956) describes this in his *Psychological Commentaries* as a conscience that exists alongside our acquired conscience, which was created by our upbringing in the local environment and has been strongly informed by the ethics of our cultural background. He also explains that *true conscience* means to feel everything together that exists in the shadow, as well as the light, indicating a depth of insight that spans the whole scale of our human expressions and personality. Hence, both true conscience and consciousness are equal parts of one whole; but that is an idea of such complexity that goes beyond the remit of this book.

What is important for us to understand is that compassion lives in the centre – in the still-point in the middle – where true actions emerge. These actions based on conscious effort follow three directions of work simultaneously. Inner work leads to *real* understanding of ourselves. Work with others leads to a genuine understanding that we are no different when it comes to suffering, struggles and frictions than anybody else, which in turn leads to a deep sense of empathy for others, the world around us and ourselves. Work for the greater good, through which we gradually neutralise the suffering that is continuously generated by the small parts in ourselves, leads to the diminishment of 'I' and gives rise to real compassion in which everything we meet in life becomes meaningful.

In all, the seed of compassion that lies within us does not grow by simply creating and demonstrating a feeling of compassion for others. It can only flourish when we get out of our own way, walk the talk and put things into action. It is the action fuelled by the force of meaning that alters us into what we are supposed to be. That is, as much as the gradual emergence of compassion makes this sometimes challenging process of altering truly bearable for us, so does genuine compassion for others have a profoundly soothing effect on their struggles and sufferings.

Experiment

1. Perform a selfless deed several times a week, regardless of your state of mind.
2. Observe what resists, what changes and what you actually gain.

References

Ashar, Y.K., Andrews-Hanna, J.R., Dimidjian, S., Wager, T.D. (in press) Towards a neuroscience of compassion: a brain systems-based model and research agenda. In: Greene, J. (ed.), *Positive Neuroscience Handbook.* Oxford University Press. http://wagerlab.colorado.edu/files/papers/Ashar_et_al_Neurosci_of_Compassion_in_press.pdf (accessed 8 Dec. 2015).

Federman, J. (1999). The politics of compassion. Dissertation, University of Southern California.

Nicoll, M., Gurdjieff, G. and Ouspensky, P. (1956). *Psychological Commentaries.* London: Stuart & Watkins.

Spikins, P., Rutherford, H. and Needham, A. (2010). From homininity to humanity: compassion from the earliest archaics to modern humans. *Time and Mind*, 3(3): 303–325.

Szasz, T. (1994). *Cruel Compassion: psychiatric control of society's unwanted.* New York: Wiley.

Solace stillness – at the end of life and the final transition 29

A contribution by Ann-Margaret Whittle BSc MA CST MCSS BFRP

Recognising our mortality and redirecting focus

> *Being mortal is about the struggle to cope with the constraints of our biology, with the limit set by genes and cells and flesh and bone.*
>
> Atul Gawande (2014)

Gawande continues saying that 'medical science has given us remarkable power to push against these limits, and the potential value of this power was the reason why I became a doctor'. He concludes: 'But again and again, I have seen the damage we do in medicine when we fail to acknowledge that such power is finite and always will be.'

Maybe it was in childhood, at the death of a beloved family pet, or at the funeral of a favourite grandmother, when you first recognised your own mortality? Maybe it was after a particularly challenging medical diagnosis, or even at a significant birthday that felt like a rite of passage? When we have that recognition then we have a choice. We can snuggle it away into the darkly opaque pouch of the 'shadow' and stuff it down, or we can meditate upon it as part of the wonders and mysteries of life itself.

Eventually, we know that we have to take responsibility for our own death and dying, and there are some wonderfully inspirational ways of doing that.

My way of choice is to look at nature and join with her in the continuously changing cycles and rhythms of the earth. With the burgeoning of the light and rising of the sap in early spring to the dying of the leaves and the deep dark return in autumn and winter, being in touch with the natural ebb and flow of Mother Earth is a wonderful teacher in approaching our own mortality.

We will all have to die, and recognising that awesome knowledge gives us the authority to begin our own inner work sooner rather than later. For we cannot too soon make those decisions that will enhance our ultimate wellbeing.

They will involve keeping fit, balancing work and home and, when the time is right, streamlining our life to become more congruent in aligning our goals and our body, heart, mind and spirit with our ultimate focus.

Taking responsibility for our own death means companioning our own inner wisdom and developing the awareness of what kind of death we want. Creating a calm and focused space in our lives will involve tying up loose ends, nurturing the relationships we want to keep, fulfilling the commitments that are important to us and always focusing on the positives as we age. We will cut a swathe through the negatives usually attributed to ageing and agree that it is good to be less tired, to have more leisure time to be creative, to keep in touch with friends and so on. Eckhart Tolle calls this time of life 'the return'. I would just love for folk to be able to see these years not as a downhill saddening descent into frailty and decline, but as an investment and a bonus, a time to offer useful practical help to others, to volunteer our skills, as many do, offering something extra to life and creating positive outcomes.

If death comes prematurely, through accident, injury or illness, then the pathway is different and we need to find the right support, state our needs and embrace the tension that often arises through the desire of the medical profession to save us at any cost and our own innate instinct when it is time for us to let go.

There are several inspirational books on this dilemma and one of my favourites is by Michael Kearney (2009). He retells the story of the Greek god of healing, Asklepios. Although his natural father was the great Apollo, he was actually brought up by his stepfather, Chiron. Now Chiron had a wound in his body that would never

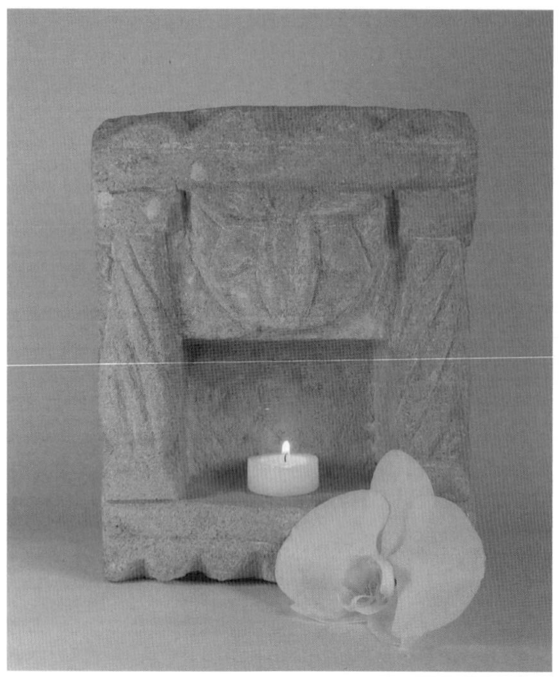

Figure 29.1

Time of return

heal. Chiron taught Asklepios about suffering and the ability to 'be with' those who would never get better. In the Asklepion temple at Pergamon there were bedrooms (you can still find them in the ruins) where the chronically sick would go in order to dream. Then in that deep inner space they would either find their way back to health or through the dream come to a place of peace around their death. Dr Kearney likens the heroic Apollo to the radical medical model that is concerned with relieving pain, as opposed to the Chiron/Asklepios focus on alleviating inner suffering, which has to be worked through and accepted on our journey towards dying and the transition at death.

Therapists who have worked on themselves will recognise that concept of the 'wounded healer' and how those who have gone deeply into embracing their own suffering are best able to 'be with' those who suffer at the end of life. Kearney talks about the presence of Chiron in the life of Asklepios reminding us that:

> *... with healing, who we are as human beings and how we are with the other in the incurable wound of his or her suffering is far more important than anything we might do or say.*
>
> Kearney (2009) *A Place of Healing*

Developing stillness in preparation for the transition

> *Often we forget that the dying are losing their whole world: their house, their job, their relationships, their body and their mind – they're losing everything. All the losses we could possibly experience in life are joined together in one overwhelming loss ...*
>
> Sogyal Rinpoche (1992)
> *The Tibetan Book of Living and Dying*

If you have never read this amazing book I do invite you to do so. Although Sogyal Rinpoche is a Master in the Tibetan Buddhist tradition, his descriptions and stories are so illuminating and immediately recognisable that I find the book quite hard to put down.

Finding stillness at the end of life requires a pathway that leads away from fear and panic towards love and surrender: a pathway that brings peace of heart. Some of the fears that may keep loved ones from that peace are belief in religious traditions about death and punishment, or fear of total oblivion, of the unknown, or even not wanting to meet an old adversary on the other side. It may be the fear of leaving their family without enough money, or of dying without forgiveness from someone they can never meet again.

Some fears can be resolved by practical intervention, making a will or asking a relative for help. Harder to come to terms with are the soul wounds where deep anger or resentment, remorse, grief, bitterness or loss of faith leach away our strength. In this situation, those who have dealt with their own soul wounds are the best help and comfort, whoever they may be – nurse, therapist, soul midwife or friend.

One of my friends was ready to let go. She had written her will, sorted out all the practicalities of her funeral, but had a deep grief that now she would never know what it meant to be a grandmother. After some discussion she decided she would leave a memory bag for the grandchild she would never see, full of storybooks she had loved, songs, pictures of her, facts about her life and a tape welcoming her grandchild into the world. When I met her the prognosis was that she had 9 to 15 months to live, but now three years later she is still amazing and looks after her granddaughter at least one day every week.

I believe that the real value of stillness for anyone at the end of life is to give enough time for each one of us to identify that place of healing inside where a measure of acceptance and peace may be felt. As death approaches, most people want to be able to go into that inner space and find their own way. We do turn our face to the wall as the end approaches, physically and metaphorically, and if it is hard for loved ones to accept this then it can become a dilemma for the dying person. Giving someone permission to go may be heart-wrenching but is a true act of love. Often it is when the family have gone off to find a coffee or talk to the doctor that the dying person takes the opportunity to leave without fuss or any pressure to stay.

Being with the dying

> *We can do no great things – only small things with great love.*
>
> Mother Teresa of Calcutta

Every time I repeat this phrase out loud my heart opens at the truth of it. Mother Teresa knew (of course she knew) that this work is a path of service and seeking any kind of 'job satisfaction' as the world knows it has no place here. It took me some time working as a volunteer in the cancer unit of a major hospital to really come to know that inside each of my cells!

In the pandemonium that is a hospital ward, it is practically impossible to deliver the therapy that you have been asked to give. That used to bother me terribly when I was asked for CranioSacral Therapy and the distractions and disruptions made it so frustrating and difficult. But of course that was *my* need, not that of the sick or dying person.

Then life intervened, and I had to spend five days on one of the wards as a patient. Two of my colleagues came on separate days to sit with me and give me treatment. They could only get to my right arm but the quality of their touch and their total commitment to being present taught me all I needed to learn. Whenever I go up to that same ward to work I remember them with deep gratitude.

Through working as a volunteer therapist in a hospital environment for 10 years, I have come to believe that there are three main skills that are really important when working with the very sick and dying: to be able to listen, to be able to touch appropriately and to be able to wait whilst remaining fully present.

To be able to listen

This involves opening the ears of the heart with no expectations and no judgement, and without the head constantly formulating responses that remove our own attention from the other person. We listen to what is said and to what is not said equally. Here the body language of leaning in and nodding encouragement is much more useful than any words. Felicity Warner (2013) and Christopher Johns (2004) both have vast experience of being with the dying and excellent advice and ideas are to be had from their books listed at the end of this chapter.

To be able to touch appropriately

We have so many forms of touch in our interactions together – hugs, shaking hands, a light kiss on the cheek, to a deep tissue massage – but touching the dying is an especially sacred act of love. It is entirely unconditional. It requires nothing back from the other person and needs to match their needs to perfection: not too heavy, but firm enough to inspire confidence and with a consistency that is constant and brings peace and calm. Holding a hand or an arm is the best place to begin, taking care to ask permission. Then gently begin to match a very light pressure to correspond with the physical response of the other's tissues. Everyone will be different and gradually it will become second nature to you to hold the other person appropriately whilst checking what is comfortable for them.

To be able to wait whilst remaining fully present

This is the skill of 'keeping vigil'. It is more than just sitting or waiting; it is being a positive and energetic presence who accompanies the other on their path. This can be the catalyst that offers the dying person the peace of heart to find their own inner space within themselves whereby they may move on.

I find that a simple meditation or personal spiritual focus is very useful at this time. It keeps me present and supports the other person. I find it beneficial to consciously see the friend connected above their bed to their own higher power, or to what Sogyal Rinpoche calls 'the clear light', whilst sitting silently with them as they sleep or drift in and out of consciousness. This is particularly useful on a noisy ward or in a busy hospice or care home.

I had a friend, let's call him Peter, with whom I would sit whilst his wife took the dog for a walk and got a breath of air. One day when I arrived he whispered to me, 'Will you do the magic?' I looked questioningly at his wife. 'Oh, he wants you to do whatever it is that you do when I go out, because it gives him so much peace.' That gave me much valuable feedback and is my meditation of choice now with those with whom I keep vigil.

The other valuable aspect of 'positive vigiling' is that it keeps us grounded and in the zone. I really want to conclude this chapter with a plea that, when involved in this kind of work, you take great care of yourself. That includes physically maintaining excellent hygiene, by washing your hands and arms meticulously, emotionally disconnecting from your friend when you leave, and writing down what you need to remember so that you can leave it on the paper. A simple physical ritual like crossing both arms over your heart with a slight bow works well for me.

You may have a favourite meditation that you can repeat as you leave. I have suggested some meditations below that you could use with your friend or that family could read and share with them as they get weaker and unable to speak or read for themselves.

They may be around finding inner peace or asking forgiveness or sending love to those far away. They may be to grandchildren yet unborn, or for healing a soul wound of the dying person around a child who was indeed born but in those days had to be given away.

They may be inspired by a photo album, or a wonderful holiday, or a garden they have nurtured. Indeed, special places in mountains or by the sea bring back serene memories, which may comfort and induce inner stillness at the end.

A therapist, carer or friend can gently tease out in conversation what is really deeply meaningful for the dying person and create a poem, a meditation or a song to read or sing whenever you see them. They serve two purposes. Firstly, it is one of the truly valuable ways of honouring their life and their contribution to your life. Secondly, it is a very gentle way of helping them come to terms with their life in the context of moving on that is inevitable for them now.

Some meditations for the end of life

Gratitude meditation template (use the words and feelings of the dying person)

I want to tell you ...

I want to tell you about my favourite things

About my sister and our holidays together

About my garden and how much I love forests and trees

And my daffodils and that special green of the leaves in spring

And the mellow rustle of those same leaves in autumn

How I love the sea best in winter when it roars and foams.

I want to tell you about my friends Sally, Jack and Suzie

And of my colleagues in the office, and how we had such a laugh

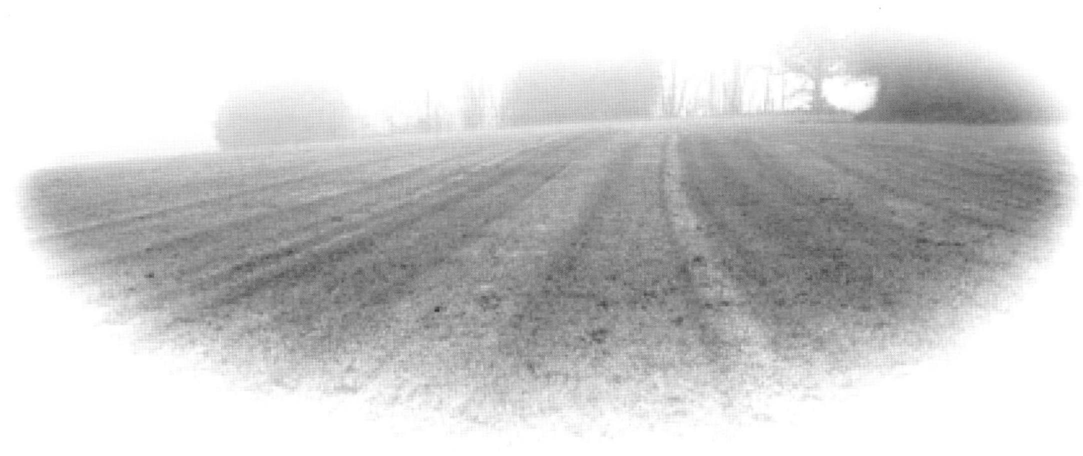

Figure 29.2
Moving on

We worked hard but enjoyed our Friday nights out.

I know they miss me now, see all my cards …

But I hope they will remember the good times

And remember to put the kettle on earlier on a Monday morning.

Template for memories of shared experience

Remember when …

Remember that holiday when the boys were small …

Speeding along the coastal road to St Tropez in our old banger.

Surfing Safari, California Girls – remember the Beach Boys tape

As we sang along at the top of our voices.

Finally, gazing at the millionaires' yachts in the marina

Right on the quay ...

We feasted on buckwheat pancakes and drank that delicious cider!

Meditation template for the end of life

You are safe ...

So now, Thomas, as you settle gently into your body, just become aware again of your breathing. There is no hurry, you have all the time in the world as we sit here together, the air drifting in and the air drifting out, gently and peacefully.

And as you do so you are drawn to a really beautiful space inside your body; it may be in your heart or in your tummy. And in that space you know that there is only peace and calm and stillness and that there you are safe. You are very safe, you are always safe.

This is your own special place where you are always safe and connected to the deepest part of your being. Just feel how it feels, so calm and peaceful, restful and still.

For this is a magical place where sound and shapes have a special meaning for you. This is your own inner sanctuary and you can visit it whenever you like. Here you can be your own true self and connect with that most mystical and spiritual part of your inner being: the part of you that is always light and free and at peace.

For that space is timeless and infinite and full of love – unbounded, infinite love. And that love is for you, that love is you and it completely surrounds you. So you can let go into it and feel it, experience it and know that you are safe.

Gaelic blessing

Deep peace of the running wave to you

Deep peace of the flowing air to you

Deep peace of the quiet earth to you

Deep peace of the shining stars to you

Deep peace of the gentle night to you

Moon and stars pour their healing light on you.

References and further reading

Gawande, A. (2014). *Being Mortal: illness, medicine and what matters in the end.* London: Profile Books.

Johns, C. (2004). *Being Mindful, Easing Suffering: reflections on palliative care.* London and Philadelphia: Jessica Kingsley.

Kearney, M. (2009). *A Place of Healing: working with nature and soul at the end of life.* New Orleans: Spring Journal Books.

Sogyal Rinpoche (1992). *The Tibetan Book of Living and Dying.* London: Rider Books.

Warner, F. (2013). *The Soul Midwives' Handbook.* London: Hay House.

7

On a philosophical note

'The whole book in a nutshell' explained

'The whole book in a nutshell' explained 30

I would like the book to finish on a philosophical note to honour the ancient teachings, as well as to demonstrate the depth of insight and wisdom those mystics and teachers brought into the world. The reader will soon recognise that Rumi's poem *Between voice and presence* holds and transmits the knowledge of every theme covered in this book, with only one slight difference: he was able to reduce the amount of words to four simple lines. I trust that Rumi's insight will leave the reader in a contemplative state of stillness and with imprints of the memory of stillness.

Between voice and presence

> ***There is a channel between voice and presence, a way where information flows. In disciplined silence the channel opens. With wandering talk it closes.***
>
> Rumi (Coleman Bark translation)

Rumi's writings are not only a work of poetry; they also speak of practical ways and practices that lead to inner transformation of our 'being'. The more subtle meanings in his words won't be recognised by our ordinary mind; they are aimed at different faculties of understanding that are attuned to a language of stillness.

The majority of Rumi's poems are embedded within this stillness, whose main objective is to make us pause and listen, as well as shifting us out of our ordinary state of consciousness into a more contemplative and refined state. In a state of contemplation we are obviously more receptive and open to information that can reach us through channels we would not recognise in our average state of mind in everyday life. Not for nothing does one of his famous sayings state that *'In silence there is eloquence'*, though silence is now rarely used or acknowledged as a means of direct communication in our society.

To become eloquent in the language of stillness, we need to adopt a specific kind of practice that is almost as old as humankind. By achieving a depth of silence, we become receptive enough to tune in to this universal language of stillness, from which all other languages, both spoken and unspoken, have grown.

This timeless practice is known to us today as a process of stilling and meditation, and Rumi's poetry provides us with a significant amount of material to unlock and understand how to apply this practice in our daily lives.

'Stop weaving …' he says, pointing towards the importance of pausing, and the urgent need to create an internal memory of stillness within our mind and body. He continues, *'… and watch how the pattern improves'*, emphasising the process of stillness by means of action through non-reaction. Without this, we will never be able to observe the countless patterns we create in our life, so that they can be improved, properly integrated into our being or ultimately transcended.

'Between voice and presence' is one of Rumi's ingenious short sayings that, in itself, gives us insight into the actual process and application of meditation and stilling practice of such depth that it can only be assimilated in small pieces of contemplative practice. Meditation is like stripping off wallpaper in a very old house. Each time we revisit the job, the next layer or level underneath is revealed. Once all the layers and coverings are removed, the house will shine with its original glory.

Our whole body–mind unit can be considered as an old house with different rooms, spaces, levels and windows. The events of life enter this great house via a continuous stream of incoming impressions and stimulus, forming and accumulating layer upon layer of new and repeating patterns on tapestries, ceilings and wall spaces, enveloping what we are in essence, and gradually creating what we have become physically, emotionally and intellectually up to the present day. This includes all our amazing capacities and talents, as well as our defects and shortcomings as an evolving human being.

Meditation could also be seen as the hammer and chisel that, with the utmost care and patience, gradually chip away all the layers, grooves and patterns that prevent the light of consciousness from illuminating the truth of what we are in essence. In philosophical terms, this whole process of experiencing and acknowledging both the conscious and non-conscious sides in us is called self-consciousness or self-realisation. The aim is to reach a level of consciousness in 'being' that possesses the whole objective truth of ourselves, as well as to experience what is not subject to change, somewhere hidden within the vastness of our internal psychological makeup.

A hint of how to ignite this process is contained in Rumi's words …

'*… voice and presence …*', which speaks about the ongoing struggle of stilling the body and mind during the initial stages of meditation. In addition, it is clearly pointing out which of our different mental faculties are involved in the process of meditation. Voice and presence represent attention and awareness respectively, interdependent inner qualities that usually oppose each other. Together they create a state in which the active part – attention – takes its seat in the foreground to be always ready to act, whilst the passive and receptive part – awareness – rests in the background just to perceive, whilst attention continues on.

In meditation, as well as in everyday life, we continuously bounce back and forth between attention and awareness. Whilst meditating, our attention is constantly attracted by the powerful pull of our thoughts, which are evoked by incoming impressions of light, sound and smell entering our allegorical seven-storey house by using the five 'open windows' of our physical senses. Just imagine for a moment how these impressions enter our mind and how they are perceived. Within a glimpse of a moment, our attention springs into action. It then starts zooming in and, once focused, it identifies with whatever thought, object or event possesses the strongest attraction. Here, our struggle lies in bringing our attention back into the house with the help of our awareness, which simply perceives and is able to be aware of the stream of incoming impressions from a non-responsive, motionless, silent and far greater perspective. Unfortunately, due to its intrinsic passiveness, as well as its inability to perceive itself and act, awareness alone is entirely helpless to take on this apparently simple undertaking.

However, Rumi is handing us the tool that takes us out of this increasing friction between awareness and attention by the word …

'*… between …*', which means neither this nor that, or the fulcrum in the middle that gives us the possibility of settling right there in the still-point between these two opposing forces, so that both are simply allowed to be. Settling there manifests a natural frictionless equilibrium between attention and awareness. Attention finds stillness and becomes pure and clear like a crystal, so that awareness finds itself reflected back by attention. Here, attention has learned how to close the shutters of all five windows, finding freedom from the continuous flow of external impressions and internal thoughts. This powerful reflective state between attention and awareness, which in time will lead to more prolonged intervals of peace of mind, is experienced as a state of 'divided attention', in which attention finally becomes attentive to awareness in the background. This linear and two-dimensional state of divided attention gives rise to …

'*There is a channel …*', which manifests as a balancing and neutralising force in the form of concentration. But before we can elaborate on this crucial point that we will all meet and cross during the process of stilling and meditation, we have to discuss the meaning of Rumi's mystical knowledge concealed in his words '*a way where information flows. In disciplined silence the channel opens, with wandering talk it closes*'.

'*… a way where information flows*' is a very significant statement in this poem, capturing the attention of the reader, and giving rise to different questions meant to ignite our curiosity and to open us up to possibilities we haven't come across or even considered before. Only a true mystic of Rumi's calibre – who undoubtedly walked the talk during his physical presence on earth eight centuries ago – in his compassionate wisdom has the capacity and authority to do that, and

MEDITATION IS TO EXPERIENCE LIFE IN A NEW WAY –
THAT IS LIFE AS A MEANS AND
NOT AS AN END

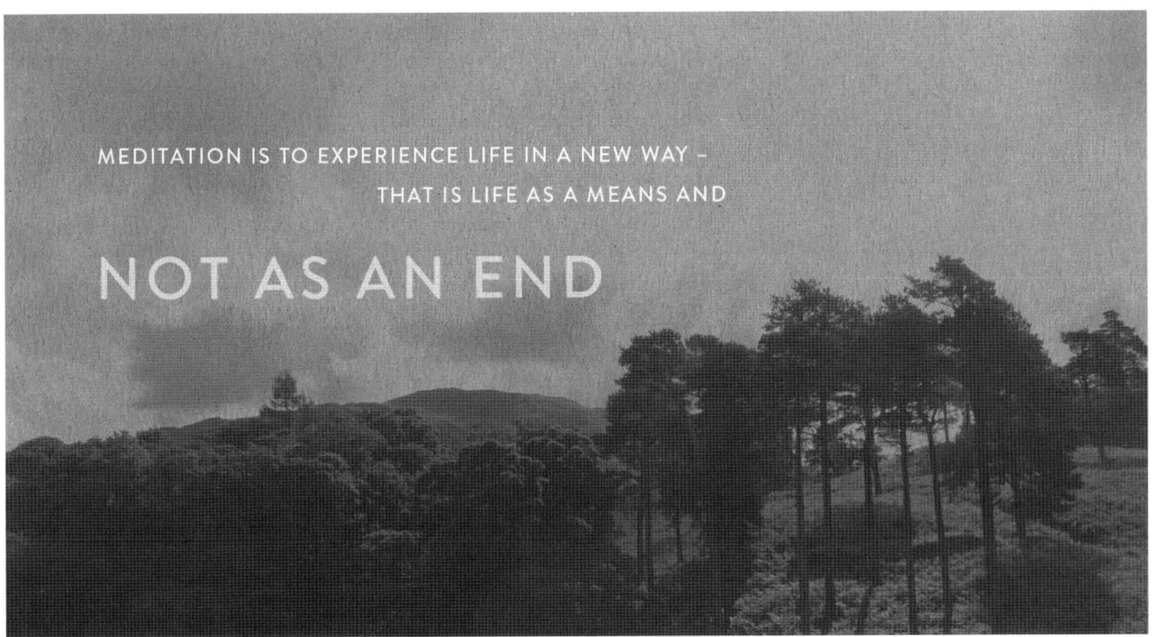

Figure 30.1

Artwork Victoria Dokas; photography Alexander Filmer-Lorch

wake us up to a greater truth. In these simple words he offers an encouraging proposition, a promise of great significance, which provides fuel in the form of unimpeachable meaning and gravitas that gradually will take us towards the realisation of our objective – that is our awakening.

In other words, *'… a way where information flows'* points towards a way of possibilities, an approach, new modality or technique by which all that has formed, crystallised, is held or has stagnated within us can be dispersed, become spacious and possibly change in the flow. We now know that there is a way that leads to a place, level or state of existence that lies above the grasp of our mind and thought. In addition, we know that this way takes us to a channel that gives us access to information we can't access in our ordinary state of mind. Rumi reveals the way to come into contact with this channel in the words …

'disciplined silence …', which hold the teachings of the process of stilling and meditation, clearly indicating by the word 'disciplined' that meditation is a process in which we will meet resistance and will experience phases of struggle and friction, and that we can't expect instant results. Rumi refers to a particular kind of effort that forms part of achieving disciplined silence, which is known in the universal teachings as 'conscious effort'. The term 'silence' in this context tells us that Rumi is not talking about a rigid discipline. The non-invasive nature of silence evokes a gradual and deepening process of stilling on all levels, in which the subtle energy of our conscious effort is directed towards remembering to remember to be aware, and being attentive to this inner stillness whilst sitting in meditation. This process will undo all doings, including all intentions, as well as gradually transcending all ideas of being the one that meditates until *'… the channel opens'*.

'… with wandering talk it closes' informs us about all the different obstacles we will face in meditation that will disrupt our conscious effort and interfere with our new studies of the language of stillness. The phrase describes the scattered nature of our mind–body–thought unit. The word 'wandering' tells us about our

different sleep-evoking states – all states that have become mechanical and habitual in us, mainly in the form of memory, and have created formations such as daydreaming, internal considering and imagining, as well as mechanical talking and identifying. These non-conscious states, which form a large part of our psychological being, don't require any kind of effort and are a strong counterforce to the conscious effort we put into our stilling practice. As is the case with awareness and attention, the active force of conscious effort bounces back against the passive force of non-conscious effort.

At this point we can go back and start elaborating on the meaning of *'There is a channel …'* and *'… the channel opens …'*. Allegorically, the channel stands for the 'vertical scale' or the 'scale of eternity', which according to the universal teachings comprises the scale of consciousness and our own individual scale of being. At this stage in meditation, attention (voice) and awareness (presence) come into perfect balance through the continuous application of stilling and meditation, merging through the power of concentration. This frictionless triad gives rise to a deep and whole state of meditation, in which our relative state of consciousness expands, all that is 'in formation' transcends, and higher knowledge of transformation will be unveiled and communicated by the omnipresent language of stillness.

And on this philosophical note, nothing more needs to be said than this: what you are left with is worth contemplating deeply within yourself in stillness and silence.

Alexander Filmer-Lorch

INDEX

A

B

C

D

Q

R

S

T

U

V

W

X

Y

Z